The Anatomy Answer Book

4000 Questions and Answers for Pre-Exam Review

W.K. Metcalf, MD, PhD

Emeritus Professor and Chairman
Department of Genetics, Cell Biology, and Anatomy
University of Nebraska Medical Center
Omaha, Nebraska

JONES AND BARTLETT PUBLISHERS
Sudbury, Massachusetts
BOSTON TORONTO LONDON SINGAPORE

World Headquarters
Jones and Bartlett Publishers
40 Tall Pine Drive
Sudbury, MA 01776
978-443-5000
info@jbpub.com
www.jbpub.com

Jones and Bartlett Publishers Canada
2406 Nikanna Road
Mississauga, ON L5C 2W6
CANADA

Jones and Bartlett Publishers International
Barb House, Barb Mews
London W6 7PA
UK

Jones and Bartlett's books and products are available through most bookstores and online booksellers. To contact Jones and Bartlett Publishers directly, call 800-832-0034, fax 978-443-8000, or visit our website www.jbpub.com.

Substantial discounts on bulk quantities of Jones and Bartlett's publications are available to corporations, professional associations, and other qualified organizations. For details and specific discount information, contact the special sales department at Jones and Bartlett via the above contact information or send an email to specialsales@jbpub.com.

Library of Congress Cataloging-in-Publication Data
Metcalf, William Kenneth.
The anatomy answer book : 4000 questions and answers for pre-exam review / W. Kenneth Metcalf.
p. ; cm.
ISBN 0-7637-3059-9 (pbk.)
1. Human anatomy—Examinations, questions, etc.
[DNLM: 1. Anatomy—Examination Questions. QS 18.2 M588a 2005] I. Title.
QM32.M417 2005
611′.0076—dc22
2005004540

Production Credits
Acquisitions Editor: Jack Bruggeman
Production Director: Amy Rose
Editorial Assistants: Kylah Goodfellow McNeill, Katilyn Crowley
Production Assistant: Kate Hennessy
Marketing Manager: Ed McKenna
Manufacturing and Inventory Coordinator: Therese Brauer
Composition: Auburn Associates, Inc.
Cover Design: Kristin E. Ohlin
Printing and Binding: Courier-Stoughton
Cover Printing: Courier-Stoughton

Printed in the United States of America
09 08 07 06 05 10 9 8 7 6 5 4 3 2

Dedication

To my wife, Norah, with whom I learned anatomy for the first time, and who now, seven children and over fifty years later, still shares my enthusiasm for helping students to learn and to understand anatomy.

Table of Contents

Preface

The philosophy of this book is the result of more than half a century of teaching anatomy to medical, physical therapy, and other health professional students and of observing the continual addition of new material to the anatomy curriculum. This increase in the amount of material in the anatomy curriculum has resulted in a substitution of memorization in place of understanding.

In the weeks prior to comprehensive examinations, students are desperately trying to review vast quantities of only partially understood material in a limited amount of time. They find traditional review books of multiple-choice questions far too time-consuming for such rapid review.

Accordingly, this text is presented in a simple question-and-answer format. It can be used as a self-testing manual by covering the answers while reading the questions. Or, for more rapid review, the questions and answers can simply be read as statements of fact. Points of major importance—hopefully, those most likely to turn up in examinations or of significant value in clinical situations—are often reviewed more than once in different formats. The design of this anatomy review text has been developed and tested in the Department of Genetics, Cell Biology, and Anatomy at the University of Nebraska Medical Center over the last several years and has been almost universally praised by the students.

It must be stressed that this is not a formal review, but a compressed one. A plethora of formal anatomy review texts are available to students. This rapid-review format assumes that the reader has some basic knowledge of anatomy and merely wishes to refresh his or her knowledge base before an examination. It is, frankly, a pre-examination cram book.

United States Medical Licensing Examinations (USMLE) contain increasing numbers of X-rays, CT Scans, MRIs, and line drawings. For this reason, and because visualization is the key to learning anatomy, questions on such material play a major role in this text.

Because this is a pre-examination review book, no references are given. The anatomical facts presented in the text have been culled from 50 or more years of preparation and examination of dissections, preparation, and presentation of lectures, and assisting of students in the anatomy laboratory. The line drawings have all been redrawn from original sketches personally prepared for lecture presentations or for handouts.

In the preparation of this review, numerous anatomy texts have been consulted to check the author's memory. A list of those most often used is appended as a short bibliography. Undoubtedly, the author's view of anatomy has been most influenced by the 27th edition of *Gray's Anatomy: Descriptive and Applied* (1938) that was used when the author was a medical student in the Anatomy Department of the Medical School, King's College, University of Durham, Newcastle-on-Tyne, Northumberland, UK.

Finally, it would be ungracious not to acknowledge the valuable contributions to the author's understanding of anatomy that have been made by colleagues too numerous to mention.

Bibliography

McMinn, R. M. H., and Hutchings, R. T. *Color Atlas of Human Anatomy*, 2d ed. Chicago: Year Book Medical Publishers, 1988.

Netter, F. H. *Atlas of Human Anatomy,* 3d ed. Carlstadt, NJ: Icon Learning Systems, 2002.

Rohen, J. W., and Yokochi, C. *Color Atlas of Anatomy*, 2d ed. Tokyo: Igaku-Shoin, 1988.

Vidic, B., and Suarez, F. R. *Photographic Atlas of the Human Body*. St. Louis: C. V. Mosby, 1984.

Williams, P. L., editor. *Gray's Anatomy. The Anatomical Basis of Medicine and Surgery,* 38th ed. Edinburgh: Churchill Livingston, 1995.

Kopf-Maier, P., editor. *Wolf-Heidegger's Atlas of Human Anatomy,* 5th ed. Basel, Switzerland: Karger, 2000.

About the Author

WILLIAM KENNETH METCALF
MB, BS (MD), University of Durham, United Kingdom
MD (PhD), University of Bristol, United Kingdom
Professor and Chairman Emeritus, Department of Genetics, Cell Biology, and Anatomy, University of Nebraska Medical Center

Previous appointments

Professor and Chairman, Department of Anatomy, University of Nebraska Medical Center
Professor, Department of Anatomy, University of Iowa
Reader, Department of Anatomy, University of Bristol, UK
Clinical Assistant, Department of Medicine, Bristol United Hospitals, Bristol, UK
Visiting Professor, Department of Anatomy, University of South Carolina at Columbia
Distinguished Visiting Professor, Department of Anatomy, University of Adelaide, Australia
External Examiner in Anatomy, University of Lagos, Nigeria
External Examiner in Anatomy, University of Ibadan, Nigeria
External Examiner in Anatomy, University of Benin, Nigeria
External Examiner in Anatomy, University of Kuwait, Kuwait
Specialist in Venereology and in Dermatology, Royal Army Medical Corp.

Teaching awards

Alpha Omega Alpha/American Association of Medical Colleges Robert J. Glaser Distinguished Teacher Award in 1991
More than two dozen student and university-wide teaching awards in both the UK and the USA

Chapter 1

The Back

THE VERTEBRAL COLUMN, THE SPINAL CORD, AND THE NERVE ROOTS

Q. The bones that together constitute the vertebral column are. . .

A. The seven cervical vertebrae; the twelve thoracic vertebrae; the five lumbar vertebrae; the five sacral vertebrae, which are fused to form the sacrum; and the three coccygeal vertebrae, which are likewise fused to form the coccyx.

Q. In Figure 1-1, identify A.

A. The vertebral body. The anterior longitudinal ligament extends from the occipital bone of the skull to the sacrum. It is attached to the anterior surface of all of the vertebral bodies.

Q. The attachments of the posterior longitudinal ligament are . . .

A. The posterior rim of each intervertebral disc and the adjacent margins of each vertebral body. Thc postcrior longitudinal ligament extends from the second cervical vertebra to the sacrum.

Q. In Figure 1-1, identify B.

A. The left pedicle of the vertebral (neural) arch.

Q. In Figure 1-1, identify C.

A. The transverse process of the vertebral arch. In the lateral view, the articular facet for the tubercle of the corresponding rib can be identified at **F**.

Q. In Figure 1-1, identify D.

A. The left lamina of the vertebral arch.

Superior Aspect

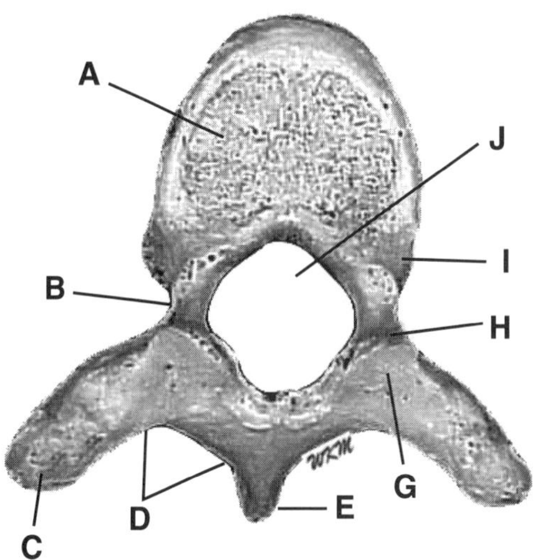

Left Lateral Aspect

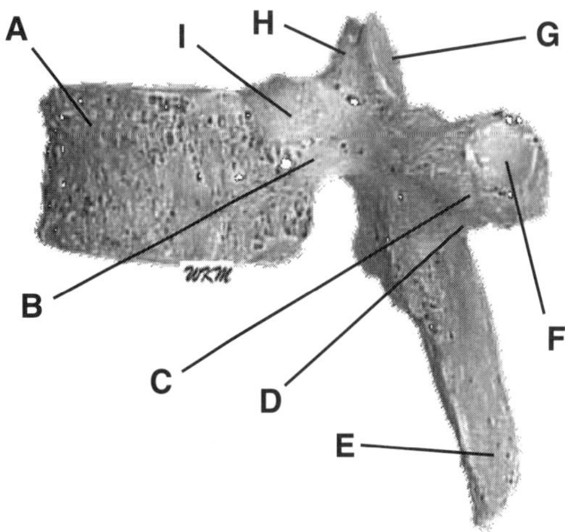

Figure 1-1 Typical Thoracic Vertebra

Q. The ligaments that connect the laminae of adjacent vertebrae are . . .

A. The ligamenta flava.

Q. In Figure 1-1, identify E.

A. The vertebral spine, the spinous process.

Q. In Figure 1-1, identify F.

A. The facet for articulation with the tubercle of the corresponding rib.

Q. The ligaments that connect individual spinous processes are named . . .

A. The interspinous ligaments.

Q. The ligament that connects all of the spinous processes is named . . .

A. The supraspinous ligament. In the cervical region, the ligamentum nuchae is a thickened, specialized, elastic segment of the supraspinous ligament. It helps maintain extension of the neck without unnecessary muscle activity.

Q. In Figure 1-1, identify G.

A. The superior articular facet for articulation with the inferior articular facet of the vertebra above it. It forms the posterior surface of the superior articular process, **H**.

Superior Aspect

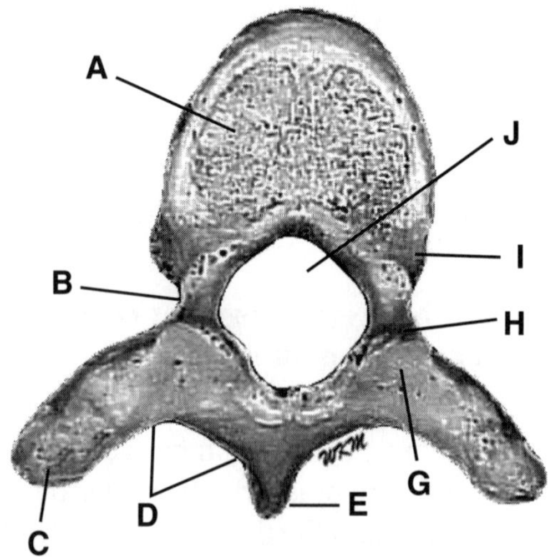

Left Lateral Aspect

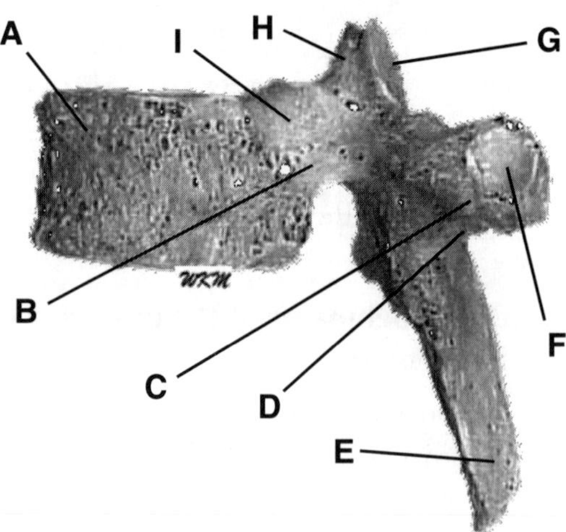

Figure 1-1 Typical Thoracic Vertebra

Q. In Figure 1-1, identify I.

A. The facet for articulation with the head of the corresponding rib. This facet is, of course, only present on thoracic vertebrae.

Q. In Figure 1-1, identify J.

A. The vertebral canal.

Q. The deep muscles of the back lie in the deep depressions situated on either side of the vertebral spines. Their nerve supply is . . .

A. The posterior primary rami of the spinal nerves. They are mixed nerves. They also carry sensory fibers to the skin over the deep muscles of the back.

Q. The deep muscles of the back can be subdivided into three layers. The most superficial layer is . . .

A. The splenius muscle group. It consists of the splenius capitis muscle and the splenius cervicis muscle.

Q. The splenius capitis muscle and the splenius cervicis muscle both turn the face to . . .

A. The ipsilateral side. This action can be deduced by the obliquely upward and lateral direction of their fibers.

Q. The second and much bulkier layer of muscles is essentially vertical. It is named . . .

A. The erector spinae (sacrospinalis) muscle. It is a powerful muscle, which extends the vertebral column with very little, if any, rotational action.

Q. The deepest group of the deep muscles of the back is the transversospinalis muscle group. The small muscles in this group run obliquely, upwards and medially, from the individual transverse processes to the spines of the vertebrae above them. Their action is to . . .

A. Rotate the vertebral column to the contralateral side.

Q. The medial part of the erector spinae muscle is deficient in the upper cervical region. Hence, in this region, immediately deep to the superficial layer, which consists of the splenius capitis and the splenius cervicis muscles, lie the superior, much enlarged, cervical segments of the transversospinalis group of muscles. They form . . .

A. The semispinalis capitis muscle and the semispinalis cervicis muscle. The former is attached to the medial part of the occipital bone, and the latter is attached to the spinous processes of the cervical vertebrae.

Q. The semispinalis capitis and the semispinalis cervicis muscles arise from . . .

A. The transverse processes of the lower six cervical vertebrae and the upper six thoracic vertebrae.

Q. The fibers of the semispinalis capitis and semispinalis cervicis muscles run . . .

A. Upwards and medially.

Q. The semispinalis muscle group rotates the head to . . .

A. The contralateral side. In addition, it assists in extension of the head.

Q. A large cutaneous nerve emerges from the posterior surface of the semispinalis capitis muscle, just above the superior margin of the splenius capitis muscle. This nerve is . . .

A. The greater occipital nerve. It supplies the skin over the occipital region of the scalp, posterior to lambda. It originates from the posterior primary ramus of the second cervical nerve.

THE MENINGES, THE SPINAL CORD, AND THE NERVE ROOTS

Q. The vertebral canal is occupied by the spinal cord, surrounded by its meninges. The outer meninx is known as . . .

A. The dura mater. It is largely protective in function.

Q. The dura mater is separated from the neural arch and the vertebral bodies by . . .

A. The vertebral venous plexus and a small quantity of fat. In the skull, the dura mater is firmly adherent to the periosteum, which is, itself, firmly adherent to the cranial bones.

Q. The two inner layers of the meninges, the arachnoid mater and the pia mater, are separated by . . .

A. The subarachnoid space. It contains the cerebrospinal fluid and the arteries and veins that supply the spinal cord.

Q. The cerebrospinal fluid is secreted by . . .

A. The choroid plexi in the lateral ventricles, the third ventricle, and the fourth ventricle.

Q. The pia mater is firmly adherent to the surface of the spinal cord. The arachnoid mater is kept in contact with the dura mater by . . .

A. The pressure of the cerebrospinal fluid.

Q. The ventral (motor) nerve roots and the dorsal (sensory) nerve roots, which are ensheathed in pia mater, cross the subarachnoid space. They leave the vertebral canal through the intervertebral foramina in prolongations of the subarachnoid space, surrounded by the arachnoid mater and the dura mater. Each motor nerve root and each sensory nerve root unites to form a mixed spinal nerve within . . .

A. The tubular prolongation of the dura mater. This prolongation of the subarachnoid space also contains the posterior nerve root ganglion of the spinal nerve.

Q. The mixed spinal nerves, therefore, are formed in . . .

A. The intervertebral foramina. In the intervertebral foramina, they divide to form the anterior primary rami and the posterior primary rami.

Q. The spinal cord is maintained in a central position in the subarachnoid space by . . .

A. The ligamentum denticulatum. This structure is a series of attachments of pia mater, covered by arachnoid mater, to the inside of the dura mater. It lies between the ventral and the dorsal nerve roots.

Q. In the adult, the spinal cord extends down the vertebral canal to . . .

A. The level of the disk between the first lumbar vertebra and the second lumbar vertebra.

Q. In the adolescent and the adult, a lumbar puncture is performed at the level of . . .

A. The iliac crest. This level usually corresponds to the interval between the third and fourth lumbar spines. It is well below the inferior end of the spinal cord. The interval between the second lumbar spine and the third lumbar spine also may be utilized with safety. A second attempt at this level is sometimes necessary if the vertebral venous plexus is penetrated during the first attempt and a blood-stained sample of cerebrospinal fluid results.

Q. In neonates, the spinal cord extends down the vertebral canal to . . .

A. The level of the disk between the second and third lumbar vertebrae. Therefore, in the neonate, lumbar punctures must not be performed higher than the interval between the third and the fourth lumbar spines.

Q. Structures that will be pierced by a midline lumbar puncture are . . .

A. The skin and the superficial fascia, the supraspinous ligament, the interspinous ligament, the ligamentum flavum, the dura mater, and the arachnoid mater. The needle then enters the subarachnoid space, and a sample of the cerebrospinal fluid can be obtained.

Q. The conus medullaris is . . .

A. A short conical tapering of the lower end of the spinal cord.

Q. The filum terminale interna is . . .

A. A fibrous continuation of the conus medullaris to the second sacral vertebrae. At this point, it fuses with the overlying meninges, forming the coccygeal ligament, the filum terminale externa. The coccygeal ligament continues to the coccyx.

Q. The cauda equina is formed of . . .

A. The ventral and the dorsal nerve roots of the lumbar and the sacral segments of the spinal cord. From their origin from the spinal cord, each runs inferiorly through the subarachnoid space to its respective intervertebral foramen.

Q. The inferior end of the subarachnoid space lies . . .

A. At the level of the second sacral vertebra. This level is important because it is essential not to penetrate the subarachnoid space when administering epidural anesthesia through the sacral hiatus. This procedure is frequently used during surgery on the lower extremity, the anal canal, and the anus and during childbirth.

Q. In Figure 1-2, identify A.

A. The posterior column of grey matter. Its cells receive sensory information from the dorsal, the posterior, nerve roots.

Q. In Figure 1-2, identify B.

A. The dorsal nerve root of a spinal nerve. It contains only sensory fibers.

Q. In Figure 1-2, identify C.

A. A dorsal root ganglion. Dorsal root ganglia lie in the intervertebral foramina. They contain the cell bodies of sensory nerve fibers. Sensory ganglia do not have synapses.

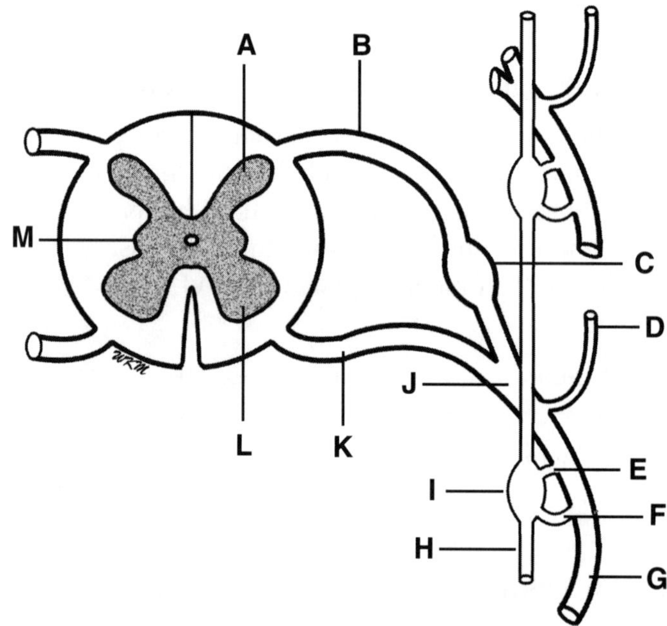

Figure 1-2 The Thoracic Spinal Cord, Transverse Section

Q. In Figure 1-2, identify D.

A. A posterior primary ramus of a mixed spinal nerve. It contains both motor and sensory fibers.

Q. In Figure 1-2, identify E.

A. A grey ramus communicantes. It carries postganglionic sympathetic fibers from the sympathetic ganglion to the mixed spinal nerve.

Q. In Figure 1-2, identify F.

A. A white ramus communicantes. It carries preganglionic fibers from the lateral grey column to the sympathetic ganglion, where they will synapse.

Q. In Figure 1-2, identify G.

A. The anterior primary ramus of a mixed spinal nerve. It contains both motor and sensory fibers.

Q. Anterior primary rami supply . . .

A. All of the voluntary muscles of the body, except the deep muscles of the back, both sternocleidomastoid muscles, and both trapezius muscles. The sensory fibers supply the skin of most of the body below the face. They do not supply the skin over the deep muscles of the back.

Q. The skin of the face and most of the scalp is supplied by . . .

A. The trigeminal (the fifth cranial) nerve.

Q. The trapezius muscle and the sternocleidomastoid muscle are supplied almost entirely by . . .

A. The spinal accessory (the eleventh cranial) nerve.

Q. In Figure 1-2, identify H.

A. The sympathetic trunk composed of connecting sympathetic ganglia. It carries both pre- and postsynaptic fibers to different segments of the body.

Q. In Figure 1-2, identify I.

A. A sympathetic chain ganglion. It contains synapses of motor sympathetic fibers. Each presynaptic axon synapses with a number of secondary neurons. Hence, sympathetic activity tends to be fairly generalized.

Q. In Figure 1-2, identify J.

A. A mixed spinal nerve. The motor and the sensory nerve roots join as they emerge from the intervertebral foramina.

Q. In Figure 1-2, identify K.

A. The ventral nerve root of a spinal nerve. It contains motor fibers to voluntary muscles. In addition, in the thoracic and the upper two lumbar segments of the spinal cord, it contains autonomic (sympathetic) motor fibers.

Q. In Figure 1-2, identify L.

A. The anterior grey column. It contains the somata (the cell bodies) of the somatic motor nerve fibers of the anterior nerve roots.

Q. In Figure 1-2, identify M.

A. The lateral grey column. It contains the somata (the cell bodies) of the autonomic neurons. They will synapse in the sympathetic chain ganglia.

THE VERTEBRAE, REGIONAL CHARACTERISTICS

Q. The skeletal structure of the back is . . .

A. The vertebral column.

Q. Excluding the "tail," the caudal vertebrae (usually three) that fuse to form the coccyx in the human vertebral column, there are . . .

A. Twenty-nine vertebrae: seven cervical vertebrae, twelve thoracic vertebrae, five lumbar vertebrae, and five fused sacral vertebrae.

Q. The cervical, thoracic, and lumbar vertebral bodies are separated by . . .

A. The intervertebral discs.

Q. The central part of each intervertebral disc is semi-fluid. It is called . . .

A. The nucleus pulposus.

Q. The periphery of each intervertebral disc is a fibrous ring. This ring is called . . .

A. The annulus fibrosus.

Q. A "slipped" disc results from . . .

A. Herniation of the nucleus pulposus through a degenerating or damaged annulus fibrosus.

Q. This herniation commonly occurs . . .

A. Posteriorly or posterolaterally.

Q. Posterolateral herniation is likely to compress . . .

A. The appropriate spinal nerve. Usually the nerve involved is the one immediately below the affected disc.

Q. The discs most commonly affected are . . .

A. The lower two cervical discs and the lower two lumbar discs.

Q. After pain in the appropriate spinal region, the commonest, and often the most severe, symptoms are . . .

A. Pain and paresthesia in the shoulder with cervical disc herniation or down the back of the leg with lumbar disc herniation. The latter symptom is often called *sciatica.*

Q. In Figure 1-3, the structure that articulates at A is . . .

A. The dens of the axis.

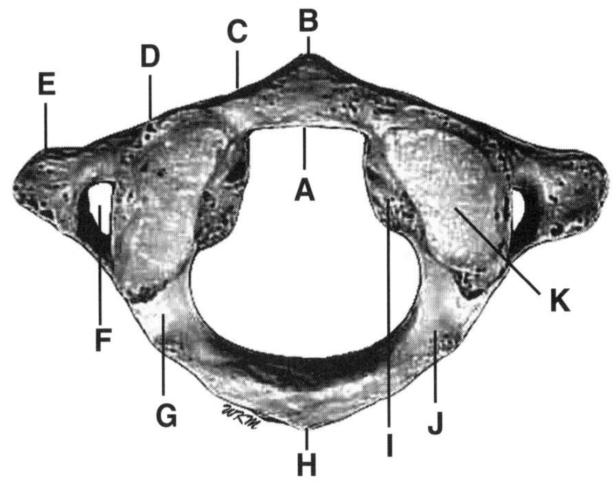

Figure 1-3 The Atlas, Superior Aspect

Q. In Figure 1-3, identify B.

A. The anterior tubercle of the atlas.

Q. Attached to the anterior tubercle of the atlas is . . .

A. The anterior longitudinal ligament.

Q. In Figure 1-3, identify C.

A. The anterior arch of the atlas.

Q. Attached to the anterior arch of the atlas is . . .

A. The anterior atlanto-occipital membrane.

Q. In Figure 1-3, identify D.

A. The left lateral mass of the atlas.

Q. In Figure 1-3, identify E.

A. The left transverse process of the atlas. Each process, both right and left, can be felt by deep palpation between the ipsilateral mastoid process and the angle of the mandible.

Q. The cervical vertebra with the longest transverse processes is . . .

A. The seventh cervical vertebra. The transverse process of the atlas is almost as long.

Q. The cervical vertebra that is most useful for gender determination is . . .

A. The atlas.

Q. The measurement of the atlas used for gender determination is . . .

A. The total atlantal width. In males, the total atlantal width is usually greater than 75 mm (3 inches). The total atlantal width is smaller in females.

Q. In Figure 1-3, identify F.

A. The left foramen transversarium. It transmits the vertebral artery and the vertebral vein.

Q. The vertebral artery traverses the foramina transversaria of all the cervical vertebrae except that of . . .

A. The seventh cervical vertebra. This foramen transversarium is only traversed by the vertebral vein.

Q. The vertebral artery originates from . . .

A. The first part of the subclavian artery.

Q. The vertebral artery terminates, after entering the skull through the foramen magnum, by joining with its counterpart to form . . .

A. The basilar artery.

Q. In Figure 1-3, the structures in groove G are . . .

A. The left vertebral artery and the left vertebral venous plexus and the suboccipital (the first cervical) nerve.

Q. The first cervical nerve terminates by dividing into . . .

A. Dorsal and ventral, anterior and posterior, primary rami. Unlike the other spinal nerves, it has no significant cutaneous component.

Q. In Figure 1-3, identify H.

A. The posterior tubercle of the atlas.

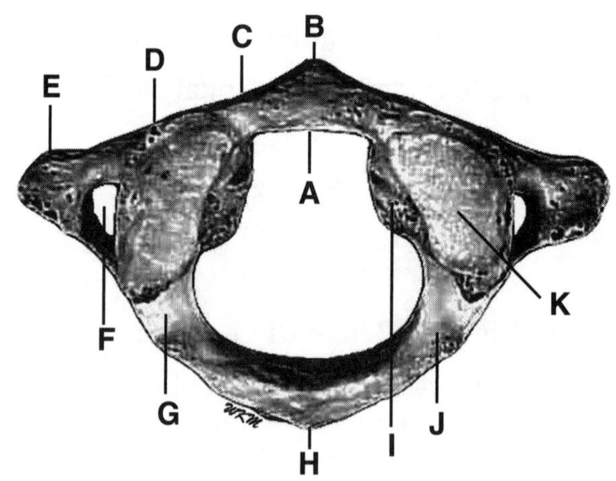

Figure 1-3 The Atlas, Superior Aspect

Q. In Figure 1-3, the ligament attached at I is . . .

A. The transverse ligament of the atlas.

Q. In Figure 1-3, identify J.

A. The posterior arch of the atlas.

Q. Attached to the posterior arch of the atlas is . . .

A. The posterior atlanto-occipital membrane.

Q. In Figure 1-3, identify K.

A. The right superior occipital articular facet.

Q. The joints mainly responsible for the nodding of the head (i.e., "saying yes") are . . .

A. The atlanto-occipital joints.

Q. In Figure 1-4, identify A.

A. The dens, the odontoid process.

Q. The ligament attached to the dens is . . .

A. The apical ligament. Superiorly, it is attached to the anterior margin of the foramen magnum.

Q. In Figure 1-4, identify B.

A. The body of the axis.

Q. In Figure 1-4, identify C.

A. The facet for the inferior facet of the atlas.

Q. The joints mainly responsible for the rotation of the head (i.e., "saying no") are . . .

A. The atlanto-axial joints.

Q. In Figure 1-4, identify D.

A. The left foramen transversarium of the axis.

Q. In Figure 1-4, identify E.

A. The left transverse process of the axis. It is much smaller than that of the atlas. It cannot be palpated.

Q. In Figure 1-4, identify F.

A. The left pedicle of the neural arch of the axis.

Q. In Figure 1-4, identify G.

A. The left lamina of the neural arch of the axis.

Q. In Figure 1-4, identify H.

A. The spinous process of the axis. It is much stouter than the other cervical or even than thoracic spines.

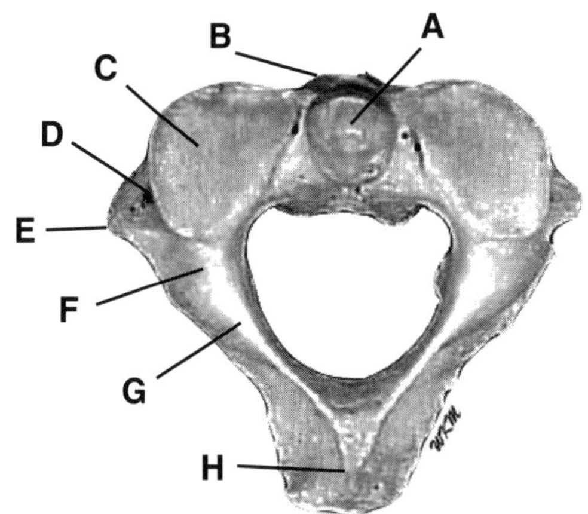

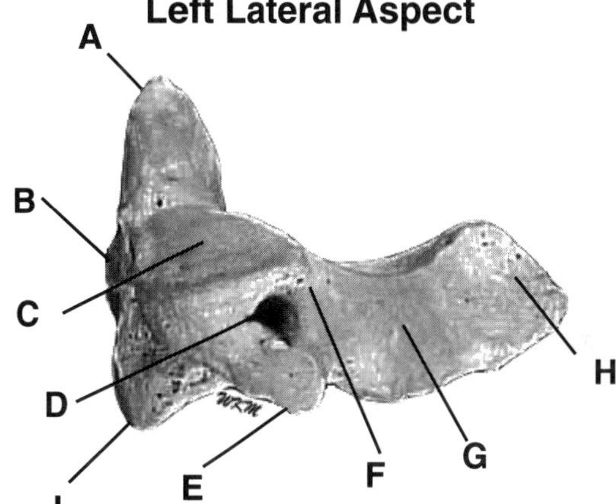

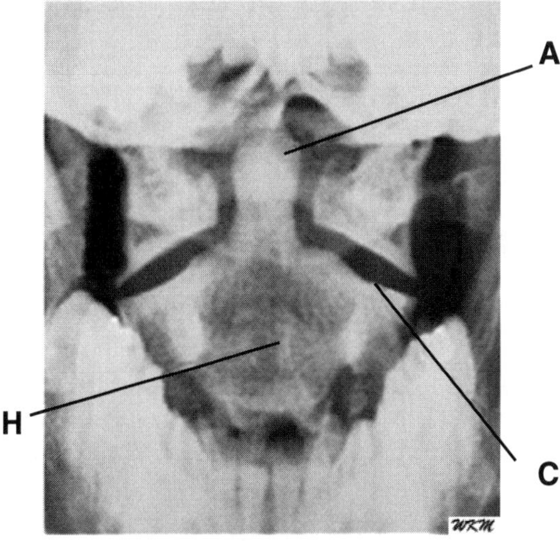

Figure 1-4 The Axis

Q. The pedicles of the neural arch of the axis form the inferior boundaries of . . .

A. The intervertebral foramina between the atlas and the axis.

Q. The nerves that pass through the intervertebral foramina between the atlas and the axis are . . .

A. The second cervical nerves. They immediately divide into anterior and posterior primary rami. The posterior primary rami, after supplying some deep muscles of the back, will become the greater occipital nerves. These nerves supply the skin over the occipital region.

Q. In Figure 1-5, identify A.

A. The vertebral body. Note that, like vertebral bodies C3 through C7, it is flattened anteroposteriorly.

Q. In Figure 1-5, identify B.

A. The anterior tubercle of the left transverse process.

Q. In Figure 1-5, identify C.

A. The left foramen transversarium. Both the vertebral vein and the vertebral artery pass through the foramina transversaria of the upper six cervical vertebrae. The seventh cervical vertebra, however, usually only carries the vertebral vein.

Q. In Figure 1-5, identify D.

A. The posterior tubercle of the left transverse process.

Q. In Figure 1-5, identify E.

A. The left superior articular process.

Q. In Figure 1-5, identify F.

A. The left inferior articular process.

Q. In Figure 1-5, identify G.

A. The left lamina of the neural arch.

Q. In Figure 1-5, identify H.

A. The spinous process of the vertebral arch.

Q. In Figure 1-5, identify I.

A. The left pedicle of the vertebral arch.

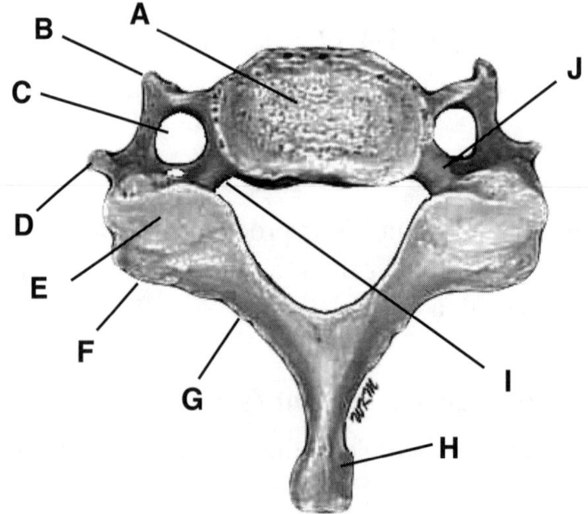

Figure 1-5 The Seventh Cervical Vertebra, Superior Aspect

Q. In Figure 1-5, identify J.

A. The right superior intervertebral notch.

Q. In Figure 1-6, identify A.

A. The superior vertebral notch for a thoracic segmental nerve.

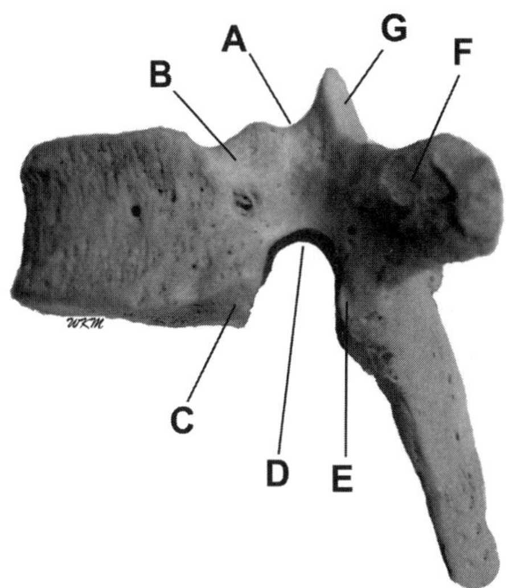

Figure 1-6 Typical Thoracic Vertebra, Left Lateral Aspect

Q. In Figure 1-6, identify B.

A. The superior costal facet. The heads of the second through the tenth ribs each articulate with two vertebral bodies and the intervertebral disc, which lies between them. The first rib articulates only with the first thoracic vertebra and the disc between the seventh cervical vertebra and the first thoracic vertebra. The eleventh and twelfth ribs each have a complete facet on the body of their corresponding vertebra.

Q. In Figure 1-6, identify C.

A. The inferior costal facet.

Q. In Figure 1-6, identify D.

A. The inferior vertebral notch. It forms the superior margin of the intervertebral foramen through which the corresponding mixed spinal nerve emerges.

Q. In Figure 1-6, identify E.

A. An inferior articular facet. It articulates with the superior articular facet of the next inferior vertebra.

Q. In Figure 1-6, identify F.

A. A costotubercular facet. It articulates with the tubercle of the corresponding rib. This facet is only present on the first through the tenth thoracic vertebra. The eleventh and twelfth ribs are "floating." They do not articulate with the transverse processes of their corresponding vertebra.

Q. In Figure 1-6, identify G.

A. The superior articular facet. It lies on the posterior surface of the superior articular process, facing posteriorly and slightly laterally. Due to the orientation of these zygapophyseal joints, vertebral rotation can occur only in the cervical and the thoracic regions of the vertebral column. It cannot occur in the lumbar region.

Q. In Figure 1-7, identify A.

A. The vertebral body of the third lumbar vertebra. Note that, unlike a typical thoracic vertebra, the transverse diameter of the lumbar vertebral body is somewhat greater than its anteroposterior dimension.

Q. In Figure 1-7, identify B.

A. The left pedicle. It is directed almost directly posteriorly.

Q. In Figure 1-7, identify C.

A. The transverse process. This vertebra has the longest transverse processes of any vertebra.

Q. In Figure 1-7, identify D.

A. The left inferior articular process. Note that the facet faces almost directly laterally. This prevents any significant rotation of the lumbar segment of the vertebral column.

Q. In Figure 1-7, identify E.

A. The spinous process.

Q. In Figure 1-7, identify F.

A. The superior articular process. Note that the facet faces medially.

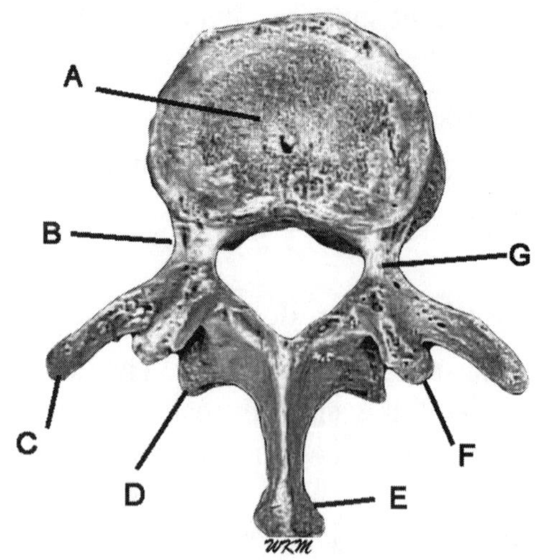

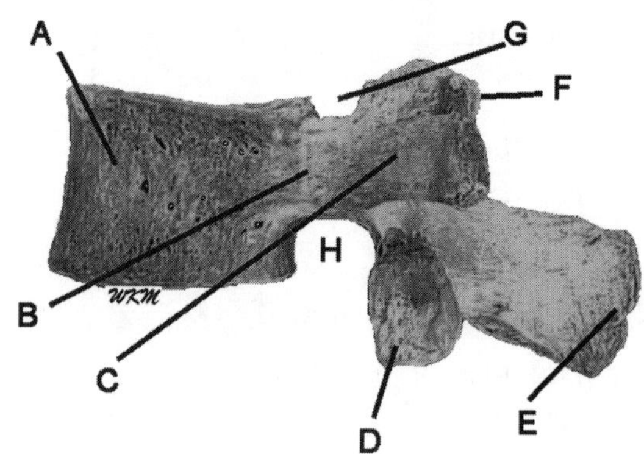

Figure 1-7 The Third Lumbar Vertebra

Q. The normal lumbar lordosis results from . . .

A. The greater anterior thickness of the intervertebral discs and the vertebral bodies.

Q. The wedging of both the intervertebral discs and the vertebral bodies is most pronounced in . . .

A. The third, fourth, and fifth lumbar segments.

Q. Lumbar lordosis is greater in . . .

A. Females. It also increases during pregnancy.

Q. The movement of the lumbar vertebrae that is restricted by the orientation of their articular facets is . . .

A. Rotation.

Q. In Figure 1-7, identify G.

A. The superior vertebral notch.

Q. In Figure 1-7, the structure that lies in the inferior vertebral notch H is . . .

A. The left third lumbar nerve. Except in the cervical region, the spinal nerve occupies the inferior notch of the corresponding vertebra.

Q. The major structure that lies in contact with the body of the third lumbar vertebra is . . .

A. The aorta. It bifurcates on the anterior surface of the body of the fourth lumbar vertebra.

Q. The segment of the bowel that crosses the aorta anterior to the body of the third lumbar vertebra is . . .

A. The third part of the duodenum.

Q. The muscle that lies in the angle between the lumbar vertebral bodies and their transverse processes, and originates from them, is . . .

A. The psoas major muscle.

Q. The features that distinguish the male sacrum from the female sacrum are all based on two major functional requirements. These are . . .

A. The necessity of increasing the transverse diameter of the female pelvic cavity and the increased robustness necessary in the male pelvis. The female sacrum is wider, shorter, and more triangular than the male sacrum. It also has a greater curvature, which results in an increase in the anteroposterior diameter of the mid-cavity of the female pelvis.

Q. Larger articular facets for articulating with the ilium are present in . . .

A. The male. This facilitates the transfer of greater stress. The smaller facets in the female allow greater rotation of the sacrum during childbirth. This rotation increases the anteroposterior diameter of the maternal pelvic outlet to allow exit of the fetal head from the pelvic cavity.

Q. The transverse measurement of the sacrum is greater in . . .

A. The female. It increases the transverse diameter of the pelvis inlet and facilitates entry of the fetal head into the pelvic inlet and its subsequent passage through the pelvis.

Q. The longitudinal measurement of the sacrum is greater in . . .

A. The male. The shortness of the sacrum in the female helps to increase the anteroposterior diameter of the pelvic outlet.

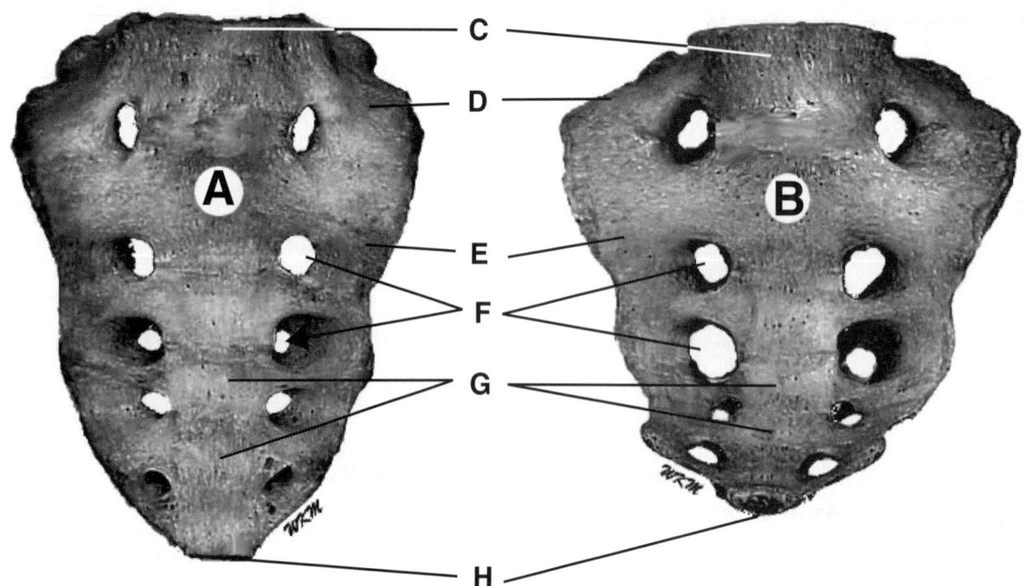

Figure 1-8 The Male Sacrum and the Female Sacrum, Anterior Aspect

Q. Identify the sex of the two sacra depicted in Figure 1-8.

A. A is male. B is female.

Q. In Figure 1-8, identify C.

A. The sacral promontory. The prominence of this structure is the major factor determining the anteroposterior diameter of the pelvic inlet. This is only of importance in the female. The smaller the prominence, the greater the anteroposterior diameter of the female pelvis.

Q. In Figure 1-8, identify D.

A. The ala. Each has an articular facet on its lateral aspect for articulation with the ilium. These are often called auricular (earlike) facets due to their shape.

Q. In Figure 1-8, identify E.

A. The lateral mass.

Q. The lateral mass of the sacrum is formed by . . .

A. Fusion of the transverse processes of the original five sacral vertebrae.

Q. In Figure 1-8, identify F.

A. The pelvic sacral foramina.

Q. The structures passing through the sacral foramina are . . .

A. The anterior primary rami of the sacral nerves. They are accompanied by the lateral sacral arteries.

Q. In Figure 1-8, identify G.

A. The vertebral bodies of two fused sacral vertebrae. The lines of fusion between individual vertebrae can be clearly seen.

Q. In Figure 1-8, identify H.

A. The articular facet for the coccyx.

Q. The two major structures that lie in contact with the anterior surface of the sacrum are . . .

A. The piriformis muscle and the sacral plexus of nerves. They are covered anteriorly by the pelvic peritoneum.

Q. The sacral plexus is formed by the union of . . .

A. The lumbo-sacral trunk and the anterior primary rami of the first, second, and third sacral nerves and part of the fourth sacral nerve.

Q. The lumbo-sacral trunk is formed from . . .

A. The anterior primary rami of the fifth lumbar nerve and part of the anterior primary ramus of the fourth lumbar nerve.

Q. The somatic components of the sacral plexus innervate . . .

A. The muscles and skin of the posterior aspect of the thigh and the muscles and skin of the leg and foot.

Q. The autonomic components of the sacral plexus provide . . .

A. Parasympathetic nerve supply to the reproductive tract, the urinary tract, and the gastrointestinal tract from the splenic flexure of the colon to the rectum.

Q. In Figure 1-9, identify A.

A. The sacral promontory.

Q. In Figure 1-9, identify B.

A. The body of the first sacral vertebra.

Q. In Figure 1-9, identify C.

A. The left pedicle of the neural arch.

Q. In Figure 1-9, the structure that lies in the superior vertebral notch of the left pedicle of the neural arch is . . .

A. The left fifth lumbar spinal nerve.

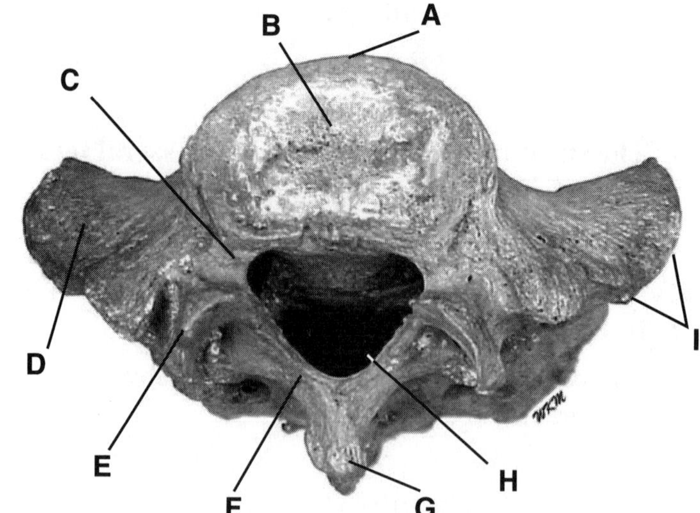

Figure 1-9 The Female Sacrum, Superior Aspect

Q. In Figure 1-9, identify D.

A. The left ala of the sacrum.

Q. In Figure 1-9, identify E.

A. The left superior articular process. Its facet faces posteromedially.

Q. In Figure 1-9, identify F.

A. The left lamina of the sacrum.

Q. In Figure 1-9, identify G.

A. The spine of the first piece of the sacrum.

Q. In Figure 1-9, identify H.

A. The vertebral canal.

Q. In Figure 1-9, identify I.

A. The facet for articulation with the right ilium.

RADIOLOGY OF THE BACK

Q. In Figure 1-10, identify A.

A. The angle of the mandible.

Q. In Figure 1-10, identify B.

A. The transverse process of the second cervical vertebra. Note that in a regular AP X-ray of the cervical spine, the arches, the lateral masses, and the transverse processes of the atlas and the odontoid process, the dens, of the axis are all obscured by the body of the mandible. This problem can be avoided by taking the X-ray with the mandible moving.

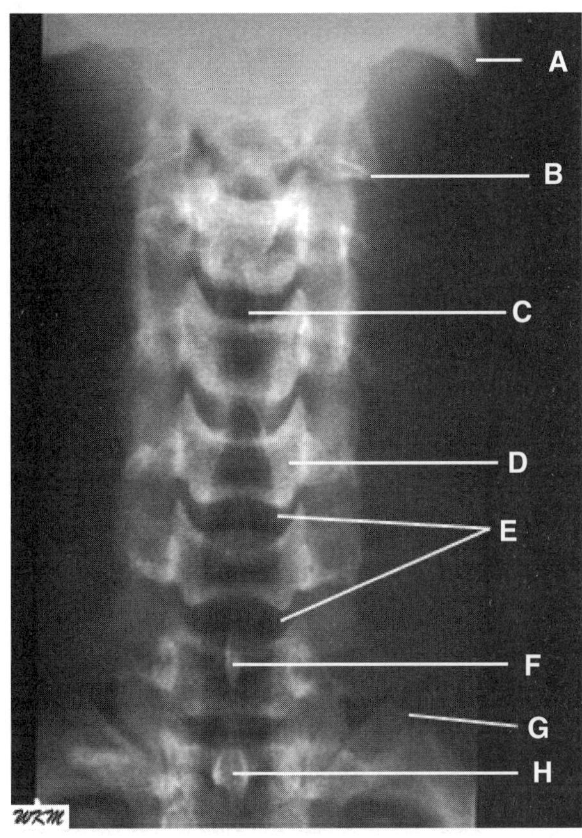

Figure 1-10 AP X-ray of the Cervical Spine

Q. In Figure 1-10, identify C.

A. The intervertebral space between the third cervical vertebra and the fourth cervical vertebra.

Q. In Figure 1-10, identify D.

A. The body of the fifth cervical vertebra.

Q. In Figure 1-10, the dark area indicated by E is . . .

A. Air in the trachea. Note that the air space narrows superiorly at the glottis.

Q. In Figure 1-10, identify F.

A. The spine of the seventh cervical vertebra.

Q. In Figure 1-10, identify G.

A. The first rib.

Q. In Figure 1-10, identify H.

A. The spine of the first thoracic vertebra.

Q. In Figure 1-11, identify A.

A. The mastoid process.

Q. In Figure 1-11, identify B.

A. The odontoid process of the second cervical vertebra, the axis.

Q. In Figure 1-11, identify C.

A. The posterior tubercle of the atlas.

Q. In Figure 1-11, identify D.

A. The spine of the axis, the second cervical vertebra.

Q. In Figure 1-11, identify E.

A. The zygapophyseal joint between the inferior articular facet of the third cervical vertebra and the superior articular facet of the fourth cervical vertebra.

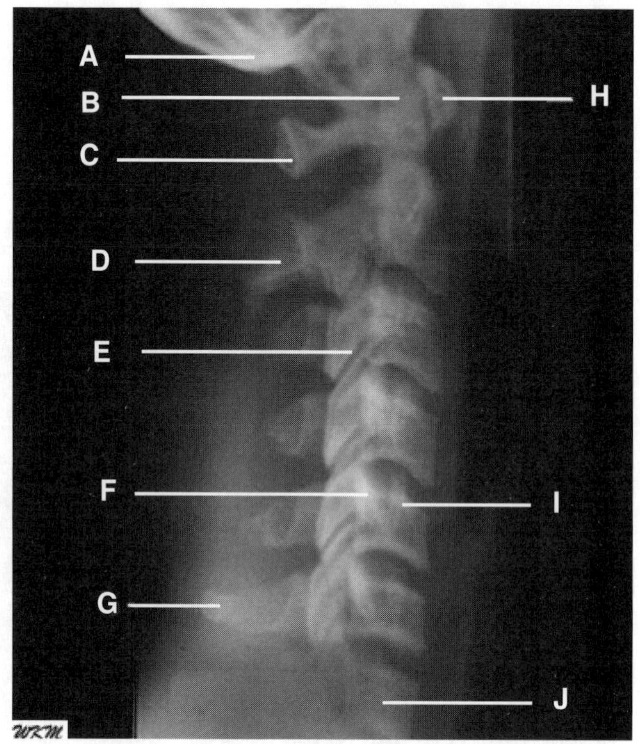

Figure 1-11 Lateral X-ray of the Cervical Spine

Q. In Figure 1-11, identify F.

A. The posterior tubercle of the transverse process of the fifth cervical vertebra.

Q. In Figure 1-11, identify G.

A. The spinous process of the sixth cervical vertebra.

Q. In Figure 1-11, identify H.

A. The anterior arch of the atlas.

Q. In Figure 1-11, identify I.

A. The anterior tubercle of the transverse process of the fifth cervical vertebra.

Q. In Figure 1-11, identify J.

A. The body of the seventh cervical vertebra.

Q. In Figure 1-12, identify A.

A. The posterior arch of the atlas.

Q. In Figure 1-12, identify B.

A. The spine of the axis.

Q. The cervical vertebral spines that can be palpated relatively easily are . . .

A. The second cervical spine and the seventh cervical spine.

Q. In Figure 1-12, identify C.

A. The intervertebral foramen for the fifth cervical nerve. It lies between the fourth cervical vertebra and the fifth cervical vertebra.

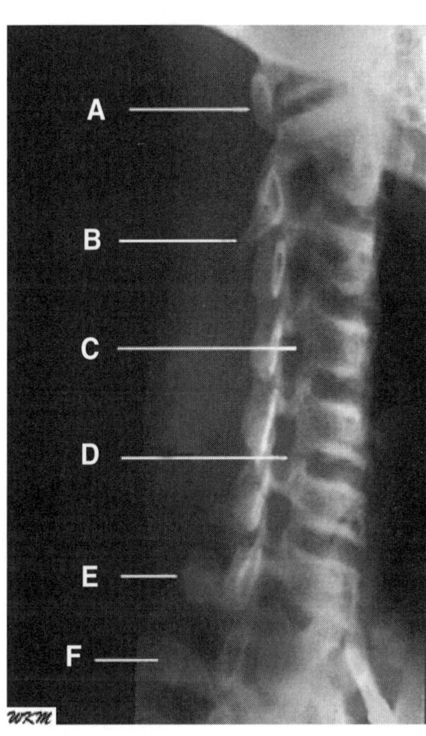

Figure 1-12 Oblique X-ray of the Cervical Spine

Q. The cutaneous distribution of the fifth cervical nerve is . . .

A. The skin over the shoulder and down the lateral side of the arm.

Q. In Figure 1-12, identify the space indicated by D.

A. A joint of Luschka. These are not true joints, but narrow fissures between the posterolateral aspects of adjacent cervical vertebrae. Note their close relationship to the intervertebral foramina, and hence to the cervical nerves that lie therein. Osteophytic outgrowths in this location are common in the elderly. The resulting pressure on the cervical nerves can result in severe neuritic pain over the distribution of the affected nerves.

Q. In Figure 1-12, identify E.

A. The spine of the seventh cervical vertebra.

Q. In Figure 1-12, identify F.

A. The spine of the first thoracic vertebra. Note that in this individual it is the vertebra prominens. More commonly, the seventh cervical spine is more prominent.

Q. In Figure 1-13, identify A.

A. The spinal cord.

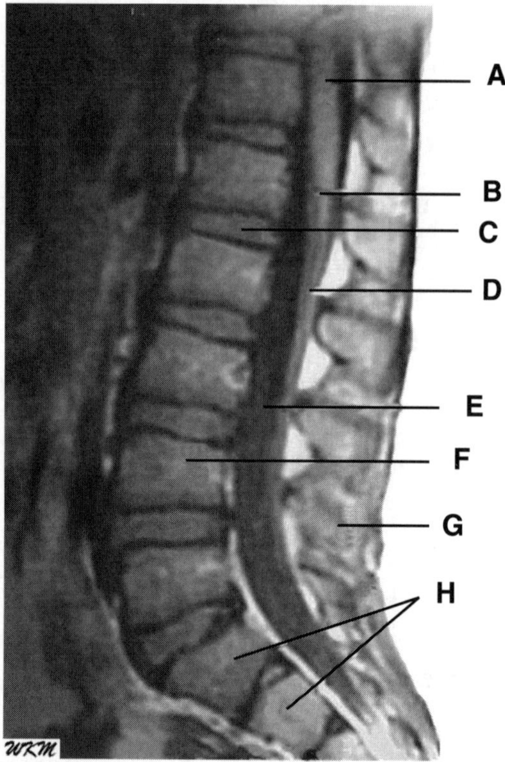

Figure 1-13 Lateral MRI of the Spinal Cord

Q. In Figure 1-13, identify B.

A. The conus medullaris.

Q. In Figure 1-13, identify C precisely.

A. The intervertebral disk between the first lumbar vertebra and the second lumbar vertebra.

Q. The spinal cord becomes the conus medullaris at the level of . . .

A. The disk between the first and second lumbar vertebrae.

Q. In Figure 1-13, identify D.

A. The filum terminale interna. It is the part of the filum terminale that lies in the subarachnoid space.

Q. In Figure 1-13, identify E.

A. The subarachnoid space.

Q. In Figure 1-13, identify F.

A. The fourth lumbar vertebra.

Q. In Figure 1-13, identify G.

A. The fourth lumbar spine.

Q. The preferred site for performing a lumbar puncture is in the interspinous space between . . .

A. The third and fourth lumbar spines.

Q. In Figure 1-13, identify H.

A. The first and second pieces of the sacrum.

Q. In Figure 1-14, identify A.

A. The ilium.

Q. In Figure 1-14, identify B.

A. The ala of the sacrum.

Q. In Figure 1-14, identify C.

A. The first sacral nerve.

Q. In Figure 1-14, identify D.

A. The dural sac.

Q. In Figure 1-14, identify E.

A. The epidural space.

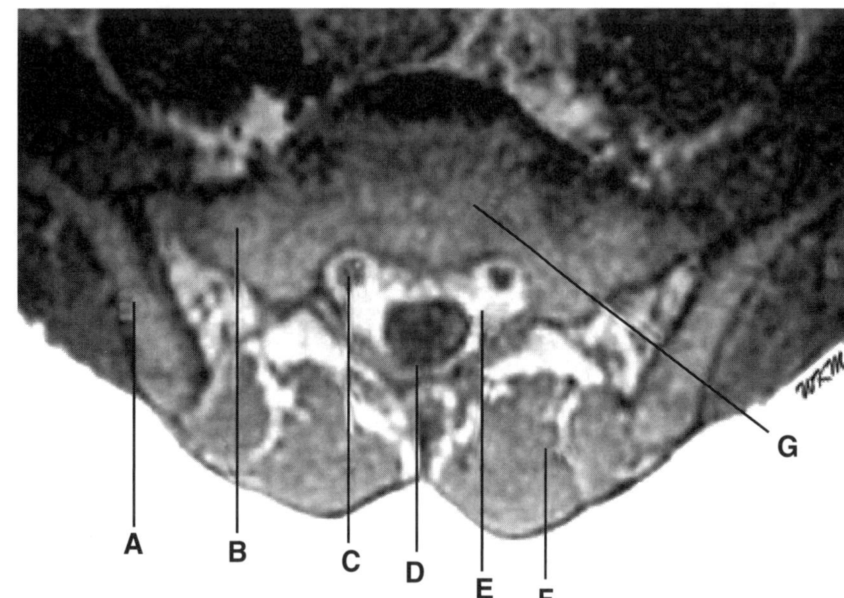

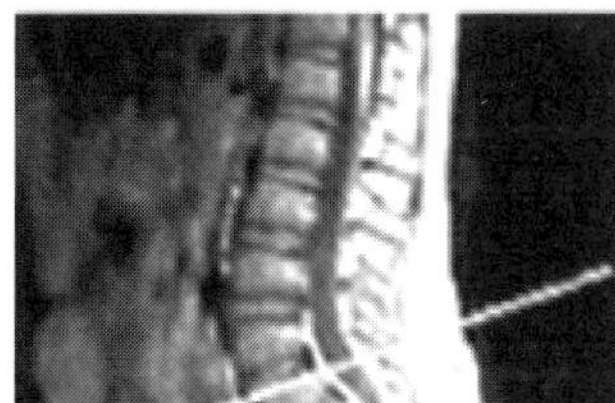

Figure 1-14 Transverse MRI of the Sacral Canal

Q. In Figure 1-14, identify F.

A. The sacrospinalis (the erector spinae) muscle.

Q. In Figure 1-14, identify G.

A. The body of the sacrum.

Chapter 2

The Upper Limb

THE SCAPULAR REGION

Q. In Figure 2-1, identify A.

A. The acromion.

Q. In Figure 2-1, identify B.

A. The spine of the scapula.

Q. In Figure 2-1, identify C.

A. The superior angle of the scapula.

Q. In Figure 2-1, identify D.

A. The supraspinous fossa. The supraspinatus muscle arises from it.

Q. In Figure 2-1, identify E.

A. The medial (dorsal) border of the scapula.

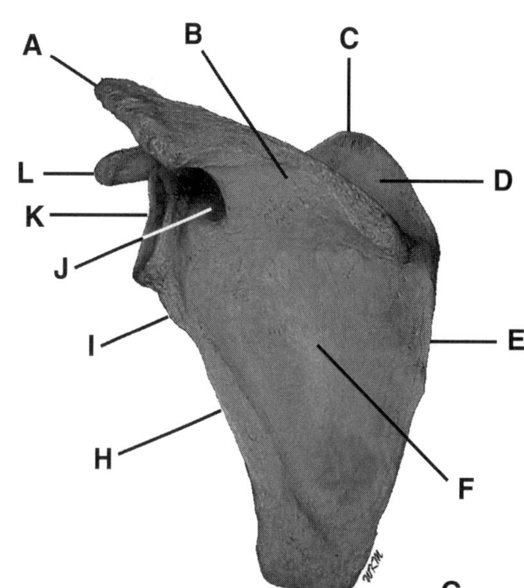

Figure 2-1 The Left Scapula, Posterior Aspect

Q. In Figure 2-1, identify F.

A. The infraspinous fossa.

Q. In Figure 2-1, identify G.

A. The inferior angle of the scapula.

Q. In Figure 2-1, identify H.

A. The lateral border of the scapula.

Q. In Figure 2-1, identify I.

A. The infraglenoid tubercle. The long head of the triceps muscle arises from it.

Q. In Figure 2-1, identify J.

A. The spinoglenoid notch. The suprascapular artery and the suprascapular nerve pass through it to reach the infraspinatus muscle.

Q. In Figure 2-1, identify K.

A. The glenoid fossa. Together with the head of the humerus, it forms the glenohumeral joint, the major component of the shoulder mechanism.

Q. In Figure 2-1, identify L.

A. The coracoid process. It is better seen from the anterior aspect of the bone.

Q. The external occipital protuberance is . . .

A. The bony prominence on the back of the skull. It is also known as the inion. It provides attachment for the upper end of the ligamentum nuchae (the nuchal ligament).

Q. The vertebra prominens is . . .

A. The spine of the seventh cervical vertebra. Occasionally, the spine of the first thoracic vertebra is more prominent.

Q. The spine of the scapula lies at the level of . . .

A. The third thoracic spine, when the subject is standing normally.

Q. The inferior angle of the scapula is normally at the level of . . .

A. The seventh thoracic spine.

Q. The fourth lumbar spine lies on . . .

A. The supracristal plane. This plane is situated at the highest point of the iliac crests. The interval between the third and the fourth lumbar spines is normally chosen for lumbar puncture.

Q. Only one of the following three bony points cannot be readily palpated: the superior angle of the scapula, the spine of the scapula, and the inferior angle of the scapula. The bony point that cannot be readily palpated is . . .

A. The superior angle of the scapula. It is covered by the thick muscle fibers of the trapezius muscle.

Q. Four muscles, the trapezius muscle, the levator scapulae muscle, the rhomboid major muscle, and the rhomboid minor muscle, connect the scapula directly to the vertebral column. They are all supplied entirely by the anterior primary rami of spinal nerves except for . . .

A. The trapezius muscle. It receives its major innervation from the spinal accessory (11th cranial) nerve. The nerve is accompanied down the anterior surface of the muscle by the superficial branch of the transverse cervical artery. The trapezius muscle also receives a few fibers from the anterior primary rami of the third and fourth cervical spinal nerves.

Q. The trapezius muscle arises from the superior nuchal line, the ligamentum nuchae, and the spines of all of the thoracic vertebrae. It is inserted into the upper border of the spine of the scapula and into the posterior border of the lateral one-third of the clavicle. The major action of the trapezius muscle is to . . .

A. Elevate the shoulder. It also assists in rotating the scapula when the arm is raised above the shoulder. Shrugging the shoulder is the best way to test the spinal accessory nerve.

Q. The latissimus dorsi muscle arises, deep to the trapezius muscle, from the spines of the lower six thoracic vertebrae, from the thoracodorsal fascia, and from the posterior part of the iliac crest. It is inserted into the floor of the bicipital groove on the humerus. Its major actions are . . .

A. Adduction and medial rotation of the humerus. It is one of the muscles used in arm wrestling.

Q. The nerve supply of the latissimus dorsi muscle is . . .

A. The thoracodorsal nerve. It arises from the posterior cord of the brachial plexus.

Q. The teres major muscle arises from the dorsal surface of the inferior angle of the scapula. It is inserted into the medial lip of the intertubercular sulcus of the humerus. Together with the latissimus dorsi muscle, it forms the posterior axillary fold. The nerve supply of the teres major muscle is . . .

A. The lower subscapular nerve, which originates from the C5 and C6 cervical nerves. It arises from the posterior cord of the brachial plexus.

Q. The rhomboid major muscle arises from the spines of the second through the fifth thoracic vertebrae, deep to the trapezius muscle. It is inserted into . . .

A. The medial border of the scapula, between the inferior angle and the base of the spine.

Q. The rhomboid minor muscle arises from the spines of the seventh cervical vertebra and the first thoracic vertebra, deep to the trapezius muscle. It is inserted into . . .

A. The medial border of the scapula at the base of its spine, just superior to the rhomboid major muscle.

Q. The nerve supply of the rhomboid major and rhomboid minor muscles is . . .

A. The dorsal scapular nerve. It arises from the anterior primary rami of the fourth and fifth cervical nerves. The nerve is accompanied on the deep surface of these muscles by the deep branch of the transverse cervical artery.

Q. The transverse cervical artery is a branch of . . .

A. The thyrocervical trunk. It is a branch of the third part of the subclavian artery.

Q. The levator scapulae muscle is attached to the medial border of the scapula, between the attachment of the rhomboid minor muscle and the superior angle of the scapula. It can be easily distinguished from the rhomboid minor muscle because it winds around . . .

A. The side of the neck. It originates from the transverse processes of the first four cervical vertebrae and then winds posteriorly and inferiorly around the side of the neck to reach the scapula.

Q. The nerve supply of the levator scapulae muscle is from . . .

A. The anterior primary of the third and fourth cervical nerves.

Q. In Figure 2-2, identify A.

A. The spine of the scapula.

Q. In Figure 2-2, identify B.

A. The coracoid process of the scapula.

Q. In Figure 2-2, identify C.

A. The lateral end of the clavicle.

Q. In Figure 2-2, identify D.

A. The acromioclavicular joint. Note that it is a plane joint; its long axis runs anteroposteriorly.

Q. In Figure 2-2, identify E.

A. The acromion, the point of the shoulder.

Q. In Figure 2-2, identify F.

A. The greater tubercle of the humerus.

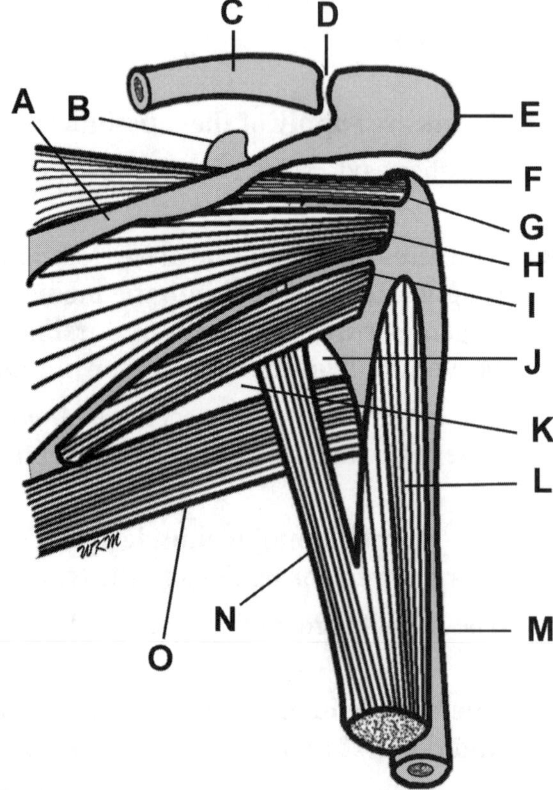

Figure 2-2 The Shoulder, Posterior Aspect

Q. In Figure 2-2, identify G.

A. The supraspinatus muscle. It arises from the supraspinous fossa of the scapula and is inserted into the greater tubercle of the humerus. It is essential for initiating arm abduction.

Q. The nerve supply of the supraspinatus muscle is . . .

A. The suprascapular nerve. It reaches the muscle through the suprascapular notch of the scapula, inferior to the transverse scapular ligament.

Q. In Figure 2-2, identify H.

A. The infraspinatus muscle. It arises from the infraspinous fossa of the scapula. It is inserted into the greater tubercle of the humerus, and, like the supraspinatus muscle, is supplied by the suprascapular nerve. It is a lateral rotator of the humerus.

Q. In Figure 2-2, identify I.

A. The teres minor muscle. It arises from the lateral border of the scapula and is attached to the greater tubercle of the humerus, inferior to the infraspinatus muscle. It is a lateral rotator of the arm and, together with the deltoid muscle, is supplied by the axillary nerve.

Q. In Figure 2-2, identify J.

A. The quadrangular space. The axillary nerve and the posterior circumflex humeral artery pass through it.

Q. In Figure 2-2, identify K.

A. The triangular space. The circumflex branch of the subscapular artery passes through it.

Q. In Figure 2-2, identify L.

A. The lateral head of the triceps muscle. It arises from a ridge on the posterior surface of the shaft of the humerus. The medial head of the triceps muscle, arising from the posterior surface of the humerus, is covered, posteriorly, by the lateral head and the long head of the muscle and is therefore not visible in this view.

Q. The nerve supply of the triceps is . . .

A. The radial nerve. It is the larger of the two terminal branches of the posterior cord of the brachial plexus.

Q. In Figure 2-2, identify M.

A. The shaft of the humerus.

Q. In Figure 2-2, identify N.

A. The long head of the triceps muscle. Note that it separates the teres major muscle from the teres minor muscle. It also separates the triangular space from the quadrangular space.

Q. In Figure 2-2, identify O.

A. The teres major muscle. Note that it forms the inferior border of both the quadrangular space and the triangular space.

Q. In Figure 2-3, identify A.

A. The subclavian artery.

Q. The subclavian artery becomes the axillary artery at . . .

A. The outer border of the first rib.

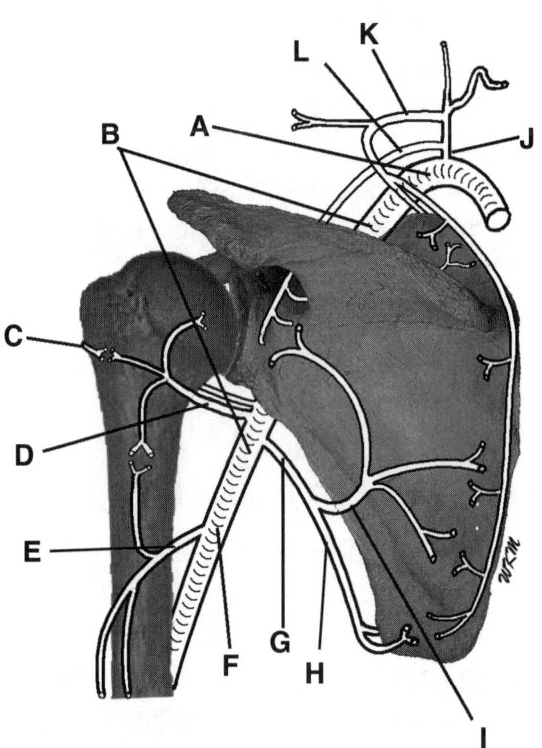

Figure 2-3 The Anastomosis Around the Scapula, Posterior Aspect

Q. In Figure 2-3, identify B.

A. The axillary artery.

Q. The axillary artery becomes the brachial artery after leaving the axilla by crossing . . .

A. The latissimus dorsi muscle and the teres major muscle.

Q. In Figure 2-3, identify C.

A. The anterior circumflex humeral artery.

Q. The most important function of the anterior circumflex humeral artery is to supply . . .

A. The tendon of the long head of the biceps muscle in the intertubercular sulcus. Interruption or arteriosclerosis of this vessel, usually later in life, results in ischemia and subsequent rupture of this tendon. This rupture results in an obvious swelling of the muscle belly when flexion of the forearm is attempted.

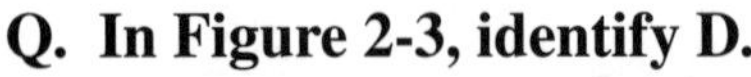

Q. In Figure 2-3, identify D.

A. The posterior circumflex humeral artery.

Q. The posterior circumflex humeral artery leaves the axilla by passing through . . .

A. The quadrangular space.

Q. The posterior circumflex artery is accompanied through the quadrangular space by . . .

A. The axillary nerve. The axillary nerve supplies the deltoid muscle, the teres minor muscle, and the skin over the deltoid muscle.

Q. In Figure 2-3, identify E.

A. The profunda brachii artery. It is a branch of the brachial artery and accompanies the radial nerve in the spiral groove on the posterior surface of the humerus.

Q. In Figure 2-3, identify F.

A. The brachial artery. It terminates by dividing into the radial and ulnar arteries, approximately half an inch (1 cm) below the elbow.

Q. In Figure 2-3, identify G.

A. The subscapular artery. It arises from the third part of the axillary artery and terminates by dividing into the circumflex scapular artery and the thoracodorsal artery.

Q. In Figure 2-3, identify H.

A. The thoracodorsal artery. It accompanies the thoracodorsal nerve.

Q. In Figure 2-3, identify I.

A. The circumflex scapular artery. It is a terminal branch of the subscapular artery. It supplies the infraspinatus muscle and the teres minor muscle.

Q. In Figure 2-3, identify J.

A. The thyrocervical trunk. It arises from the third part of the subclavian artery and gives rise to the suprascapular artery, the transverse cervical artery, the ascending cervical artery, and the inferior thyroid artery.

Q. The branches of the thyrocervical trunk that participate in the anastomosis around the scapula are . . .

A. The suprascapular artery and the deep branch of the transverse cervical artery.

Q. In Figure 2-3, identify K.

A. The transverse cervical artery. It divides into a transverse superficial branch and a deep descending branch. The latter also divides into superficial and deep branches.

Q. In Figure 2-3, identify L.

A. The suprascapular artery. It passes above the transverse scapular ligament to reach the supraspinatus muscle and the infraspinatus muscle. The suprascapular nerve passes below the transverse scapular ligament between the ligament and the scapula.

Q. In Figure 2-4, identify A.

A. The anatomical neck of the humerus.

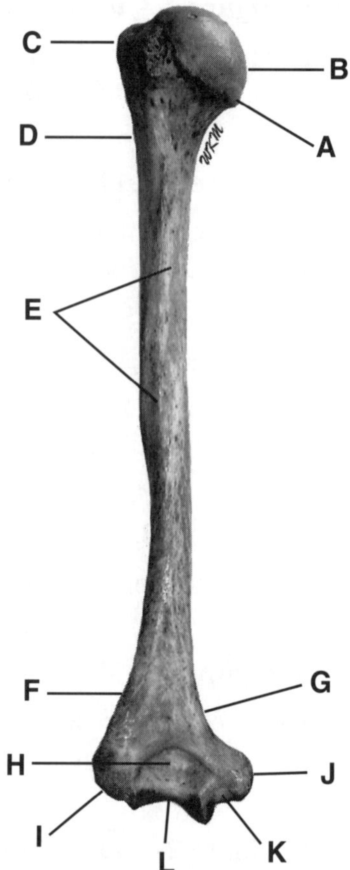

Figure 2-4 The Left Humerus, Posterior Aspect

Q. In Figure 2-4, identify B.

A. The head of the humerus.

Q. In Figure 2-4, identify C.

A. The greater tubercle (greater tuberosity) of the humerus.

Q. In Figure 2-4, identify D.

A. The surgical neck of the humerus. This is the region most commonly fractured by indirect violence. The axillary nerve is closely related to its medial aspect and is therefore frequently injured in such fractures.

Q. In Figure 2-4, identify E.

A. The musculospiral groove. This area is in close relationship with the radial nerve, because the latter winds around the shaft of the humerus. The radial nerve is vulnerable to external pressure in this area and is liable to be involved in fractures of the shaft of the humerus.

Q. In Figure 2-4, identify F.

A. The lateral supracondylar ridge.

Q. In Figure 2-4, identify G.

A. The medial supracondylar ridge.

Q. In Figure 2-4, identify H.

A. The olecranon fossa.

Q. In Figure 2-4, identify I.

A. The lateral epicondyle.

Q. In Figure 2-4, identify J.

A. The trochlear notch. It is the area that articulates with the ulna.

Q. In Figure 2-4, identify K.

A. The groove for the ulnar nerve. At this point, the ulnar nerve is vulnerable to external trauma. When stimulated, a tingling sensation may be felt down the medial side of the forearm and hand, hence the common appellation of "funny bone" for this part of the elbow.

Q. In Figure 2-4, identify L.

A. The prominent medial epicondyle.

Q. The bony prominence that can be felt through the deltoid muscle immediately inferior to the acromion in the anatomical position is . . .

A. The greater tubercle of the humerus. It is separated from the acromion by a bursa, appropriately named the subacromial bursa.

Q. The deltoid muscle is inserted into the deltoid tuberosity, approximately halfway down the lateral aspect of the humerus. Its superior attachment (i.e., its origin) is from . . .

A. The anterior border of the lateral one-third of the clavicle, the tip of the acromion, and the inferior border of the spine of the scapula.

Q. The most important function of the deltoid muscle is . . .

A. Abduction of the arm. Its posterior fibers contribute significantly to lateral rotation of the humerus. Its anterior fibers contribute, less importantly, to medial rotation of the humerus.

Q. The nerve supply of the deltoid muscle is . . .

A. The axillary nerve. It is one of the two terminal branches of the posterior cord of the brachial plexus.

Q. Other structures supplied by the axillary nerve are . . .

A. The teres minor muscle and the skin over the deltoid muscle. The branch to the skin is the upper lateral cutaneous nerve of the arm.

Q. The axillary nerve reaches the deltoid muscle by circling . . .

A. The surgical neck of the humerus. As it passes through the quadrangular space, it is accompanied by the posterior circumflex humeral artery, which is a lateral branch of the third part of the axillary artery.

Q. A "square shoulder" following an injury indicates . . .

A. Anterior dislocation of the head of the humerus. Because the greater tubercle of the humerus no longer displaces the deltoid muscle laterally, the rounded contour of the normal shoulder is lost.

Q. The bony prominence that can be felt immediately inferior to the lateral one-third of the clavicle is . . .

A. The coracoid process of the scapula. The lesser tubercle of the humerus can be felt immediately inferior to the coracoid process.

THE PECTORAL REGION

Q. In Figure 2-5, identify A.

A. The head of the humerus.

Q. The three rotator cuff muscles, which are attached to the greater tubercle of the humerus, are . . .

A. The supraspinatus muscle, the infraspinatus muscle, and the teres minor muscle.

Q. In Figure 2-5, identify B.

A. The greater tubercle of the humerus.

Q. In Figure 2-5, identify C.

A. The lesser tubercle (lesser tuberosity) of the humerus.

Q. The muscle that is inserted into the lateral lip of the intertubercular sulcus is . . .

A. The pectoralis major muscle. The latissimus dorsi muscle attaches to the floor of the intertubercular sulcus (the bicipital groove) between the pectoralis major muscle and the teres major muscle.

Q. In Figure 2-5, identify D.

A. The intertubercular sulcus (the bicipital groove). It is occupied by the tendon of the long head of the biceps. The tendon of the latissimus major muscle is inserted into its floor.

Q. In Figure 2-5, identify E.

A. The medial lip of the intertubercular sulcus.

Q. In Figure 2-5, identify F.

A. The lateral lip of the intertubercular sulcus (the bicipital groove).

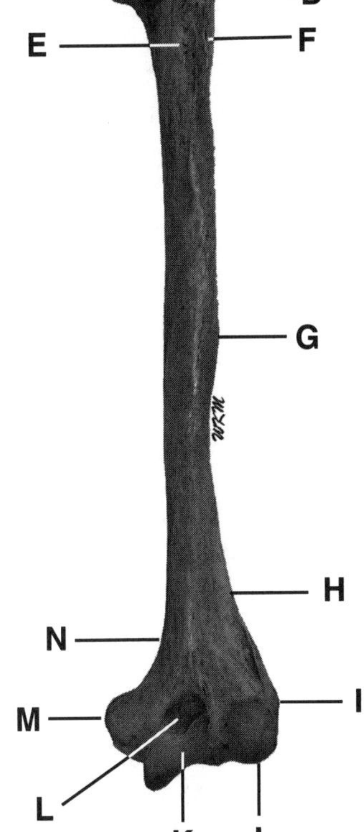

Figure 2-5 Left Humerus, Anterior Aspect

Q. In Figure 2-5, identify G.

A. The deltoid tuberosity. It is formed by the attachment of the deltoid muscle.

Q. In Figure 2-5, identify H.

A. The lateral supracondylar ridge. The lateral intermuscular septum is attached to it.

Q. In Figure 2-5, identify I.

A. The lateral epicondyle.

Q. In Figure 2-5, identify J.

A. The capitulum (capitellum). It articulates with the head of the radius.

Q. In Figure 2-5, identify K.

A. The trochlea. It articulates with the trochlear notch of the ulna.

Q. In Figure 2-5, identify L.

A. The coronoid fossa for the coronoid process of the ulna.

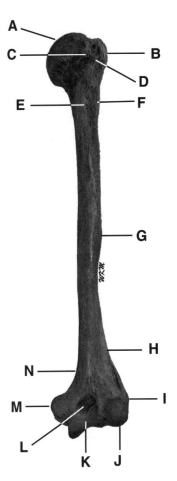

Q. The muscle that is attached to the medial lip of the intertubercular sulcus is . . .

A. The teres major muscle.

Q. In Figure 2-5, identify M.

A. The medial epicondyle. The ulnar nerve lies posterior to it.

Q. The rotator cuff muscle that is attached to the lesser tubercle of the humerus is . . .

A. The subscapularis muscle.

Q. In Figure 2-5, identify N.

A. The medial supracondylar ridge.

Q. In Figure 2-6, identify muscle A.

A. The subclavius muscle. It acts as a cushion between the subclavian artery and the clavicle.

Q. In Figure 2-6, identify muscle B.

A. The deltoid muscle. It causes the rounded contour of the shoulder.

Q. In Figure 2-6, identify muscle C.

A. The subscapularis muscle. It forms most of the posterior wall of the axilla.

Q. In Figure 2-6, identify muscle D.

A. The teres major muscle. Together with the latissimus dorsi muscle, it forms the posterior axillary fold.

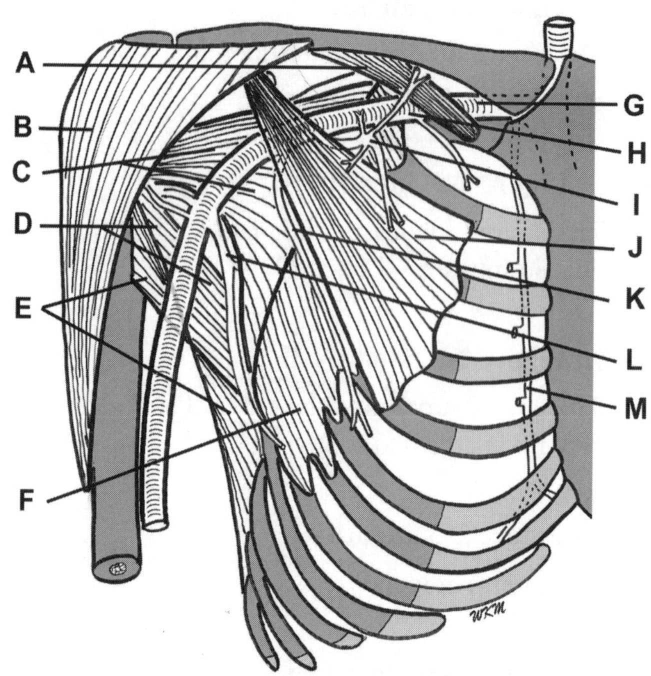

Figure 2-6 The Pectoral Region and Axilla

Q. In Figure 2-6, identify muscle E.

A. The latissimus dorsi muscle. It winds around the lower border of the teres major muscle, posterior to the axillary artery, and is inserted into the floor of the intertubercular sulcus.

Q. In Figure 2-6, identify muscle F.

A. The serratus anterior muscle. Its multiple origins, from the second to the eighth ribs, give its anterior border a serrated appearance. It forms the medial wall of the axilla.

Q. In Figure 2-6, identify artery G.

A. The subclavian artery. On the right side, it originates from the innominate artery, posterior to the sternoclavicular joint.

Q. In Figure 2-6, identify artery H.

A. The axillary artery. At the outer border of the first rib, the subclavian artery continues as the axillary artery.

Q. In Figure 2-6, identify artery I.

A. The thoracoacromial (acromiothoracic) trunk. It arises from the axillary artery, posterior to the pectoralis minor muscle. It emerges superior to the pectoralis minor muscle and divides into four branches to supply the muscles of the upper part of the pectoral region.

Q. In Figure 2-6, identify muscle J.

A. The pectoralis minor muscle. It originates from the coracoid process of the scapula and attaches to the second, third, fourth, and fifth ribs near their junction with their costal cartilages. The pectoralis minor muscle is used, arbitrarily, to divide the axillary artery into three parts.

Q. In Figure 2-6, identify artery K.

A. The lateral thoracic artery. It runs to the chest wall under cover of the anterior axillary fold. It is one of the major arteries that supply the breast. It enlarges during pregnancy and lactation.

Q. In Figure 2-6, identify artery L.

A. The subscapular branch of the third part of the axillary artery. It terminates by dividing into the circumflex scapular artery, which supplies the infraspinatus muscle and the teres minor muscle, and the thoracodorsal artery, which supplies the lower posterior axillary wall.

Q. In Figure 2-6, identify artery M.

A. The internal thoracic artery. Its three large mammary branches are represented, as are its two terminal branches, the superior epigastric artery and the musculophrenic artery.

Q. The pectoralis major muscle has two distinct components. They are . . .

A. A clavicular head and a sternocostal head.

Q. The two heads of the pectoralis major muscle fuse and are inserted into . . .

A. The lateral lip of the intertubercular sulcus (the bicipital groove) of the humerus.

Q. The clavicular head of the pectoralis major receives its nerve supply from . . .

A. The lateral pectoral nerve from the lateral cord of the brachial plexus. It does not pierce the pectoralis minor muscle, but passes through the clavipectoral fascia, superior to the muscle.

Q. The type of activity that would be weakened if the lateral pectoral nerve were severed during a biopsy of the axillary lymph nodes in staging carcinoma of the breast is. . .

A. Medial rotation of the humerus when the arm is raised above the head. This movement occurs when brushing or combing the hair.

Q. The sternocostal head of the pectoralis major receives its nerve supply from . . .

A. The medial pectoral nerve. It arises from the medial cord of the brachial plexus. This nerve contains fibers from the lower roots of the plexus. It penetrates the pectoralis minor muscle to reach and supply the pectoralis major muscle.

Q. The major actions of the pectoralis major are . . .

A. Adduction and medial rotation of the humerus, such as occurs in arm wrestling.

THE MAMMARY GLAND AND LYMPHATIC DRAINAGE

Q. The breast is a modified sebaceous gland. It therefore lies in the superficial fascia of the pectoral region extending from . . .

A. The second to the sixth ribs.

Q. A significant part of the female breast extends into the axilla. It is referred to as . . .

A. The axillary tail.

Q. The lymphatics from the lobules of the breast first drain centripetally to the subareolar lymphatic plexus. From this plexus, the majority of the lymph drains centrifugally into . . .

A. The anterior (pectoral) group of the axillary lymph nodes. However, lymph from the medial portion of the breast drains into the mediastinal nodes, which lie along the internal thoracic veins.

Q. Lymph from the anterior (pectoral) group of axillary nodes drains into . . .

A. The apical group of axillary lymph nodes.

Q. The lateral group of axillary lymph nodes also drains into the apical group of axillary nodes. The lateral group of axillary lymph nodes lies along . . .

A. The axillary vein.

Q. The lateral group of axillary lymph nodes receives lymph from . . .

A. The upper limb. However, lymph from the lateral side of the upper limb follows the cephalic vein and reaches the apical lymph nodes directly. Lymph drainage from the back passes through the posterior (subscapular) lymph nodes before reaching the apical group.

THE BRACHIAL PLEXUS

Q. In Figure 2-7, the components of the brachial plexus indicated by A are . . .

A. The roots of the plexus. They are the anterior (ventral) primary rami of the indicated spinal nerves.

Q. In Figure 2-7, the components of the brachial plexus indicated by B are . . .

A. The superior, middle, and inferior trunks of the plexus.

Q. The trunk of the brachial plexus that contains fibers from only one anterior primary ramus is . . .

A. The middle trunk. It carries fibers from the anterior primary ramus of C7. All anterior primary rami, except C1, are mixed nerves. They contain both motor and sensory fibers.

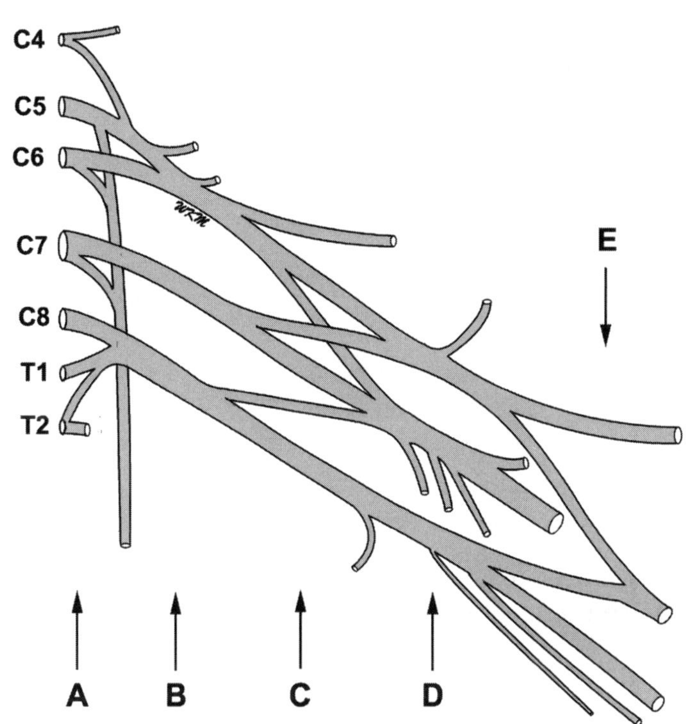

Figure 2-7 The Brachial Plexus, Formation

Q. In Figure 2-7, the components of the brachial plexus indicated by C are . . .

A. The divisions of the plexus. Each trunk divides into anterior and posterior divisions posterior to the clavicle. Note that fibers from all three posterior divisions unite to form the posterior cord.

Q. The anterior divisions of the upper and middle trunks unite to form . . .

A. The lateral cord of the brachial plexus.

Q. In Figure 2-7, the components of the brachial plexus indicated by D are . . .

A. The cords of the plexus. They form the first part of the plexus, which lies inferior to the clavicle. They are named the lateral, the posterior, and the medial cords. These names correspond to their relationship to the second part of the axillary artery.

Q. The medial cord of the brachial plexus is formed by . . .

A. The anterior division of the inferior trunk of the brachial plexus.

Q. In Figure 2-7, the branches of the brachial plexus indicated by E are . . .

A. The terminal branches.

Q. In Figure 2-8, identify A.

A. The nerve to the levator scapulae muscle. It carries fibers from the fourth and fifth anterior primary rami to the levator scapulae muscle.

Q. In Figure 2-8, identify B.

A. The dorsal scapular nerve. It supplies both the rhomboid major muscle and the rhomboid minor muscle. It carries fibers from the fifth and the sixth anterior primary rami.

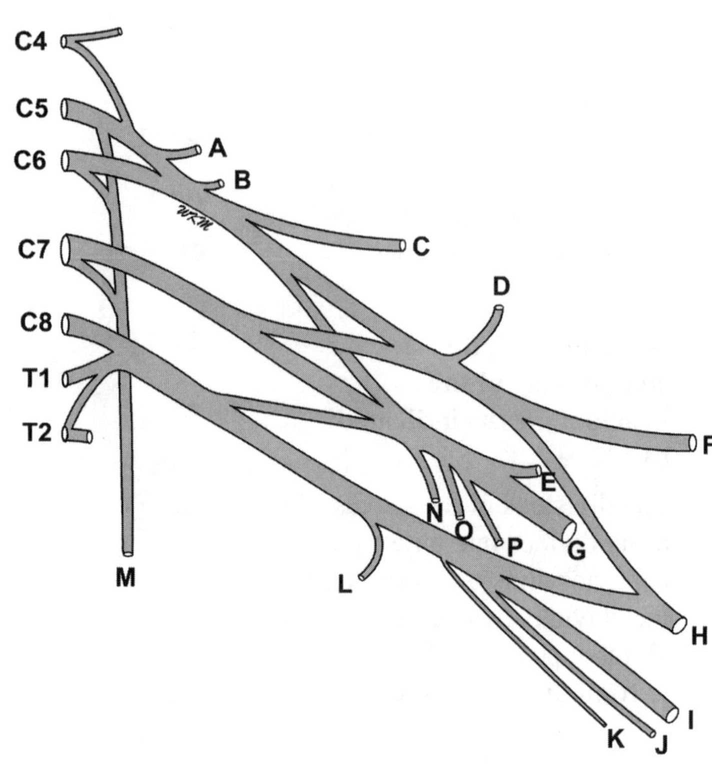

Figure 2-8 The Brachial Plexus, Branches

Q. In Figure 2-8, identify C.

A. The suprascapular nerve. It carries fibers from the fifth and the sixth anterior primary rami to the supraspinatus muscle and the infraspinatus muscle.

Q. In Figure 2-8, identify D.

A. The lateral pectoral nerve. It supplies the clavicular head of the pectoralis major muscle.

Q. In Figure 2-8, identify E.

A. The axillary nerve. Via the upper lateral cutaneous nerve of the arm, it carries fibers from the fifth and the sixth anterior primary rami to the teres minor muscle, the deltoid muscle, and the skin over the deltoid muscle.

Q. In Figure 2-8, identify F.

A. The musculocutaneous nerve. It carries fibers from the fifth and the sixth anterior primary rami to the anterior group of muscles of the arm and continues as the lateral cutaneous nerve of the forearm.

Q. In Figure 2-8, identify G.

A. The radial nerve. It supplies all of the muscles on the posterior surface of the arm and the forearm. It also supplies the brachioradialis muscle.

Q. In Figure 2-8, identify H.

A. The median nerve. It supplies most of the muscles on the anterior surface of the forearm and five muscles on the radial side of the hand. These latter five muscles are the three muscles of the thenar eminence—the flexor pollicis brevis muscle, the abductor pollicis brevis muscle, and the opponens pollicis muscle—plus the lateral two lumbrical muscles.

Q. In Figure 2-8, identify I.

A. The ulnar nerve. It supplies two muscles on the ulnar side of the front of the forearm: the flexor carpi ulnaris muscle and the ulnar half of the flexor digitorum profundus muscle. In the hand, it supplies those muscles that are not supplied by the median nerve.

Q. In Figure 2-8, identify J.

A. The medial antebrachial cutaneous nerve. It supplies the skin of the medial side of the forearm.

Q. In Figure 2-8, identify K.

A. The medial brachial cutaneous nerve. It supplies the skin of the medial side of the arm.

Q. In Figure 2-8, identify L.

A. The medial pectoral nerve. It supplies the sternocostal head of the pectoralis major muscle and the pectoralis minor muscle.

Q. In Figure 2-8, identify M.

A. The long thoracic nerve, C5, C6, and C7. It supplies the serratus anterior muscle. It is accompanied by the lateral thoracic artery. A lesion of this nerve, usually resulting from axillary node dissection, will cause a "winged" scapula.

Q. In Figure 2-8, identify N.

A. The upper subscapular nerve. It supplies the upper part of the subscapularis muscle. It also sends a small articular branch to the glenohumeral articulation.

Q. In Figure 2-8, identify O.

A. The thoracodorsal nerve. It accompanies the thoracodorsal artery to the latissimus dorsi muscle. The latissimus dorsi muscle is supplied by both the thoracodorsal nerve and the thoracodorsal artery.

Q. In Figure 2-8, identify P.

A. The lower subscapular nerve. It supplies the lower part of the subscapularis muscle and the teres major muscle. The upper subscapular nerve, the thoracodorsal nerve, and the lower subscapular nerve are all branches of the posterior cord of the brachial plexus.

THE AXILLA

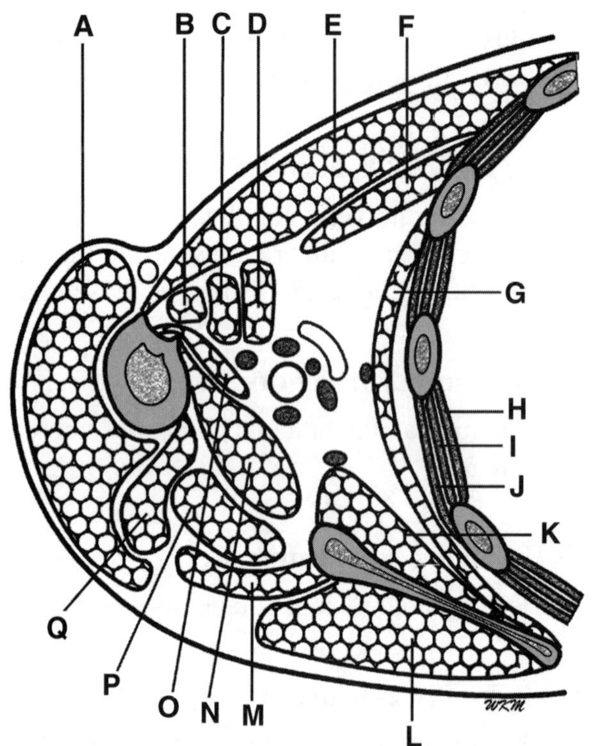

Figure 2-9 The Axilla, Horizontal Section: Muscles

Q. In Figure 2-9, identify muscle A.

A. The deltoid muscle. It is the major abductor of the humerus. In addition, its posterior fibers are lateral rotators of the humerus; its anterior fibers are medial rotators of the humerus.

Q. In Figure 2-9, identify muscle B.

A. The long head of the biceps muscle. It becomes tendinous as it ascends in the intertubercular sulcus to its origin from the supraglenoid tubercle of the scapula.

Q. In Figure 2-9, identify muscle C.

A. The short head of the biceps muscle. It arises, together with the coracobrachialis muscle, from the coracoid process of the scapula.

Q. In Figure 2-9, identify muscle D.

A. The coracobrachialis muscle. It is inserted halfway down the medial side of the shaft of the humerus.

Q. In Figure 2-9, identify muscle E.

A. The pectoralis major muscle. It inserts on the lateral lip of the intertubercular sulcus. With the pectoralis minor muscle, it forms the anterior wall of the axilla.

Q. In Figure 2-9, identify muscle F.

A. The pectoralis minor muscle. It arises from the second, third, and fourth costal cartilages. Its fibers converge to be inserted on the coracoid process of the scapula.

Q. In Figure 2-9, identify muscle G.

A. The serratus anterior muscle. It forms the medial wall of the axilla. It arises from the second through the eighth ribs and inserts on the medial border of the scapula.

Q. In Figure 2-9, identify muscle H.

A. An innermost intercostal muscle. It is a vestigial remnant of the transversus thoracis muscle.

Q. In Figure 2-9, identify muscle I.

A. An internal intercostal muscle. The internal intercostal muscles are probably largely expiratory in action.

Q. In Figure 2-9, identify muscle J.

A. An external intercostal muscle. The intercostal muscles are important muscles of respiration. The external intercostals are probably mainly inspiratory in action.

Q. In Figure 2-9, identify muscle K.

A. The subscapularis muscle. It is inserted into the lesser tubercle of the humerus. It is one of the four rotator cuff muscles responsible for the stability of the glenohumeral joint. The other rotator cuff muscles are the supraspinatus muscle, the infraspinatus muscle, and the teres minor muscle.

Q. In Figure 2-9, identify muscle L.

A. The infraspinatus muscle. It is one of the three lateral rotators of the humerus. The other two lateral rotators are the posterior fibers of the deltoid muscle and the teres minor muscle.

Q. In Figure 2-9, identify muscle M.

A. The teres minor muscle. It is difficult to separate from the infraspinatus muscle; however, it is innervated by the axillary nerve, whereas the infraspinatus muscle is supplied by the suprascapular nerve.

Q. In Figure 2-9, identify muscle N.

A. The teres major muscle. It is inserted into the medial lip of the intertubercular sulcus and is supplied by the lower subscapular nerve.

Q. In Figure 2-9, identify muscle O.

A. The tendon of the latissimus dorsi muscle. It winds around the teres major muscle to attach to the floor of the intertubercular sulcus. It is supplied by the thoracodorsal nerve and is one of the three powerful medial rotators of the humerus.

Q. In Figure 2-9, identify muscle P.

A. The long head of the triceps muscle. It arises from the infraglenoid tubercle on the scapula.

Q. In Figure 2-9, identify muscle Q.

A. The lateral head of the triceps muscle. It arises from an oblique ridge on the back of the humerus.

Q. In Figure 2-10, identify vein A.

A. The cephalic vein. It lies in the deltopectoral groove. After the cephalic vein penetrates the clavipectoral fascia, it terminates in the axillary vein.

Q. In Figure 2-10, identify nerve B.

A. The musculocutaneous nerve. This nerve lies on the lateral side of the axillary artery. It supplies the three muscles on the front of the arm: the biceps brachii muscle, the coracobrachialis muscle, and the brachialis muscle. The biceps brachii and the brachialis muscles are powerful flexors of the forearm. The biceps brachii muscle is also the most powerful supinator of the forearm. The musculocutaneous nerve continues as the lateral antebrachial cutaneous nerve, supplying the skin of the lateral side of the forearm.

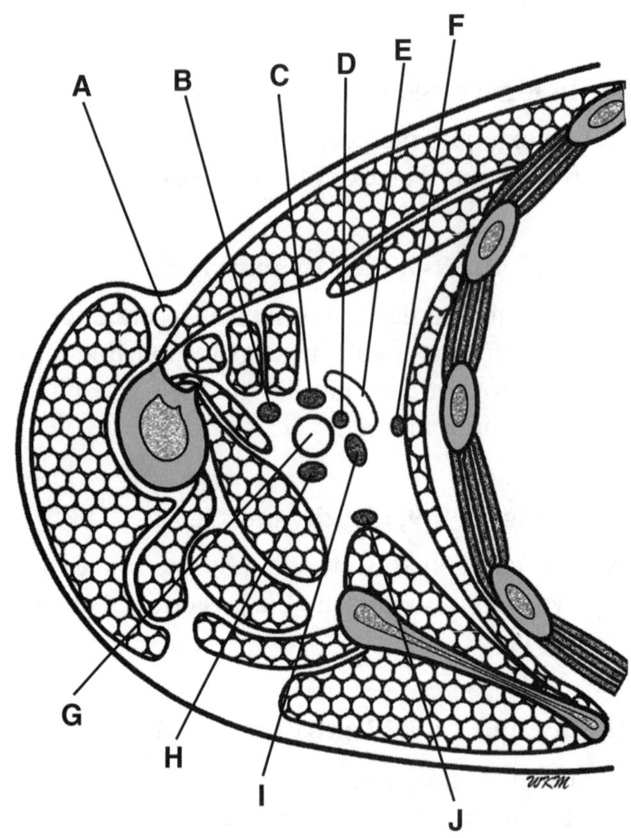

Figure 2-10 The Axilla, Horizontal Section: Vessels and Nerves

Q. In Figure 2-10, identify nerve C.

A. The median nerve. It lies anterior to the axillary artery. With the exception of the brachioradialis muscle, it supplies all of the muscles on the lateral side of the forearm and five muscles on the radial side of the hand. It also supplies the skin on the lateral side of the front of the forearm and hand.

Q. In Figure 2-10, identify nerve D.

A. The medial antebrachial cutaneous nerve.

Q. In Figure 2-10, identify vein E.

A. The axillary vein.

Q. In Figure 2-10, identify nerve F.

A. The long thoracic nerve. It arises from the fifth, sixth, and seventh anterior primary rami (the roots of the brachial plexus). It supplies the serratus anterior muscle.

Q. In Figure 2-10, identify artery G.

A. The third part of the axillary artery.

Q. The branches of the third part of the axillary artery are . . .

A. The subscapular artery, the posterior circumflex humeral artery, and the anterior circumflex humeral artery.

Q. In Figure 2-10, identify nerve H.

A. The radial nerve.

Q. The radial nerve supplies . . .

A. All of the muscles on the posterior aspect of the arm and the forearm. These are all extensor muscles of the forearm and wrist. The radial nerve also supplies the brachioradialis muscle.

Q. In Figure 2-10, identify nerve I.

A. The ulnar nerve.

Q. The ulnar nerve supplies . . .

A. The flexor carpi ulnaris muscle, the ulnar half of the flexor digitorum profundus muscle, and all of the small muscles of the hand with the exception of the three muscles of the thenar eminence and the lateral two lumbrical muscles.

Q. In Figure 2-10, identify nerve J.

A. The thoracodorsal nerve. It supplies the latissimus dorsi muscle.

THE ARM AND THE CUBITAL FOSSA

Q. The arm is described as having two fibromuscular compartments. They are . . .

A. The anterior and the posterior compartments of the arm.

Q. The anterior and the posterior compartments of the arm are separated by . . .

A. The medial and the lateral intermuscular septa. These are well developed just above the elbow. They are attached to the medial and the lateral supracondylar ridges.

Q. The muscles in the anterior compartment of the arm are . . .

A. The biceps muscle, the coracobrachialis muscle, and the brachialis muscle.

Q. The nerve supply of the coracobrachialis muscle, the biceps muscle, and the brachialis muscle is . . .

A. The musculocutaneous nerve.

Q. The muscles in the posterior compartment of the arm are . . .

A. The medial head, the long head, and the lateral head of the triceps muscle.

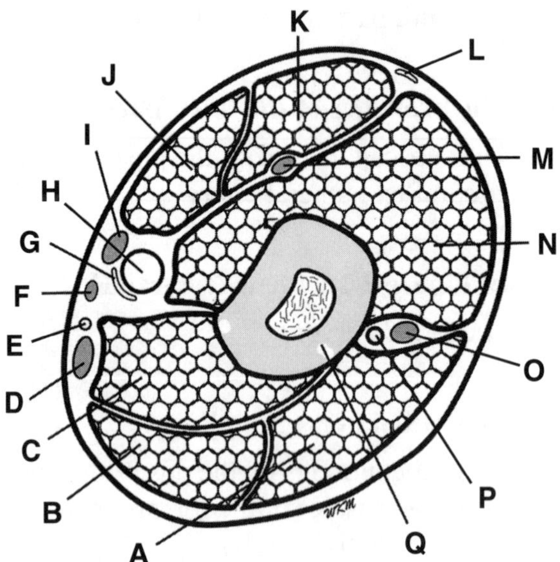

Figure 2-11 The Left Arm, Transverse Section of the Lower Third

Q. In Figure 2-11, identify A.

A. The lateral head of the triceps muscle.

Q. In Figure 2-11, identify B.

A. The long head of the triceps muscle.

Q. In Figure 2-11, identify C.

A. The medial head of the triceps muscle.
Together, the three heads of the triceps are the only major extensors of the elbow joint.

Q. In Figure 2-11, identify nerve D.

A. The ulnar nerve. It pierces the medial intermuscular septum and enters the forearm posterior to the medial epicondyle of the humerus.

Q. In Figure 2-11, identify the artery E.

A. The superior ulnar collateral artery. It accompanies the ulnar nerve, posterior to the medial epicondyle.

Q. In Figure 2-11, identify nerve F.

A. The medial antebrachial cutaneous nerve.

Q. In Figure 2-11, identify G.

A. The brachial vein. It lies anteromedial to the brachial artery. Veins are thin walled and often collapse after death, hence the characteristic shape seen in this diagram.

Q. In Figure 2-11, identify H.

A. The brachial artery. Because they have thick elastic walls, arteries are circular in section.

Q. In Figure 2-11, identify I.

A. The median nerve. It accompanies the brachial artery through the cubital fossa, lying on its medial side.

Q. In Figure 2-11, identify J and K.

A. The short head of the biceps muscle and the long head of the biceps muscle, respectively. Because the biceps muscle is inserted into the bicipital tuberosity of the radius, it is a powerful flexor and supinator of the forearm.

Q. In Figure 2-11, identify vein L.

A. The cephalic vein.

Q. In Figure 2-11, identify nerve M.

A. The musculocutaneous nerve. It supplies the biceps muscle, the brachialis muscle, and the coracobrachialis muscle. It then continues as the lateral antebrachial cutaneous nerve to supply the skin of the lateral side of the forearm.

Q. In Figure 2-11, identify N.

A. The brachialis muscle. It is a powerful flexor of the forearm. It arises from most of the anterior surface of the humerus and inserts into the coronoid process of the ulna.

Q. In Figure 2-11, identify nerve O.

A. The radial nerve. It is accompanied by the profunda brachii artery.

Q. In Figure 2-11, identify artery P.

A. The profunda brachii artery.

Q. In Figure 2-11, identify Q.

A. The shaft of the humerus.

Q. The superficial veins lie in . . .

A. The superficial fascia. They perforate the deep fascia to reach the deep veins.

Q. The superficial veins are accompanied by . . .

A. Lymphatic channels.

Q. In Figure 2-12, identify vein A.

A. The cephalic vein. It is labeled both in the arm and in the forearm. It traverses the deltopectoral groove to pierce the clavipectoral fascia and join the axillary vein. It originates at the lateral end of the dorsal venous arch of the hand.

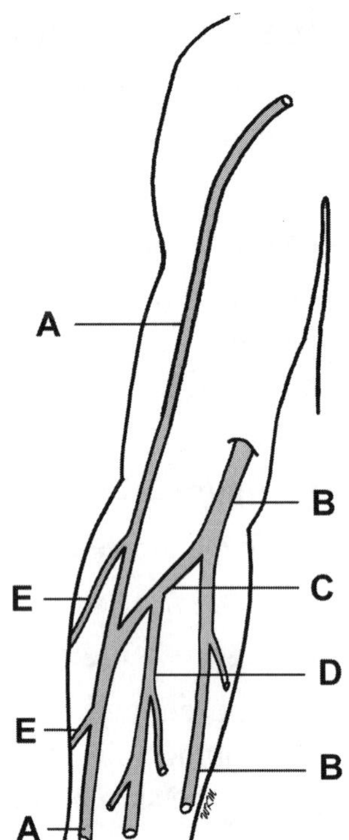

Figure 2-12 The Superficial Veins; Right Upper Limb

Q. In Figure 2-12, identify vein B.

A. The basilic vein. It is labeled both in the arm and in the forearm. It can be seen perforating the deep fascia to immediately enter the brachial vein. It originates at the medial end of the dorsal venous arch of the hand.

Q. In Figure 2-12, identify vein C.

A. The median cubital vein. It is used for venipuncture.

Q. In Figure 2-12, identify vein D.

A. The median antebrachial vein.

Q. In Figure 2-12, identify veins E.

A. Accessory cephalic veins.

Q. In Figure 2-13, identify artery A.

A. The brachial artery. In the cubital fossa, it is protected superficially by the bicipital aponeurosis, the attachment of the biceps tendon to the deep fascia of the forearm and skin.

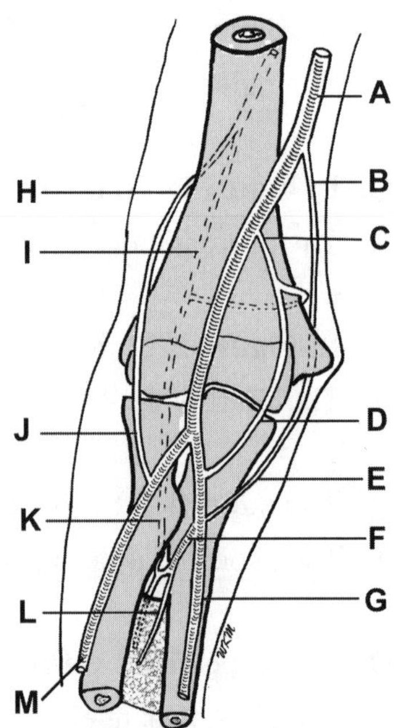

Figure 2-13 The Anastomosis Around the Right Elbow

Q. In Figure 2-13, identify artery B.

A. The superior ulnar collateral artery. It accompanies the ulnar nerve posterior to the medial epicondyle.

Q. In Figure 2-13, identify artery C.

A. The inferior ulnar collateral artery.

Q. In Figure 2-13, identify artery D.

A. The anterior ulnar recurrent artery.

Q. In Figure 2-13, identify artery E.

A. The posterior ulnar recurrent artery.

Q. In Figure 2-13, identify artery F.

A. The common interosseous artery. It divides almost immediately into anterior and posterior interosseous arteries, which descend on their respective aspects of the interosseous membrane.

Q. In Figure 2-13, identify artery G.

A. The ulnar artery. It runs down the forearm, deep to the superficial flexor muscles, on the surface of the insertion of the brachialis muscle. Subsequently, it lies on the anterior surface of the flexor digitorum profundus muscle.

Q. In Figure 2-13, identify arteries H and I.

A. They are the anterior and posterior branches of the profunda brachii artery, respectively. The anterior branch accompanies the radial nerve.

Q. In Figure 2-13, identify artery J.

A. The radial recurrent artery. It accompanies the radial nerve, passing anterior to the lateral epicondyle.

Q. In Figure 2-13, identify artery K.

A. The interosseous recurrent artery. It arises from the common interosseous artery via its posterior interosseous branch.

Q. In Figure 2-13, identify artery L.

A. The anterior interosseous artery.

Q. In Figure 2-13, identify artery M.

A. The radial artery. It runs a superficial course, deep to the deep fascia. It is palpable only at the wrist.

Q. The boundaries of the triangular cubital fossa are . . .

A. Medially, the lateral border of the pronator teres muscle; laterally, the medial border of the brachioradialis muscle. Its superior border is an arbitrary line drawn between the two epicondyles.

Q. The roof of the cubital fossa consists of the deep fascia and the superficial fascia, between which lies . . .

A. The median cubital vein. It is often used for venipuncture.

Q. The deep fascia, deep to the median cubital vein, is reinforced by . . .

A. The bicipital aponeurosis. The bicipital aponeurosis extends from the lateral side of the tendon of the biceps muscle to the deep fascia of the forearm.

Q. The bicipital aponeurosis separates the median cubital vein from . . .

A. The underlying brachial artery. This aponeurosis protects the artery from damage by inexpert phlebotomists.

Q. The floor of the cubital fossa consists of two muscles. They are . . .

A. The brachialis muscle, superiorly, and the supinator muscle, inferiorly. The latter muscle encircles the upper part of the shaft of the radius.

Q. The strong tendon of the biceps brachii muscle passes through the cubital fossa from above. It crosses the cubital fossa obliquely, from its medial to its lateral side, to be inserted into . . .

A. The posterior part of the radial tuberosity. Therefore, it is both a powerful supinator and a powerful flexor of the forearm.

Q. The brachial artery divides into the radial and ulnar arteries half an inch (1 cm), inferior to the elbow joint. As it does so, it lies between . . .

A. The tendon of the biceps muscle posteriorly, which separates it from the brachialis muscle and the elbow joint, and, anteriorly, the bicipital aponeurosis, which separates it from the median cubital vein. In the days when patients were often bled or "cupped," the aponeurosis was often called the *Grace à Dieu* ("Thanks be to God") aponeurosis, because it protected the brachial artery from injury by the knife used to open the median cubital vein.

Q. The median nerve and the brachial artery descend together through the cubital fossa, with the brachial artery lying . . .

A. Laterally. The median nerve then crosses anterior to the ulnar artery before entering the forearm between the two heads of the pronator teres muscle.

Q. Two nerves descend through the cubital fossa lateral to the brachial artery. They are . . .

A. The lateral antebrachial cutaneous nerve, anteriorly, and the radial nerve, posteriorly.

Q. As the lateral antebrachial cutaneous nerve and the radial nerve cross the elbow anteriorly, they lie between . . .

A. The brachioradialis and brachialis muscles, superiorly, and the brachioradialis and supinator muscles, inferiorly.

THE FOREARM

Q. In Figure 2-14, identify muscle A.

A. The pronator teres muscle.

Q. In Figure 2-14, identify muscle B.

A. The flexor carpi radialis muscle.

Q. The flexor carpi radialis muscle is inserted into . . .

A. The bases of the second and third metacarpal bones. The first metacarpal bone is the proximal bone of the thumb and therefore needs to have unrestricted mobility.

Q. In Figure 2-14, identify muscle C.

A. The palmaris longus muscle. It is frequently absent. It terminates in the palmar aponeurosis.

Q. In Figure 2-14, identify muscle D.

A. The flexor carpi ulnaris muscle.

Q. The flexor carpi ulnaris muscle arises from the common flexor origin, but it also arises from . . .

A. The posterior border of the shaft of the ulna. The ulnar nerve enters the forearm between the two heads of the flexor carpi ulnaris muscle.

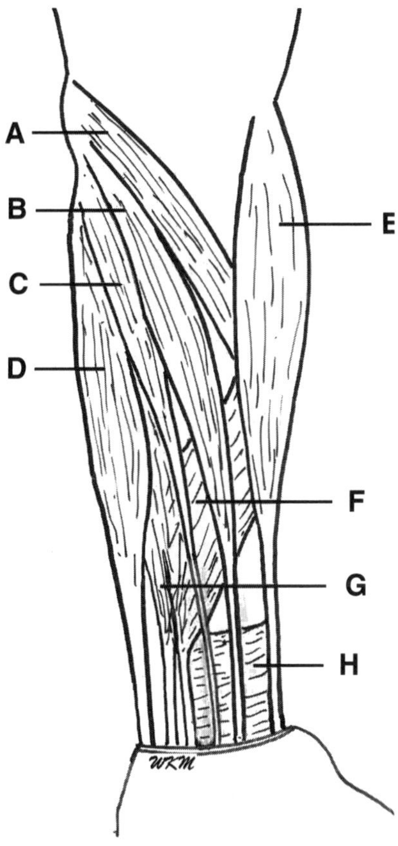

Figure 2-14 The Left Forearm, Superficial Muscles

Q. In Figure 2-14, identify muscle E.

A. The brachioradialis muscle. It is supplied by the radial nerve.

Q. In Figure 2-14, identify F and G.

A. They are, respectively, the radial head and the humeral head of the flexor digitorum superficialis muscle. The median nerve runs down the forearm deep to the radial head of this muscle.

Q. In Figure 2-14, identify muscle H.

A. The pronator quadratus muscle. It is supplied by the anterior interosseous branch of the median nerve.

Q. In Figure 2-15, identify nerve A.

A. The posterior antebrachial cutaneous nerve. It originates, with the lower lateral cutaneous nerve of the arm, from the radial nerve, as the latter lies in the spiral groove on the humerus. It supplies the skin on the posterior surface of the forearm.

Q. In Figure 2-15, identify nerve B.

A. The posterior interosseous nerve. It supplies the deep muscles on the back of the forearm.

Q. In Figure 2-15, identify nerve C.

A. The lateral antebrachial cutaneous nerve. It is a continuation of the musculocutaneous nerve. It supplies the skin on the lateral aspect of the forearm.

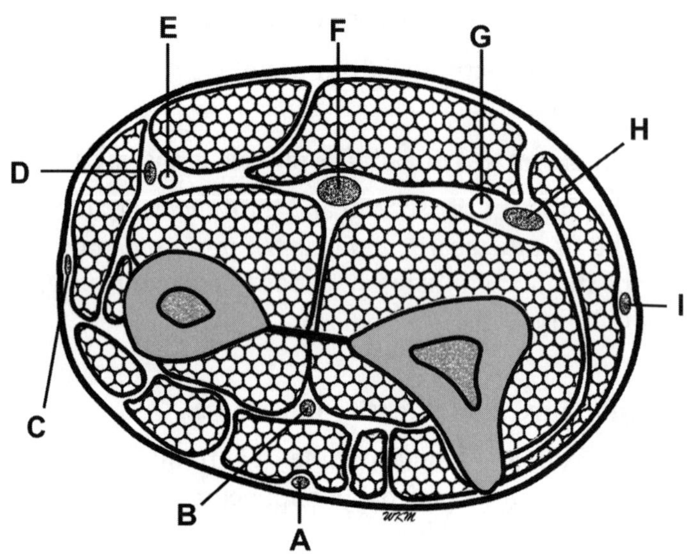

Figure 2-15 The Right Mid-Forearm, Transverse Section: Vessels and Nerves

Q. In Figure 2-15, identify nerve D.

A. The superficial (cutaneous) terminal branch of the radial nerve.

Q. In Figure 2-15, identify artery E.

A. The radial artery. At this point, it is just overlapped by the edge of the brachioradialis muscle. It soon becomes superficial.

Q. In Figure 2-15, identify nerve F.

A. The median nerve. It lies deep to the radial head of the flexor digitorum superficialis muscle.

Q. In Figure 2-15, identify artery G.

A. The ulnar artery. It accompanies the ulnar nerve, which lies medial to it.

Q. In Figure 2-15, identify nerve H.

A. The ulnar nerve. It lies between the only muscles it supplies in the forearm. These two muscles are the ulnar head of the flexor digitorum profundus muscle and the flexor carpi ulnaris muscle.

Q. In Figure 2-15, identify nerve I.

A. The medial antebrachial cutaneous nerve. It arises from the medial cord of the brachial plexus.

Q. In Figure 2-16, identify A.

A. The flexor carpi ulnaris muscle. It is inserted into the pisiform bone and continues as the pisohamate and the pisometacarpal ligaments.

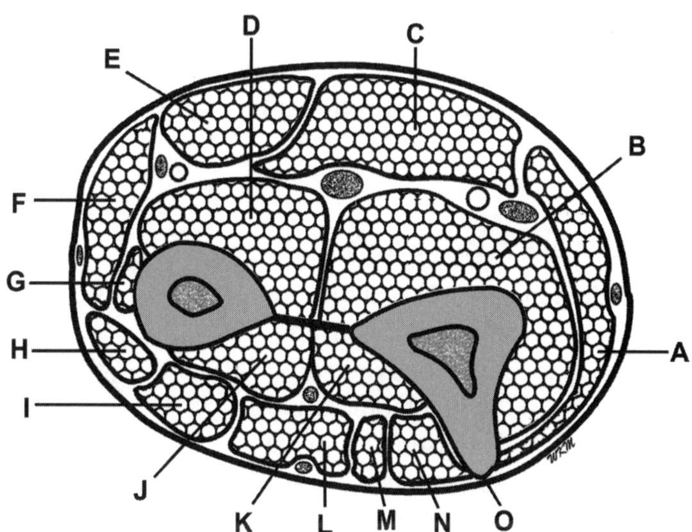

Figure 2-16 The Right Mid-Forearm, Transverse Section: Muscles

Q. In Figure 2-16, identify B.

A. The flexor digitorum profundus muscle. It is inserted into the bases of the terminal phalanges of all four fingers. Its ulnar half is supplied by the ulnar nerve; the remainder is supplied by the anterior interosseous branch of the median nerve.

Q. In Figure 2-16, identify C.

A. The flexor digitorum superficialis muscle. Note that its radial head is superficial to the median nerve. Note also that the palmaris longus muscle is absent in this figure.

Q. In Figure 2-16, identify D.

A. The flexor pollicis longus muscle. It is supplied by the anterior interosseous branch of the median nerve and is inserted into the terminal phalanx of the thumb.

Q. In Figure 2-16, identify E.

A. The flexor carpi radialis muscle. It is inserted into the bases of the second and third metacarpal bones.

Q. In Figure 2-16, identify F.

A. The brachioradialis muscle. It arises from the lateral supracondylar ridge on the humerus and is inserted into the lateral side of the distal end of the radius. It is supplied by the trunk of the radial nerve before it divides into its superficial and deep branches.

Q. In Figure 2-16, identify G.

A. The insertion of the pronator teres muscle.

Q. The pronator teres muscle arises by a superficial head from the common flexor origin on the medial epicondyle of the humerus and by a deep head from the coronoid process of the ulna. It is inserted into . . .

A. The roughened area at the most convex part of the radius, approximately at its mid-shaft.

Q. With the exceptions of the brachioradialis and the flexor carpi ulnaris muscles, the superficial muscles on the anterior surface of the forearm are supplied by . . .

A. The median nerve.

Q. In Figure 2-16, identify H.

A. The extensor carpi radialis longus muscle. It arises from the lateral supracondylar ridge, inferior to the brachioradialis muscle, and is inserted into the base of the second metacarpal bone. It receives a branch from the main trunk of the radial nerve.

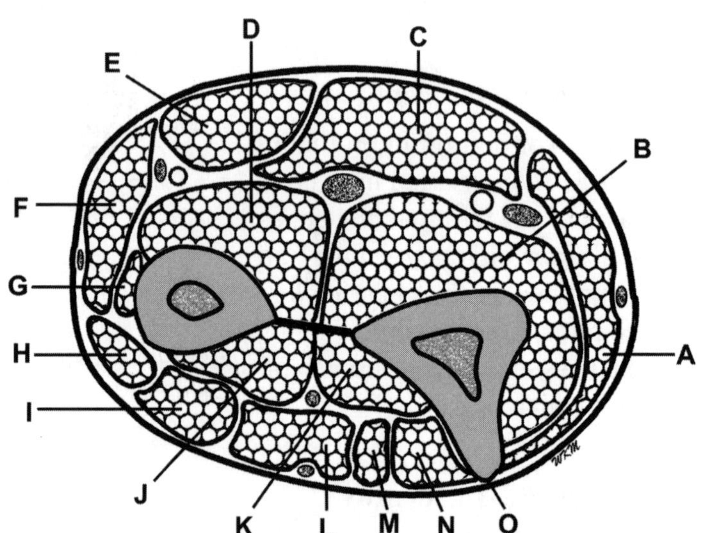

Figure 2-16 The Right Mid-Forearm, Transverse Section: Muscles

Q. In Figure 2-16, identify I.

A. The extensor carpi radialis brevis muscle. It is supplied, together with the supinator muscle, by the deep branch of the radial nerve. It is inserted into the base of the third metacarpal bone.

Q. In Figure 2-16, identify J.

A. The abductor pollicis longus muscle. It arises from the posterior surfaces of both the ulna and the radius, but at this level, only its origin from the radius can be seen. It is inserted into the base of the first metacarpal bone.

Q. Distal to the radial origin of the abductor pollicis longus muscle is the origin of the extensor pollicis brevis muscle. The extensor pollicis brevis muscle is inserted into . . .

A. The dorsal surface of the proximal phalanx of the thumb.

Q. Proximal to the radial origin of the abductor pollicis longus muscle is the insertion of the supinator muscle. Its origin is . . .

A. The supinator crest on the ulna.

Q. In Figure 2-16, identify K.

A. The extensor pollicis longus muscle. It is inserted into the base of the terminal phalanx of the thumb.

Q. In Figure 2-16, identify L.

A. The extensor digitorum muscle. Although its tendons gain attachment to the bases of each of the phalanges of the digits, their fusion with the capsules of the metacarpophalangeal joints largely limits their extensor activity to the proximal phalanges.

Q. The deep muscle arising from the posterior surface of the ulna distal to the extensor pollicis longus muscle is . . .

A. The extensor indicis muscle. It passes deep to the extensor retinaculum in the same compartment as the extensor digitorum muscle. It fuses with the ulnar side of the tendon of the extensor digitorum muscle to the index finger, posterior to the head of its metacarpal bone.

Q. In Figure 2-16, identify M.

A. The extensor digiti minimi muscle. It passes through a separate compartment of the extensor retinaculum and is joined on its ulnar side by the slip of the extensor digitorum muscle to the little finger. The tendon of the extensor digiti minimi muscle is usually split, forming two, apparently separate, tendons. The lateral of these is often mistaken for the tendon of the extensor digitorum muscle to the little finger.

Q. In Figure 2-16, identify N.

A. The extensor carpi ulnaris muscle. It is inserted into the tubercle (the styloid process) on the base of the fifth metacarpal bone.

Q. The nerve supply of the extensor carpi ulnaris muscle is . . .

A. The posterior interosseous branch of the radial nerve. All the muscles on the posterior surface of the forearm are supplied, either directly or indirectly, by the radial nerve.

Q. In Figure 2-16, identify O.

A. The subcutaneous posterior border of the shaft of the ulna. It is often broken by direct violence, a so-called "defense" fracture.

THE HAND

Q. The bones of the hand consist of . . .

A. The eight carpal bones, the five metacarpal bones, and the fourteen phalangeal bones. The thumb has only two phalanges, the remaining fingers each have three.

Q. The blood supply of the hand comes almost entirely from two arteries. They are . . .

A. The radial artery and the ulnar artery.

Q. The ulnar artery enters the hand by crossing anterior to the flexor retinaculum and lateral to the pisiform bone. It is separated from that bone by . . .

A. The ulnar nerve.

Q. As they cross the flexor retinaculum, the ulnar nerve and the ulnar artery are both protected by . . .

A. The superficial medial extension of the flexor retinaculum to the pisiform bone, anterior to the ulnar artery and nerve. The artery, however, is readily palpable at this point.

Q. Having crossed the flexor retinaculum superficially, the ulnar artery gives off a deep branch, which runs deep to the long flexors of the fingers, to join . . .

A. The termination of the radial artery. This completes the deep palmar arch.

Q. After giving off its deep branch, the ulnar artery turns laterally running deep to . . .

A. The palmar aponeurosis and superficial to the long flexor tendons. It forms the superficial palmar arch. The superficial palmar arch is completed by the superficial palmar branch of the radial artery.

Q. The superficial palmar arch gives rise to . . .

A. Three common digital branches to the index, middle, ring, and little fingers and one proper digital branch to the ulnar side of the little finger.

Q. The superficial palmar arch is completed by anastomosing with . . .

A. The small superficial palmar branch of the radial artery.

Q. At the wrist, the radial artery lies on . . .

A. The anterior surface of the lower end of the radius, inferior to the pronator quadratus muscle. It is usually more readily palpable than the ulnar artery.

Q. The radial artery then passes posteriorly, between the scaphoid bone and the tendons of . . .

A. The abductor pollicis longus muscle and the extensor pollicis brevis muscle. It then enters the anatomical snuff box.

Q. The floor of the anatomical snuff box is formed by . . .

A. The neck of the scaphoid. Tenderness in this area after a fall may indicate a fracture of the "waist" of the scaphoid bone. Fractured scaphoids are often missed on normal X-ray views of the wrist. An oblique view is necessary to visualize such fractures. Failure to immobilize the fragments may result in prolonged delay in union due to disruption of the blood supply to the proximal fragment of the scaphoid bone.

Q. The radial artery continues distally, deep to the tendon of the extensor pollicis longus muscle, to pass anteriorly between the two heads of . . .

A. The first dorsal interosseous muscle.

Q. As it reaches the palm, the radial artery gives off . . .

A. The princeps pollicis artery and the radialis indicis artery.

Q. It then continues as the deep palmar arch, passing between . . .

A. The bases of the metacarpal bones and the interossei muscles, posteriorly, and the long flexor tendons, anteriorly.

Q. The deep palmar arch gives off three palmar metacarpal arteries. These vessels unite with the three common digital arteries from the superficial palmar arch. The enlarged common digital arteries then divide to form . . .

A. The proper digital arteries of the first, second, third, and fourth fingers.

Q. The deep palmar arch terminates by joining with . . .

A. The small deep palmar branch of the ulnar artery, thus completing the deep palmar arch.

Q. Running laterally in the concavity of the deep palmar arch lies . . .

A. The deep branch of the ulnar nerve, which terminates in the adductor pollicis muscle.

Q. The majority of the muscles of the forearm are supplied from . . .

A. The seventh and eighth cervical segments of the spinal cord. The muscles of the arm are largely supplied by the fifth and sixth cervical segments. The muscles on the posterior aspect of the arm tend to be supplied by one segment lower than those on the anterior aspect.

Q. The segmental innervation of the small muscles of the hand is from . . .

A. The anterior primary ramus of the first thoracic nerve. The muscles on the thenar side of the hand also receive a contribution from the anterior primary ramus of the eighth cervical nerve.

Q. With the exception of the three muscles of the thenar eminence and the first two lumbrical muscles, which are supplied by the median nerve, the intrinsic muscles of the hand are supplied by . . .

A. The ulnar nerve. All of the intrinsic muscles of the hand, except for the palmaris brevis muscle, are supplied by the deep branch of the ulnar nerve.

Q. In Figure 2-17, identify A.

A. The abductor pollicis brevis muscle. It arises from the anterior surface of the flexor retinaculum and is inserted on the radial side of the base of the proximal phalanx of the thumb.

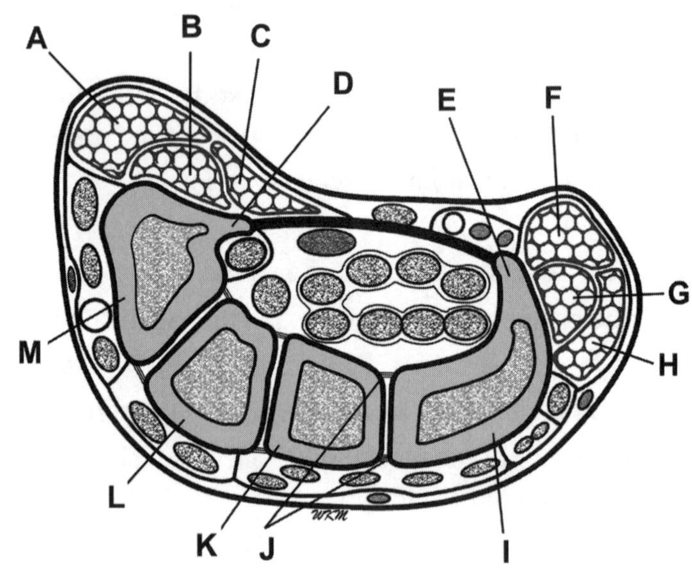

Figure 2-17 The Right Wrist, Transverse Section: Bones, Thenar Muscles, and Hypothenar Muscles

Q. In Figure 2-17, identify B.

A. The opponens pollicis muscle. It arises from the anterior surface of the flexor retinaculum and is inserted into the whole length of the shaft of the first metacarpal bone.

Q. In Figure 2-17, identify C.

A. The flexor pollicis brevis muscle. It has a superficial head, which arises from the crest of the trapezium bone, and a deep head, which arises from the anterior surface of the trapezoid bone and the capitate bone. Both heads unite and join with the tendon of the abductor pollicis brevis to be inserted into the radial side of the base of the proximal phalanx of the thumb. There is a sesamoid bone in the united tendons.

Q. The three muscles that constitute the thenar eminence are . . .

A. The abductor pollicis brevis muscle, the opponens pollicis muscle, and the flexor pollicis brevis muscle.

Q. In Figure 2-17, identify D.

A. The crest of the trapezium bone.

Q. In Figure 2-17, identify E.

A. The hook of the hamate bone.

Q. In Figure 2-17, identify F.

A. The flexor digiti minimi muscle.

Q. In Figure 2-17, identify G.

A. The opponens digiti minimi muscle.

Q. In Figure 2-17, identify H.

A. The abductor digiti minimi muscle.

Q. In Figure 2-17, identify I.

A. The hamate bone.

Q. In Figure 2-17, identify J.

A. The palmar carpal interosseous ligament and the dorsal carpal interosseous ligament.

Q. In Figure 2-17, identify K.

A. The capitate bone.

Q. In Figure 2-17, identify L.

A. The trapezoid bone.

Q. In Figure 2-17, identify M.

A. The trapezium bone.

Q. The flexor retinaculum converts the front of the carpus into a tunnel. The medial attachments of the flexor retinaculum are . . .

A. The pisiform bone and the hook of the hamate bone.

Q. The lateral attachments of the flexor retinaculum are . . .

A. The tubercle of the scaphoid bone and the crest of the trapezium bone.

Q. Attached to the flexor retinaculum superficially are . . .

A. The tendon of the palmaris longus tendon and the palmar aponeurosis.

Q. Many structures pass through the carpal tunnel; they include . . .

A. The tendons of both the flexor digitorum superficialis and the flexor digitorum profundus muscles, which share a common synovial sheath, and the tendon of the flexor pollicis longus muscle, which has its own synovial sheath. In a separate compartment, in the groove of the trapezium, lies the tendon of the flexor carpi radialis muscle, also with its own synovial sheath. Anteriorly, between the tendons and the flexor retinaculum, lies the median nerve.

Q. Repetitive overuse of these muscles causes inflammation and swelling in the carpal tunnel, compressing the median nerve, which results in "carpal tunnel syndrome." The symptoms of carpel tunnel syndrome are . . .

A. Pain and paresthesia, abnormal sensations, numbness and tingling of the radial side of the hand and the anterior surface of the radial three and a half digits and gradual weakening of fine movements of the thumb.

Q. Carpal tunnel syndrome is common among computer operators, butchers, and fish skinners. These occupations all involve . . .

A. Prolonged, repetitive movements of the wrist and fingers.

Q. The gender in which carpel tunnel syndrome occurs most frequently is . . .

A. The female gender.

Q. An increased risk of carpal tunnel syndrome occurs during pregnancy. This is probably due to . . .

A. Peripheral edema, which tends to occur in pregnancy.

Q. The muscles involved in carpal tunnel syndrome are those supplied by the median nerve in the hand distal to the carpal tunnel. The muscles involved are . . .

A. The flexor pollicis brevis muscle, the abductor pollicis brevis muscle, the opponens pollicis muscle, and the lateral two lumbrical muscles.

Q. The action of the lumbrical muscles is to assist . . .

A. The interossei muscles in flexing the metacarpophalangeal joints and extending the interphalangeal joints of the fingers. This combination of movements puts the fingers into the writing position.

Q. The nerve supply of the first (radial) two lumbrical muscles is . . .

A. The median nerve. The ulnar (medial) two lumbrical muscles are supplied by the deep terminal branch of the ulnar nerve.

Q. The segmental innervation of the small muscles of the hand is . . .

A. The first thoracic segment of the spinal cord. The muscles of the thenar eminence also receive a contribution from the eighth cervical segment of the spinal cord.

Q. The cutaneous segmental innervation of the small muscles of the hand differs. The thenar skin is supplied by . . .

A. The sixth cervical anterior primary ramus.

Q. The skin of the middle finger is supplied by . . .

A. The seventh cervical anterior primary ramus.

Q. The skin over the little finger is supplied by . . .

A. The eighth cervical anterior primary ramus.

Q. The skin of the thenar eminence and the lateral side of the palm is supplied by . . .

A. The superficial palmar branch of the median nerve.

Q. The skin of the palmar surface and the dorsal surface of the distal phalanges of the thumb and the lateral two and a half fingers is supplied by . . .

A. The terminal digital branches of the median nerve.

Q. The skin of the hypothenar eminence and of the medial side of the palm is supplied by . . .

A. The superficial palmar branch of the ulnar nerve.

Q. The skin over the medial part of the dorsum of the hand, the posterior surface of the proximal phalanx of the little finger, and the posterior surface of the medial half of the proximal phalanx of the ring finger is supplied by . . .

A. The dorsal cutaneous branch of the ulnar nerve.

Q. The skin over the lateral part of the dorsum of the hand and the dorsal surface of the proximal phalanges of the remaining fingers and of the thumb is supplied by . . .

A. The superficial (cutaneous) branch of the radial nerve.

Q. The skin on the palmar surface of the medial one and one-half fingers is supplied by . . .

A. The superficial terminal branch of the ulnar nerve.

Q. In Figure 2-18, identify A.

A. The carpal tunnel. It is formed by the flexor retinaculum and the concavity of the carpus.

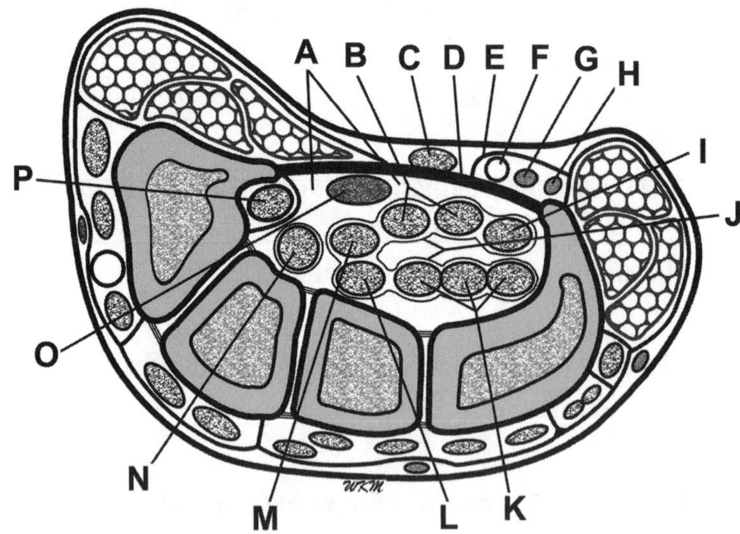

Figure 2-18 The Right Wrist, Transverse Section: The Carpal Tunnel

Q. In Figure 2-18, identify B.

A. The tendons of the flexor digitorum superficialis muscle to the middle and ring fingers. Note that they lie on a more superficial plane than the tendons of the flexor digitorum superficialis muscle to the index and little fingers.

Q. In Figure 2-18, identify C.

A. The tendon of the palmaris longus muscle. At this point it fuses with the anterior surface of the flexor retinaculum.

Q. In Figure 2-18, identify D.

A. The flexor retinaculum. It is attached laterally to the tubercle of the scaphoid bone and to the crest of the trapezium bone and medially to the pisiform bone and to the hook of the hamate bone.

Q. In Figure 2-18, identify E.

A. An extension of the antebrachial fascia. It is sometimes called the superficial part of the flexor retinaculum. It stretches from the pisiform bone and passes over the ulnar nerve and the ulnar artery to the flexor retinaculum. The canal formed, Guyon's canal, may be the site of ulnar nerve entrapment.

Q. In Figure 2-18, identify F.

A. The ulnar artery. Note that it and the ulnar nerve are superficial to the flexor retinaculum proper and do not pass through the carpal tunnel.

Q. In Figure 2-18, identify G.

A. The deep branch of the ulnar nerve. The deep branch of the ulnar nerve supplies the muscles of the hypothenar eminence and all of the deep muscles of the hand, including the third and fourth lumbrical muscles.

Q. In Figure 2-18, identify H.

A. The superficial branch of the ulnar nerve. It supplies the palmaris brevis muscle and the proper digital nerves to the medial side of the little finger and the adjacent sides of the ring and little fingers.

Q. In Figure 2-18, identify I.

A. The tendon of the flexor digitorum superficialis muscle to the little finger.

Q. In Figure 2-18, identify J.

A. The common synovial sheathes of the tendons of the flexor digitorum profundus and superficialis muscles.

Q. In Figure 2-18, identify K.

A. The three fused medial tendons of the flexor digitorum profundus muscle.

Q. In Figure 2-18, identify L.

A. The tendon of the flexor digitorum profundus muscle to the index finger. Flexion of the terminal phalanx of the index finger is possible without flexion of the terminal phalanges of the other fingers. Isolated flexion of the terminal phalanges of the other fingers cannot occur.

Q. In Figure 2-18, identify M.

A. The tendon of the flexor digitorum superficialis muscle to the index finger.

Q. In Figure 2-18, identify N.

A. The tendon of the flexor pollicis longus tendon. It has its own synovial sheath.

Q. In Figure 2-18, identify O.

A. The median nerve. It supplies a recurrent branch to the three muscles of the thenar eminence and the first two lumbrical muscles. It also supplies the skin of the palmar surface of the thumb and the skin of the adjacent sides of the thumb, index, middle, and ring fingers.

Q. In Figure 2-18, identify P.

A. The tendon of the flexor carpi radialis. It lies in a groove in the trapezium bone and is inserted into the bases of the second and third metacarpal bones.

Q. In Figure 2-19, identify A.

A. The lateral compartment of the mid-palmar space. It is also called the thenar compartment and the anterior adductor compartment of the hand. These fascial compartments are only potential spaces, but are clinically important in infections of the palm and on the dorsum of the hand.

Q. In Figure 2-19, identify B.

A. The mid-palmar septum. It extends from the shaft of the third metacarpal bone to the deep surface of the palmar aponeurosis.

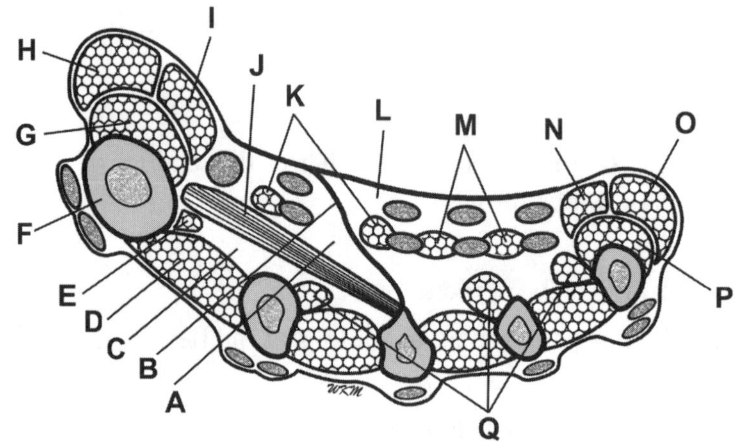

Figure 2-19 The Right Hand, Transverse Section: Intrinsic Muscles and Fascial Spaces

Q. In Figure 2-19, identify C.

A. The adductor space. If an abscess occurs in this space, it may be drained by an incision in the web between the index finger and the thumb.

Q. In Figure 2-19, identify D.

A. The first dorsal interosseous muscle. In addition to extension of the interphalangeal joints and flexion of the metacarpophalangeal joints, the dorsal interossei muscles *abduct* the digits. The palmar interossei muscles *adduct* the digits.

Q. In Figure 2-19, identify E.

A. The deep head of the flexor pollicis brevis muscle. It is supplied by the deep branch of the ulnar nerve. Because of this, it is sometimes called the first palmar interosseous muscle. This nomenclature results in there being four palmar interosseous muscles.

Q. In Figure 2-19, identify F.

A. The shaft of the first metacarpal bone.

Q. In Figure 2-19, identify G.

A. The opponens pollicis muscle. It is inserted into the shaft of the first metacarpal bone.

Q. In Figure 2-19, identify H.

A. The abductor pollicis brevis muscle. It is inserted into the radial side of the proximal phalanx of the thumb.

Q. In Figure 2-19, identify I.

A. The flexor pollicis brevis muscle. This muscle, together with the opponens pollicis muscle and the abductor pollicis brevis muscle, forms the thenar eminence and occupies the thenar space. They are all supplied by the recurrent branch of the median nerve. The flexor pollicis brevis muscle is inserted into the radial side of the base of the proximal phalanx of the thumb by a tendon, which contains a sesamoid bone.

Q. In Figure 2-19, identify J.

A. The transverse head of the adductor pollicis muscle. It is inserted, together with its oblique head, by a tendon containing a sesamoid bone into the ulnar side of the base of the proximal phalanx of the thumb.

Q. In Figure 2-19, identify K.

A. The first two lumbrical muscles. They each arise from only one tendon of the flexor digitorum profundus muscle and are supplied by the median nerve.

Q. In Figure 2-19, identify L.

A. The medial compartment of the mid-palmar space. It is separated from the lateral compartment by a septum attached posteriorly to the shaft of the third metacarpal bone.

Q. In Figure 2-19, identify M.

A. The medial two lumbrical muscles. They each arise from the adjacent sides of the flexor digitorum profundus muscle tendons and are supplied by the deep branch of the ulnar nerve.

Q. In Figure 2-19, identify N.

A. The flexor digiti minimi brevis muscle.

Q. In Figure 2-19, identify O.

A. The abductor digiti minimi muscle. This muscle, together with the flexor digiti minimi brevis muscle and the opponens digiti minimi muscle, forms the hypothenar eminence. Together they occupy the hypothenar space.

Q. In Figure 2-19, identify P.

A. The opponens digiti minimi muscle. It is inserted on the shaft of the fifth metacarpal bone.

Q. In Figure 2-19, identify Q.

A. The three palmar interosseous muscles. All of the interossei muscles, through their insertion into the dorsal expansion of the extensor tendons, extend the interphalangeal joints and flex the metacarpophalangeal joints of the fingers.

Q. In Figure 2-20, identify A.

A. The tendon of the abductor pollicis longus muscle.

Q. In Figure 2-20, identify B.

A. The tendon of the extensor pollicis brevis muscle.

Q. In Figure 2-20, identify C.

A. The superficial branch of the radial nerve.

Q. In Figure 2-20, identify D.

A. The radial artery.

Q. In Figure 2-20, identify E.

A. The tendon of the extensor pollicis longus muscle.

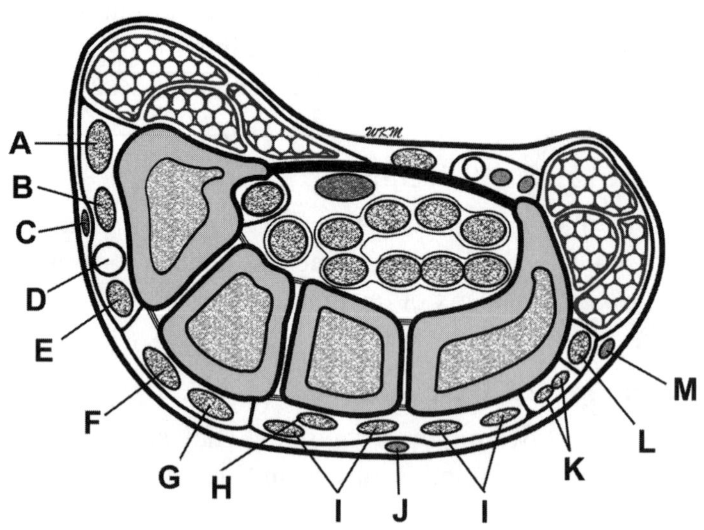

Figure 2-20 The Right Wrist, Transverse Section: Structures Crossing the Wrist Posteriorly

Q. In Figure 2-20, identify F.

A. The tendon of the extensor carpi radialis longus muscle.

Q. In Figure 2-20, identify G.

A. The tendon of the extensor carpi radialis brevis muscle.

Q. In Figure 2-20, identify H.

A. The tendon of the extensor indicis muscle.

Q. In Figure 2-20, identify the four tendons indicated by the two I's.

A. The four tendons of the extensor digitorum muscle.

Q. In Figure 2-20, identify J.

A. The terminal branch of the posterior antebrachial cutaneous nerve.

Q. In Figure 2-20, identify K.

A. The split tendon of the extensor digiti minimi muscle.

Q. In Figure 2-20, identify L.

A. The tendon of the extensor carpi ulnaris muscle.

Q. In Figure 2-20, identify M.

A. The terminal branch of the medial antebrachial cutaneous nerve.

Q. In Figure 2-21, identify A.

A. The tendon of the flexor pollicis longus muscle. It is inserted into the base of the distal phalanx of the thumb.

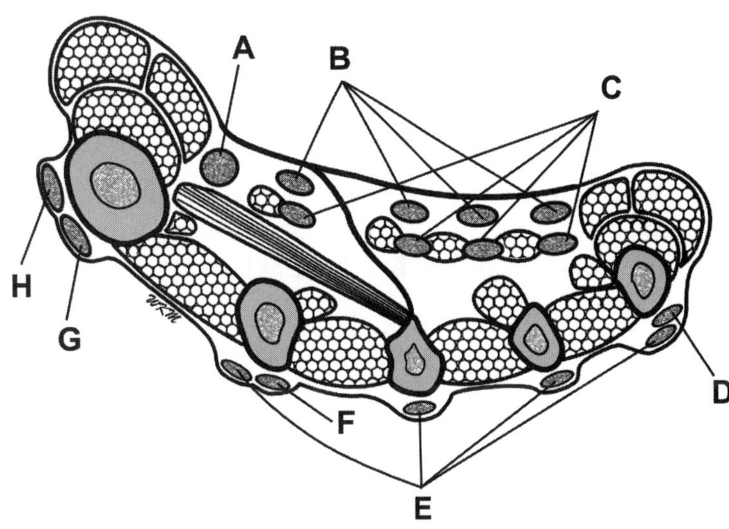

Figure 2-21 The Right Hand, Transverse Section: Tendons of the Forearm Muscles

Q. In Figure 2-21, identify B.

A. The four tendons of the flexor digitorum superficialis muscle. They are inserted into the bases of the intermediate phalanges of the fingers.

Q. In Figure 2-21, identify C.

A. The tendons of the flexor digitorum profundus muscle. They are inserted into the bases of the terminal phalanges of the fingers.

Q. In Figure 2-21, identify D.

A. The tendon of the extensor digiti minimi muscle.

Q. In Figure 2-21, identify E.

A. The tendons of the extensor digitorum muscle.

Q. In Figure 2-21, identify F.

A. The tendon of the extensor indicis muscle.

Q. In Figure 2-21, identify G.

A. The tendon of the extensor pollicis longus muscle.

Q. In Figure 2-21, identify H.

A. The tendon of the extensor pollicis brevis muscle.

THE STERNOCLAVICULAR JOINT

Q. The sternoclavicular joint is the articulation between the medial end of the clavicle and . . .

A. The manubrium sterni and the costal cartilage of the first rib.

Q. The movements that occur at the sternoclavicular joint are . . .

A. Elevation and depression, abduction and adduction; protrusion and retraction, flexion and extension. The clavicle also has to rotate approximately 30° to allow the scapula to rotate around the chest wall. Thus, it is a triaxial joint.

Q. The sternoclavicular articulation is a synovial joint. It has an intra-articular fibrocartilaginous disc, which completely subdivides the joint into two cavities. Inferiorly, the disc is firmly attached to . . .

A. The first costal cartilage.

Q. Superiorly, the disc is most firmly attached to . . .

A. The medial end of the clavicle.

Q. These attachments specifically resist . . .

A. Medial displacement of the clavicle.

Q. The strongest and the most important ligament of the sternoclavicular joint is . . .

A. The costoclavicular ligament.

Q. The majority of the fibers of the costoclavicular ligament run from . . .

A. The superior surface of the first costal cartilage, upwards and medially, to the inferior surface of the medial end of the clavicle.

Q. The movements of the clavicle that are resisted by the costoclavicular ligament are . . .

A. Elevation and medial displacement. The costoclavicular ligament is so strong that a fall on the outstretched hand often fractures the clavicle distal to the ligament, which is itself rarely torn.

Q. The clavicle is firmly attached to the coracoid process of the scapula by . . .

A. The coracoclavicular ligament.

Q. The coracoclavicular ligament consists of two parts, the conoid and the trapezoid components. The more lateral of these is the trapezoid component. Its fibers run from . . .

A. The coracoid process. The trapezoid component runs laterally, almost horizontally, to a rough ridge on the inferior aspect of the lateral end of the clavicle.

Q. Its primary function is to prevent . . .

A. Medial displacement of the scapula on the clavicle.

Q. The medial conoid component of the coracoclavicular ligament is almost vertical. Its major function is to prevent . . .

A. Downward displacement of the scapula.

Q. The facets of the acromioclavicular joint are relatively small, and the capsular ligament is relatively weak. Although the joint is reinforced superiorly by the acromioclavicular ligament, its stability depends on . . .

A. The coracoclavicular ligament. Because the capsular ligament is weak, tearing of the capsular ligament commonly occurs. The resulting condition is known as a "separated shoulder."

Q. The subsequent linear depression at the end of the clavicle is clearly visible. It will run . . .

A. Anteroposteriorly.

Q. The bony point of the shoulder is formed by . . .

A. The expanded acromial end of the spine of the scapula.

Q. The rounded curve of the shoulder is caused by . . .

A. The thick muscular fibers of the deltoid muscle. It crosses the greater tuberosity of the humerus. When the glenohumeral joint is dislocated, the head of the humerus usually lies in the subscapular fossa. Hence, the fibers of the deltoid muscle will descend vertically from the acromion, causing a "square shoulder."

THE GLENOHUMERAL JOINT

Q. The glenohumeral joint is triaxial. Its three axes of movement are . . .

A. Anteroposterior, transverse, and longitudinal along the shaft of the humerus.

Q. Abduction of the humerus at the glenohumeral joint is limited to . . .

A. A right angle.

Q. The additional 90° of abduction, which is made possible by the shoulder mechanism, is accomplished by . . .

A. Rotation of the scapula around the chest wall.

Q. The supraspinatus muscle initiates abduction of the humerus. The movement is continued by the actions of . . .

A. The deltoid muscle and other muscles that move the scapula. These muscles are principally the serratus anterior muscle and the trapezius muscle.

Q. In Figure 2-22, identify A.

A. The subscapularis muscle. It arises from the subscapular fossa of the scapula and is inserted into the lesser tubercle of the humerus.

Q. The nerve supply to the subscapular muscle is from . . .

A. The upper and lower subscapular nerves. They are branches of the posterior cord of the brachial plexus.

Q. In Figure 2-22, identify B.

A. The supraspinatus muscle. It arises from the supraspinous fossa of the scapula and is inserted into the greater tubercle of the humerus.

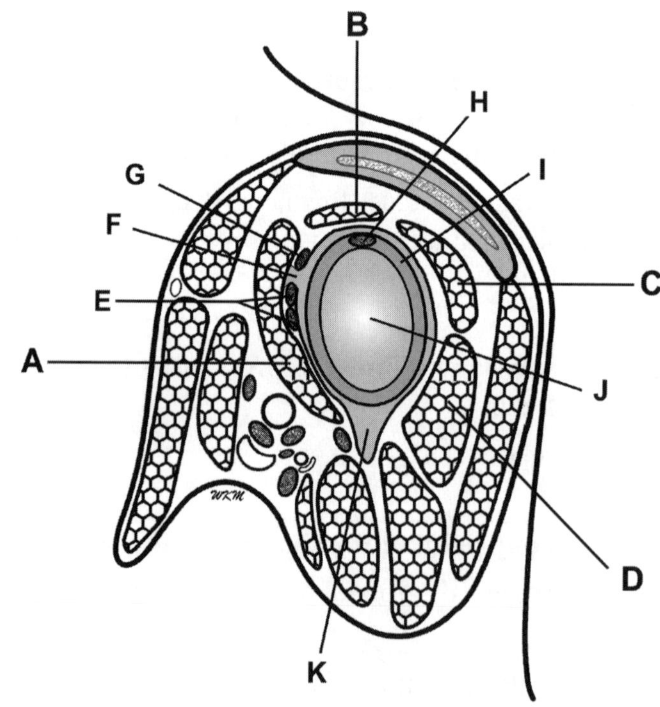

Figure 2-22 Glenohumeral Joint, Parasagittal Section: Rotator-Cuff Muscles and the Capsular Ligament

Q. In Figure 2-22, identify C.

A. The infraspinatus muscle. It arises from the infraspinous fossa of the scapula and is inserted into the greater tubercle of the humerus.

Q. The supraspinatus muscle and the infraspinatus muscle are both supplied by . . .

A. The suprascapular nerve.

Q. In Figure 2-22, identify D.

A. The teres minor muscle. It arises from the lateral border of the scapula and is inserted into the greater tubercle of the humerus.

Q. The teres minor muscle is supplied by . . .

A. The axillary nerve.

Q. The supraspinatus muscle, the infraspinatus muscle, the teres minor muscle, and the subscapularis muscle are referred to as the four "rotator-cuff" muscles. However, one of these muscles does not actually rotate the humerus. The exception is . . .

A. The supraspinatus muscle. In addition to stabilizing the joint, it initiates abduction of the humerus.

Q. In Figure 2-22, identify E.

A. The middle and inferior glenohumeral ligaments. They are merely minor thickenings in the capsule.

Q. In Figure 2-22, identify F.

A. The opening in the capsule of the glenohumeral joint, which establishes a communication between the joint and the subscapular bursa.

Q. In Figure 2-22, identify G.

A. The superior glenohumeral ligament.

Q. In Figure 2-22, identify H.

A. The tendon of the long head of the biceps muscle. It enters the capsule by passing deep to the transverse intertubercular ligament. It is attached to the supraglenoid tubercle on the scapula.

Q. The short head of the biceps muscle and the coracobrachialis muscle arise from . . .

A. The tip of the coracoid process of the scapula. They are both supplied by the musculocutaneous nerve, which also supplies the long head of the biceps muscle and the brachialis muscle.

Q. In Figure 2-22, identify I.

A. The glenoidal labrum. It is a fibrocartilaginous triangular ring, which serves to slightly deepen the glenoidal cavity for articulation with the head of the humerus.

Q. In Figure 2-22, identify J.

A. The glenoidal cavity. It is covered by hyaline articular cartilage.

Q. In Figure 2-23, identify A.

A. The combined tendinous origin of the coracobrachialis muscle and the short head of the biceps muscle. This section is lateral to the coracoid process. In this particular section, it is easy to confuse their combined origin with the origin of the pectoralis minor muscle.

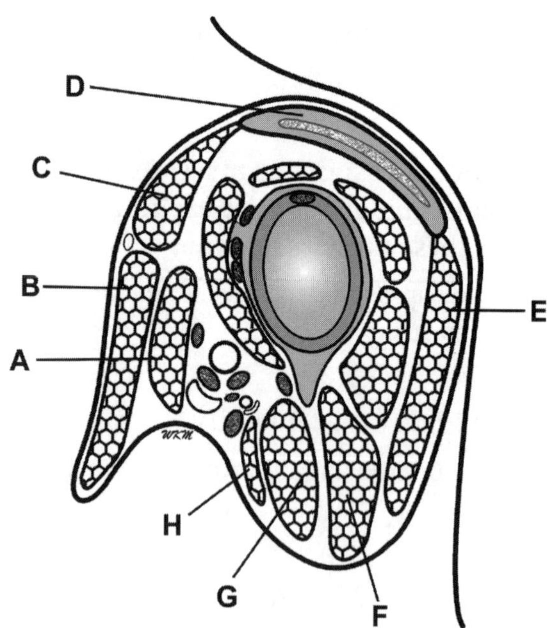

Figure 2-23 Glenohumeral Joint, Parasagittal Section: Accessory Muscles

Q. In Figure 2-23, identify B.

A. The pectoralis major muscle. It forms the anterior axillary fold and is separated from the anteromedial margin of the deltoid muscle by the deltopectoral groove, in which lies the cephalic vein.

Q. In Figure 2-23, identify C.

A. The anterior part of the deltoid muscle. It arises from the anterior margin of the acromion and the anterior border of the lateral one-third of the clavicle.

Q. In Figure 2-23, identify D.

A. The acromial process of the spine of the scapula.

Q. In Figure 2-23, identify E.

A. The posterior part of the deltoid muscle. These fibers contribute to lateral rotation of the humerus. They arise from the acromial process and the spine of the scapula.

Q. In Figure 2-23, identify F.

A. The long head of the triceps muscle. It arises from the infraglenoid tubercle on the scapula and separates the teres major muscle from the teres minor muscle.

Q. In Figure 2-23, identify G.

A. The teres major muscle. Its line of pull is too far from the glenohumeral joint for it to be part of the rotator-cuff mechanism.

Q. In Figure 2-23, identify H.

A. The latissimus dorsi muscle. It winds around the inferior border of the teres major muscle to form the posterior axillary fold.

Q. In Figure 2-24, identify vein A.

A. The axillary vein. Deep veins are usually crescent shaped in section.

Q. In Figure 2-24, identify nerve B.

A. The median nerve. Note its position between the axillary vein and the axillary artery.

Q. In Figure 2-24, identify artery C.

A. The axillary artery.

Q. In Figure 2-24, identify nerve D.

A. The musculocutaneous nerve. It is approaching the coracobrachialis muscle, which it supplies.

Q. In Figure 2-24, identify vein E.

A. The cephalic vein. It lies in the deltopectoral groove between the deltoid muscle and the pectoralis major muscle.

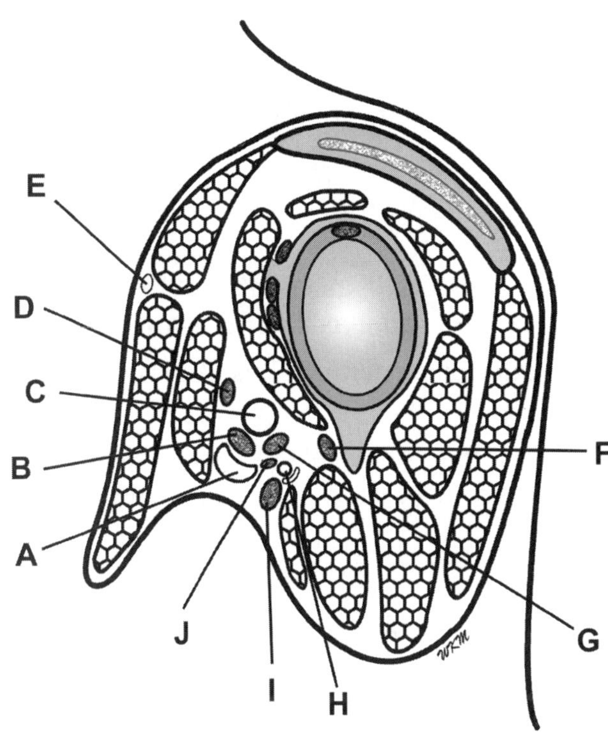

Figure 2-24 Glenohumeral Joint, Parasagittal Section: Vessels and Nerves

Q. In Figure 2-24, identify nerve F.

A. The axillary nerve. It is passing posteriorly, through the quadrangular space, to supply the teres minor muscle and the deltoid muscle.

Q. In Figure 2-24, identify nerve G.

A. The ulnar nerve. Neither it nor the median nerve supply any structure in the arm.

Q. In Figure 2-24, identify vessels H.

A. The profunda brachii artery and its venae comitantes. They accompany the radial nerve.

Q. In Figure 2-24, identify nerve I.

A. The radial nerve. It runs inferiorly to the anterior surface of the latissimus dorsi muscle.

Q. In Figure 2-24, identify nerve J.

A. The medial antebrachial cutaneous nerve. It is surprisingly large and is sometimes mistaken for the much larger ulnar nerve.

THE ELBOW JOINT

Q. The elbow joint is located between the trochlear and the capitulum of the humerus and . . .

A. The trochlear notch of the ulna and the head of the radius.

Q. The capsular ligament of the elbow joint is loose anteriorly and posteriorly, but the ulnar and radial collateral ligaments are strong. Thus, the joint is only capable of . . .

A. Flexion and extension. It is a uniaxial hinge joint.

Q. The ulnar collateral ligament is firmly attached to the medial epicondyle of the humerus superiorly. It divides into two bands inferiorly, which are attached to . . .

A. The olecranon and to the coronoid process of the ulna, respectively.

Q. The radial collateral ligament is attached superiorly to the lateral epicondyle. Inferiorly, it splits into anterior and posterior bands, which both fuse with . . .

A. The annular ligament. The bands gain attachment, together with the annular ligament, to the margins of the radial facet on the ulna.

Q. The anterior relations of the elbow joint are . . .

A. The brachialis tendon and the biceps tendon. They separate the joint from the brachial artery and the median nerve.

Q. The posterior relation of the elbow joint is . . .

A. The tendon of the triceps muscle. The anconeus muscle is posterolateral to the joint.

Q. Anterolateral to the elbow joint lie . . .

A. The brachioradialis muscle and the radial nerve.

Q. Anteromedial to the elbow joint are . . .

A. The pronator teres muscle and the long flexor muscles, which arise from the common flexor origin. The ulnar nerve lies posterior to the medial epicondyle.

Q. The superior radioulnar articulation is located between the circumference of the head of the radius and the radial notch on the ulna. It is therefore a . . .

A. Uniaxial pivot joint.

Q. The superior radioulnar articulation has only one significant ligament, which embraces the neck of the radius. It is . . .

A. The annular ligament.

Q. Until around the age of five, an unexpected pull on the hand may cause subluxation of the head of the radius. This is rare after age five, because at this age . . .

A. The head of the radius begins to ossify and is therefore no longer deformable.

THE RADIOCARPAL AND CARPOMETACARPAL JOINTS

Q. The radiocarpal (wrist) joint is a condyloid joint between the radius, a triangular disc, and . . .

A. The scaphoid bone, the lunate bone, and the triquetral bone.

Q. The ulna is separated from the radiocarpal joint by a small triangular fibrocartilaginous disc. The base of this disc is attached to . . .

A. The ulnar side of the lower end of the radius. Its apex is attached to the base of the styloid process of the ulna.

Q. The fulcrum for the pivoting of the radius around the head of the ulna during pronation and supination is . . .

A. The attachment of the apex of the fibrocartilaginous disc of the radiocarpal joint to the base of the styloid process of the ulna.

Q. Both the anterior and the posterior capsule and even the collateral ligaments of the wrist joint are relatively lax. However, the only movements that can take place are . . .

A. Flexion, extension, abduction, and adduction. Rotation is not possible.

Q. Of the movements possible at the radiocarpal articulation, the most limited is . . .

A. Abduction. The radial side of the carpus, which carries the thumb, is much more mobile, and hence more unstable than the ulnar side.

Q. Rotation at the radiocarpal articulation is prevented because . . .

A. The anteroposterior radius of curvature and the mediolateral radius of curvature of the reciprocal joint surfaces differ markedly. The joint is an ellipsoid joint. Such joints are only capable of moving around two axes; they are biaxial.

Q. The carpometacarpal joint of the thumb is a saddle-shaped condyloid synovial joint. The movements that occur at this joint are . . .

A. Flexion, extension, adduction, and abduction. The shape of the reciprocal joint surfaces causes some degree of rotation of the metacarpal bone to occur during flexion. This compound movement results in opposition of the thumb to the little finger.

Q. The movements that take place at the medial four carpometacarpal joints are . . .

A. Very limited flexion and extension.

THE METACARPOPHALANGEAL AND INTERPHALANGEAL JOINTS

Q. The metacarpophalangeal joints are . . .

A. Biaxial, condyloid, synovial articulations. Flexion, extension, abduction, and adduction can take place. However, it should be remembered that abduction of the fingers is defined as taking place from a line centered on the middle finger.

Q. The interphalangeal joints are . . .

A. Uniaxial, hinge, condyloid, synovial joints.

Q. Extension at the metacarpophalangeal and interphalangeal joints is limited by . . .

A. The collateral ligaments. These strong bands run distally and anteriorly from the proximal to the distal bone of each joint. They are somewhat laxer in the metacarpophalangeal joints to allow for abduction and adduction of the digits. Variable degrees of passive overextension can occur.

RADIOLOGY OF THE UPPER LIMB

Q. In Figure 2-25, identify A.

A. The coracoid process of the scapula.

Q. In Figure 2-25, identify B.

A. The acromial process.

Q. In Figure 2-25, identify C.

A. The head of the humerus.

Q. In Figure 2-25, identify D.

A. The greater tubercle.

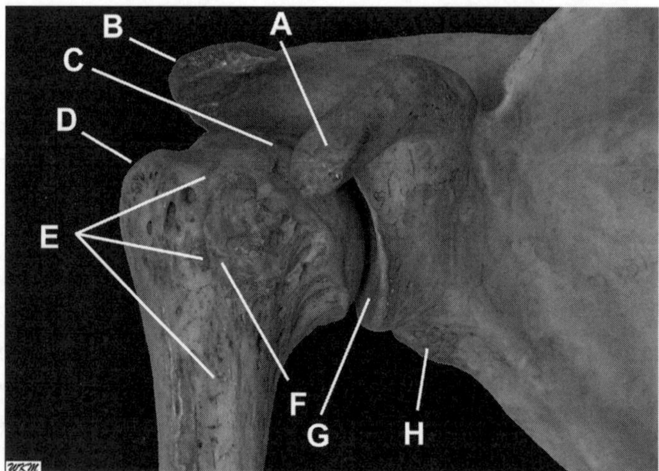

Figure 2-25 The Right Glenohumeral Articulation: The Humerus and the Scapula

Q. The three muscles that are attached to the greater tubercle of the humerus are . . .

A. The supraspinatus muscle, the infraspinatus muscle, and the teres minor muscle.

Q. In Figure 2-25, identify E.

A. The intertubercular sulcus (the bicipital groove) of the humerus. It is traversed by the long head of the biceps muscle.

Q. In Figure 2-25, identify F.

A. The lesser tubercle of the humerus. It is the humeral attachment of the subscapularis muscle.

Q. In Figure 2-25, identify G.

A. The glenoid fossa of the scapula.

Q. In Figure 2-25, identify H.

A. The infraglenoid tubercle. It is the origin of the long head of the triceps muscle.

Q. In Figure 2-26, identify A.

A. The clavicle.

Q. In Figure 2-26, identify B.

A. The coracoid process of the scapula.

Q. In Figure 2-26, identify C.

A. The acromion.

Q. In Figure 2-26, identify D.

A. The head of the humerus.

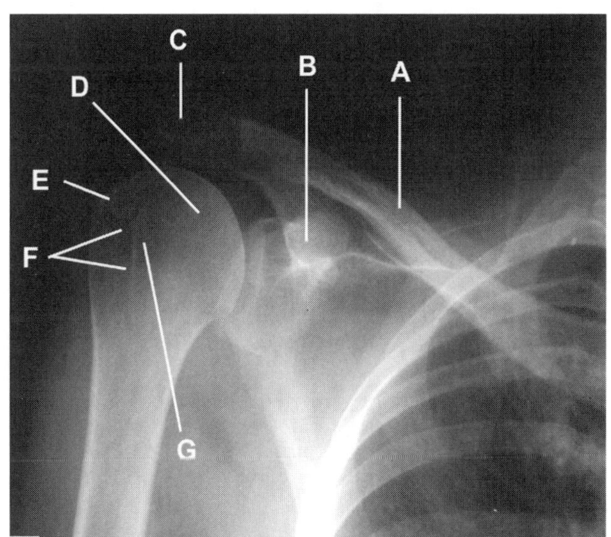

Figure 2-26 AP X-ray of the Right Shoulder

Q. In Figure 2-26, identify E.

A. The greater tubercle (greater tuberosity) of the humerus.

Q. In Figure 2-26, identify F.

A. The intertubercular sulcus.

Q. In Figure 2-26, identify G.

A. The lesser tubercle (lesser tuberosity) of the humerus.

Q. In Figure 2-27, identify A.

A. A layer of subcutaneous fat.

Q. In Figure 2-27, identify B.

A. The epiphyseal line of the head of the humerus.

Q. In Figure 2-27, identify C.

A. The deltoid muscle.

Q. In Figure 2-27, identify D.

A. The supraspinatus muscle.

Q. In Figure 2-27, identify E.

A. The acromion.

Q. In Figure 2-27, identify F.

A. The acromioclavicular joint.

Q. In Figure 2-27, identify G.

A. The acromial end of the clavicle.

Q. In Figure 2-27, identify H.

A. The glenohumeral joint.

Q. In Figure 2-28, identify A.

A. The subscapularis muscle.

Q. In Figure 2-28, identify B.

A. The head of the scapula.

Q. In Figure 2-28, identify C.

A. The infraspinatus muscle.

Q. In Figure 2-28, identify D.

A. The deltoid muscle.

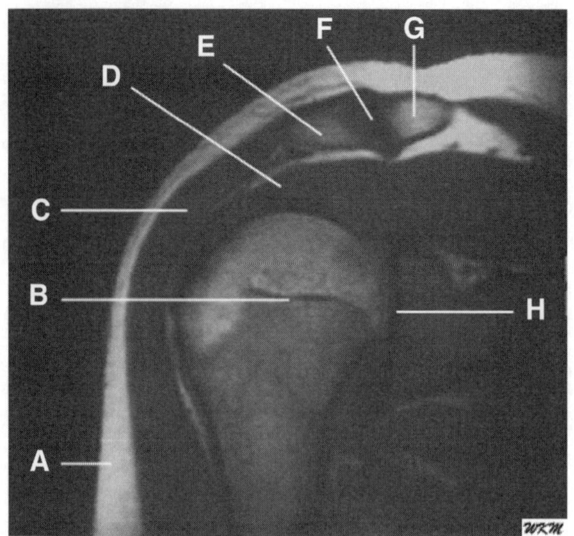

Figure 2-27 Coronal MRI of the Shoulder

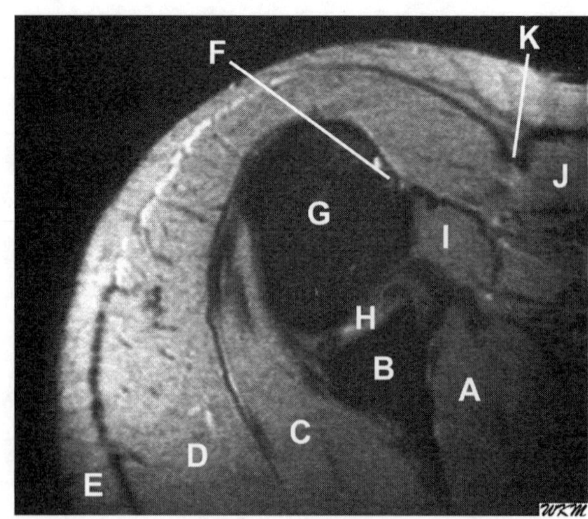

Figure 2-28 Transverse MRI of the Shoulder

Q. In Figure 2-28, identify E.

A. Subcutaneous fat.

Q. In Figure 2-28, identify F.

A. The position of the tendon of the long head of the biceps muscle.

Q. In Figure 2-28, identify G.

A. The head of the humerus.

Q. In Figure 2-28, identify H.

A. The glenohumeral joint cavity.

Q. In Figure 2-28, identify I.

A. The combined short head of the biceps muscle and the coracobrachialis muscle.

Q. In Figure 2-28, identify J.

A. The pectoralis major muscle.

Q. In Figure 2-28, identify K.

A. The cephalic vein in the deltopectoral groove.

Q. In Figure 2-29, the diagnosis is . . .

A. Anterior dislocation of the right glenohumeral joint. The common method of injury is overextension of the abducted shoulder. This causes forward displacement of the head of the humerus into the subscapular fossa. The only other type of dislocation of this joint is posteriorly into the infraspinous fossa; however, this is uncommon. It is difficult to visualize an injury that would displace the head of the humerus posteriorly. The usual cause of this latter, most unusual, displacement is a fall on the hand with the elbow extended and the shoulder at 90° of flexion.

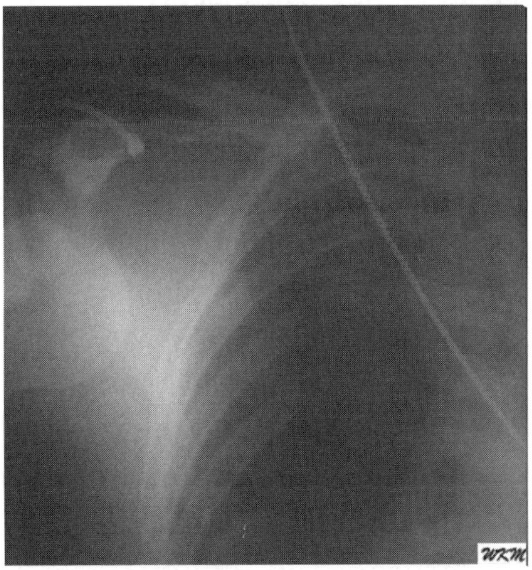

Figure 2-29 AP X-ray of the Right Shoulder

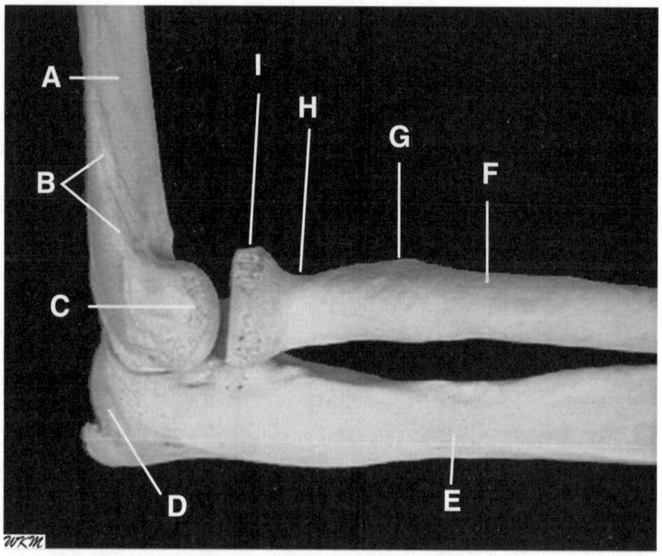

Q. In Figure 2-30, identify A.

A. The shaft of the humerus.

Q. In Figure 2-30, identify B.

A. The lateral supracondylar ridge. To it is attached the lateral intermuscular septum, which is itself perforated by the radial nerve.

Q. In Figure 2-30, identify C.

A. The lateral epicondyle of the humerus.

Figure 2-30 The Skeleton of the Right Elbow, Lateral Aspect

Q. In Figure 2-30, identify D.

A. The olecranon process of the ulna. Notice the olecranon "spur" projecting from it. This spur results from ossification in the tendon of the triceps muscle at its insertion.

Q. In Figure 2-30, identify E.

A. The shaft of the ulna.

Q. In Figure 2-30, identify F.

A. The shaft of the radius.

Q. In Figure 2-30, identify G.

A. The radial tuberosity. The tendon of the biceps is inserted into its posterior area. Anteriorly, it is separated from the tendon of the biceps muscle by a bursa.

Q. In Figure 2-30, identify H.

A. The neck of the radius. It is embraced by the annular ligament. The proximal end of the radius is not attached by ligaments, either to the humerus or to the ulna. This enables the radius to rotate freely in the annular ligament.

Q. In Figure 2-30, identify I.

A. The head of the radius.

Q. In Figure 2-31, identify A.

A. The shaft of the humerus.

Q. In Figure 2-31, identify B.

A. The superimposed medial and lateral supracondylar ridges of the humerus.

Q. In Figure 2-31, identify C.

A. The capitulum (capitellum). It is superimposed on the trochlea.

Q. In Figure 2-31, identify D.

A. The olecranon process of the ulna.

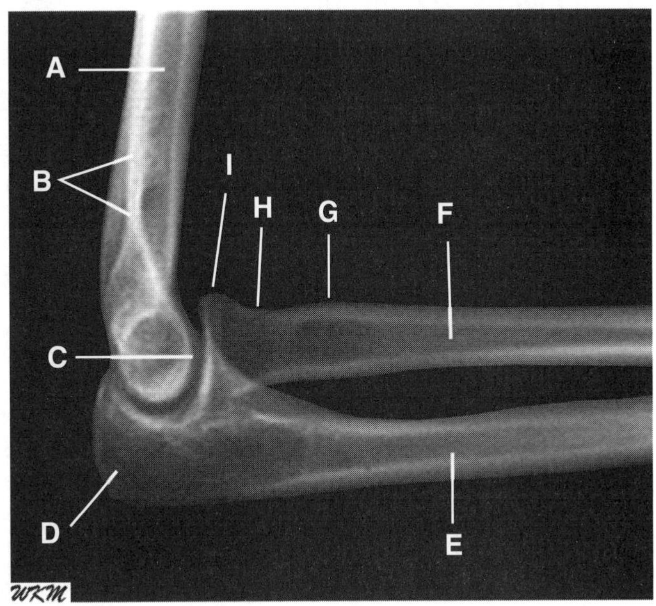

Figure 2-31 Lateral X-ray of the Elbow

Q. In Figure 2-31, identify E.

A. The shaft of the ulna. Its posterior border is subcutaneous, and hence is likely to be fractured by direct violence (a "defense" fracture).

Q. In Figure 2-31, identify F.

A. The shaft of the radius.

Q. In Figure 2-31, identify G.

A. The radial tuberosity. The tendon of the biceps brachii muscle is attached to it.

Q. In Figure 2-31, identify H.

A. The neck of the radius.

Q. The neck of the radius is enclosed by the . . .

A. The annular ligament. It is attached to the ulna and only loosely attached to the radius.

Q. In Figure 2-31, identify I.

A. The head of the radius.

Q. The radius is attached directly to the humerus by . . .

A. Its lax capsular ligament. The radial collateral ligament fuses with the annular ligament.

Q. In Figure 2-32, identify A.

A. The distal end of the shaft of the humerus.

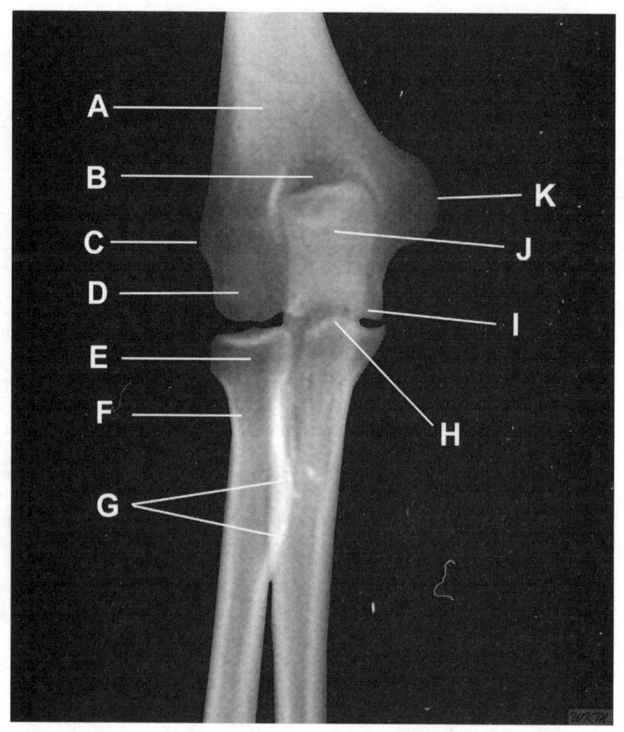

Figure 2-32 AP X-ray of the Left Elbow

Q. In Figure 2-32, identify B.

A. The olecranon fossa of the humerus.

Q. In Figure 2-32, identify C.

A. The lateral epicondyle.

Q. In Figure 2-32, identify D.

A. The capitulum (capitellum) of the humerus.

Q. In Figure 2-32, identify E.

A. The head of the radius.

Q. In Figure 2-32, identify F.

A. The neck of the radius.

Q. In Figure 2-32, identify G.

A. The radial tuberosity. It is the site of the insertion of the biceps muscle.

Q. In Figure 2-32, identify H.

A. The coronoid process of the ulna.

Q. In Figure 2-32, identify I.

A. The trochlea of the humerus.

Q. In Figure 2-32, identify J.

A. The olecranon process of the ulna.

Q. In Figure 2-32, identify K.

A. The medial epicondyle of the humerus. The ulnar nerve grooves it posteriorly.

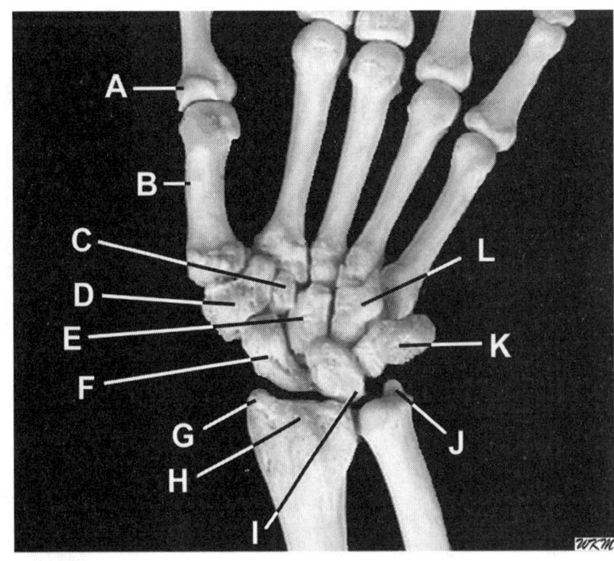

Figure 2-33 The Skeleton of the Hand, Posterior Aspect

Q. In Figure 2-33, identify A.

A. The base of the proximal phalanx of the thumb.

Q. In Figure 2-33, identify B.

A. The first metacarpal bone.

Q. In Figure 2-33, identify C.

A. The trapezoid bone.

Q. In Figure 2-33, identify D.

A. The trapezium bone.

Q. In Figure 2-33, identify E.

A. The capitate bone.

Q. In Figure 2-33, identify F.

A. The scaphoid bone. It is the most frequently fractured bone of the carpus.

Q. In Figure 2-33, identify G.

A. The styloid process of the radius.

Q. In Figure 2-33, identify H.

A. The dorsal tubercle of the radius.

Q. In Figure 2-33, identify I.

A. The lunate bone. It is the most commonly displaced carpal bone.

Q. In Figure 2-33, identify J.

A. The styloid process of the ulna.

Q. In Figure 2-33, identify K.

A. The triquetral bone. It obscures the pisiform bone, which lies anterior to it.

Q. In Figure 2-33, identify L.

A. The hamate bone.

Q. In Figure 2-34, identify A.

A. A sesamoid bone in the tendon of the flexor pollicis brevis muscle.

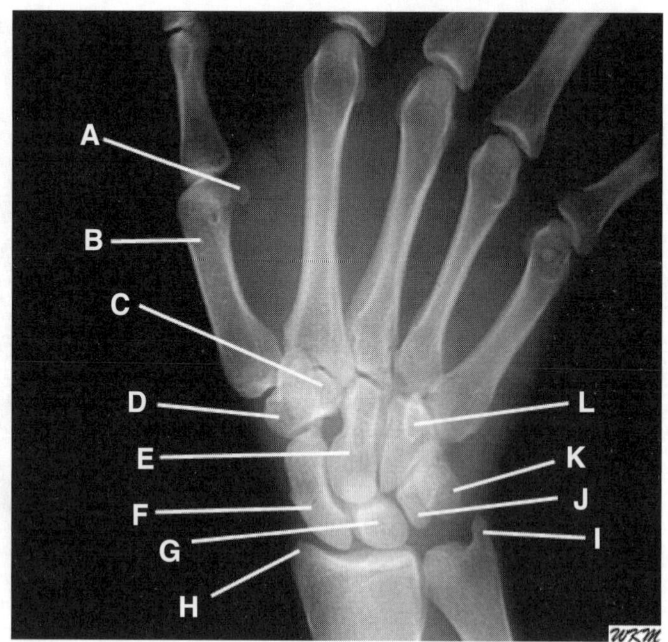

Figure 2-34 PA X-ray of the Right Wrist

Q. In Figure 2-34, identify B.

A. The first metacarpal bone.

Q. In Figure 2-34, identify C.

A. The trapezoid bone.

Q. In Figure 2-34, identify D.

A. The trapezium bone.

Q. In Figure 2-34, identify E.

A. The capitate bone.

Q. In Figure 2-34, identify F.

A. The scaphoid bone. The neck of this bone is frequently fractured by falls on the hand.

Q. Following a fracture of the scaphoid bone, the area of tenderness is situated in . . .

A. The anatomical snuff box.

Q. In Figure 2-34, identify G.

A. The lunate bone.

Q. In Figure 2-34, identify H.

A. The styloid process of the radius.

Q. In Figure 2-34, identify I.

A. The styloid process of the ulna.

Q. In Figure 2-34, identify J.

A. The triquetral bone.

Q. In Figure 2-34, identify K.

A. The pisiform bone. It is a carpal bone that functions as a sesamoid bone in the tendon of the flexor carpi ulnaris muscle.

Q. In Figure 2-34, identify L.

A. The hook of the hamate. The ulnar nerve can be palpated against the hook of the hamate.

Q. In Figure 2-35, identify A.

A. The radius. Note the bowing at the site of a greenstick fracture. Due to the incomplete degree of ossification of the long bones at this age, fractures sometimes result in bending rather than snapping of the bone, just as green sticks bend and dry sticks break.

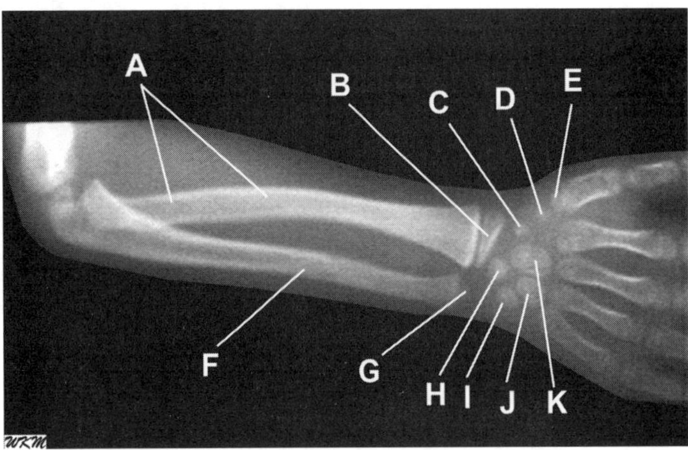

Figure 2-35 X-ray of the Forearm and Hand of a Six-Year-Old

Q. In Figure 2-35, identify B.

A. The distal epiphysis of the radius. Note that at six years of age the radial epiphysis is not yet fused with the radial shaft.

Q. In Figure 2-35, identify C.

A. The scaphoid bone. At this age, it is only partly ossified.

Q. In Figure 2-35, identify D.

A. The trapezium bone. At this age, ossification is just starting.

Q. In Figure 2-35, identify E.

A. The unfused proximal epiphysis of the first metacarpal bone.

Q. In Figure 2-35, identify F.

A. The ulna. Note the greenstick fracture of the lower third of the shaft of the bone.

Q. In Figure 2-35, identify G.

A. The distal epiphysis of the ulna. At this age, the epiphysis is only just visible.

Q. In Figure 2-35, identify H.

A. The incompletely ossified lunate bone.

Q. In Figure 2-35, identify I.

A. The incompletely ossified triquetral bone.

Q. In Figure 2-35, identify J.

A. The incompletely ossified hamate bone.

Q. In Figure 2-35, identify K.

A. The incompletely ossified capitate bone. Note the varying stages of ossification of the different bones at this age. Compare this radiograph with Figure 2-34.

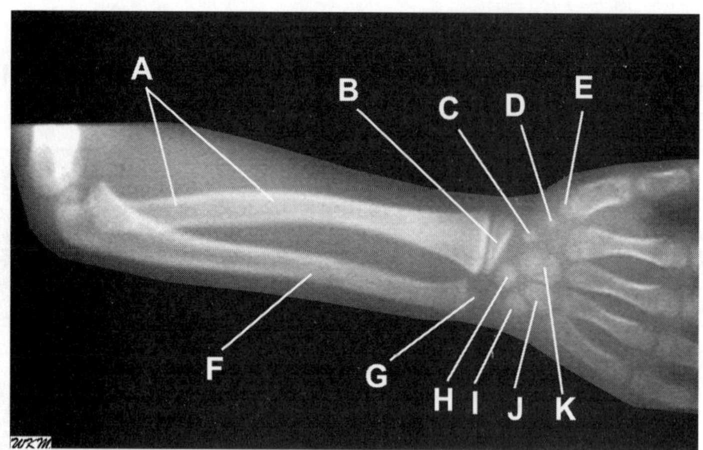

Figure 2-35 X-ray of the Forearm and Hand of a Six-Year-Old

Q. In Figure 2-36, identify A.

A. The anterior circumflex humeral artery.

Q. In Figure 2-36, identify B.

A. The posterior circumflex humeral artery.

Q. In Figure 2-36, identify C.

A. The brachial artery.

Q. In Figure 2-36, identify D.

A. The profunda brachii artery.

Q. In Figure 2-36, identify E.

A. The thoracodorsal artery.

Q. In Figure 2-36, identify F.

A. The circumflex scapular artery.

Q. In Figure 2-36, identify G.

A. The subscapular artery.

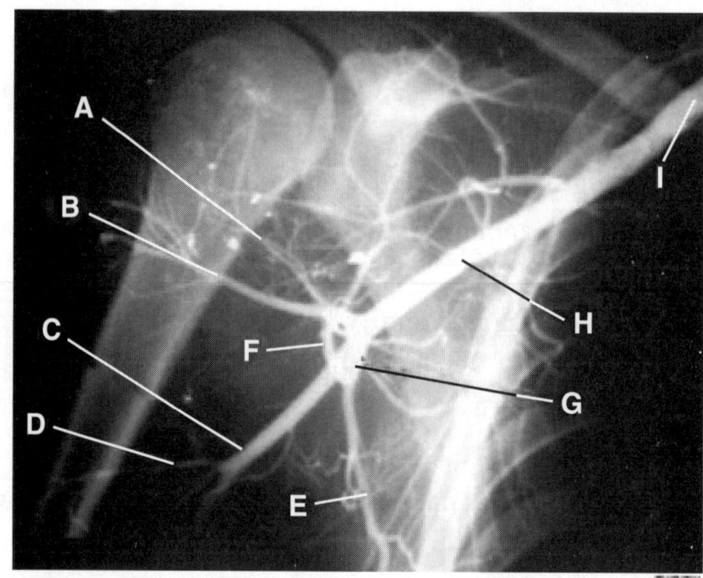

Figure 2-36 Arteriograph of the Axillary Artery

Q. In Figure 2-36, identify H.

A. The axillary artery.

Q. In Figure 2-36, identify I.

A. The subclavian artery.

Q. In Figure 2-37, identify A.

A. The anterior interosseous artery.

Q. In Figure 2-37, identify B.

A. The ulnar artery.

Q. In Figure 2-37, identify C.

A. The radial artery.

Q. In Figure 2-37, identify D.

A. The contribution of the radial artery to the deep palmar arch. It is usually much larger than shown.

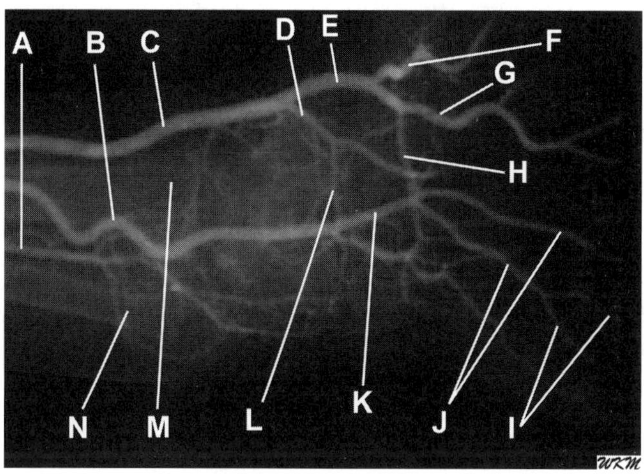

Figure 2-37 Arteriogram of the Wrist and Hand

Q. In Figure 2-37, identify E.

A. The first palmar metacarpal artery. More commonly, the princeps pollicis artery and the radialis indicis artery arise individually from the main trunk of the radial artery.

Q. In Figure 2-37, identify F.

A. The princeps pollicis artery.

Q. In Figure 2-37, identify G.

A. The radialis indicis artery. In this case, it supplies the radial contribution to the superficial palmar arch.

Q. In Figure 2-37, identify H.

A. The superficial palmar arch.

Q. In Figure 2-37, identify I.

A. Two proper digital arteries.

Q. In Figure 2-37, identify J.

A. Two common digital arteries.

Q. In Figure 2-37, identify K.

A. The continuation of the ulnar artery. It becomes the major contributor to the superficial palmar arch.

Q. In Figure 2-37, identify L.

A. The deep branch of the ulnar artery. It completes the deep palmar arch.

Q. In Figure 2-37, identify M.

A. The distal end of the radius.

Q. In Figure 2-37, identify N.

A. The distal end of the ulna.

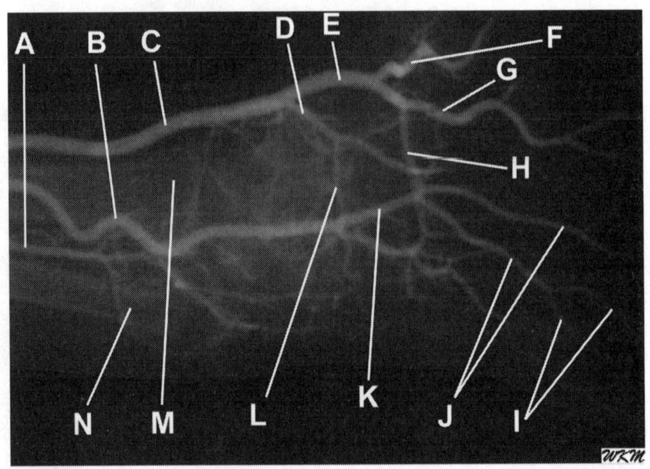

Figure 2-37 Arteriogram of the Wrist and Hand

Chapter 3

The Head and Neck

THE FACE AND THE SCALP

Q. The muscles of the face are divided into a superficial group and a deep group. The function of the superficial muscles is to move . . .

A. The skin. These muscles are situated largely in the superficial fascia and are commonly known as the "muscles of facial expression." They are important in protecting the eye, in speech, in closing the lips during mastication, and in interpersonal communication.

Q. The nerve that supplies the muscles of facial expression is . . .

A. The facial (seventh cranial) nerve.

Q. The embryonic pharyngeal arch supplied by the facial nerve is . . .

A. The second pharyngeal arch.

Q. The embryonic pharyngeal arch from which the muscles of facial expression are derived is . . .

A. The second pharyngeal arch.

Q. The deeper muscles of the face are responsible for moving . . .

A. The mandible. They are commonly known as the "muscles of mastication."

Q. The nerve supply of the muscles of mastication is . . .

A. The mandibular division of the trigeminal (fifth cranial) nerve.

Q. The embryonic pharyngeal arch that is supplied by the mandibular division of the trigeminal nerve is . . .

A. The first embryonic pharyngeal arch.

Q. The embryonic pharyngeal arch from which the muscles of mastication are derived is . . .

A. The first pharyngeal arch.

Q. The cutaneous nerve that supplies the skin of the face is . . .

A. The trigeminal (fifth cranial) nerve.

Q. The division of the trigeminal nerve that supplies the skin of the forehead and the anterior part of the scalp is . . .

A. The ophthalmic division.

Q. The area of the scalp supplied by the ophthalmic division of the trigeminal nerve extends posteriorly almost to . . .

A. Lambda. It is the site of the now-closed posterior fontanelle.

Q. The branches of the ophthalmic division of the trigeminal nerve that supply the scalp are . . .

A. The two branches of the frontal branch of the ophthalmic division of the trigeminal nerve. They are the large supraorbital nerve and the smaller supratrochlear nerve.

Q. The structures on the face that are supplied by the ophthalmic division of the trigeminal nerve are . . .

A. The cornea, the skin of the upper eyelid, and the skin of the nose. The cornea, the skin of the medial part of the upper eyelid, and the skin of the nose are supplied by suitably named branches from the nasociliary branch of the ophthalmic division of the trigeminal nerve. The skin of the lateral part of the upper eyelid is supplied by the lacrimal branch of the ophthalmic division of the trigeminal nerve.

Q. The nerve supply of the skin of the cheek is provided by . . .

A. The maxillary division of the trigeminal nerve.

Q. The branches of the maxillary nerve that supply the skin of the cheek are . . .

A. The zygomaticotemporal nerve, the zygomaticofacial nerve, and the infraorbital nerve.

Q. The cutaneous innervation over the mandible is provided by . . .

A. The mandibular division of the trigeminal nerve.

Q. The nerves involved in cutaneous innervation are . . .

A. The buccal nerve and the mental nerve. Both originate from the mandibular division of the trigeminal nerve.

Q. The major groups of the muscles of facial expression are . . .

A. The muscle surrounding the eye, the muscles surrounding the mouth, the muscles of the cheek, and the muscles involved with the nose.

Q. The facial nerve exits the skull through . . .

A. The stylomastoid foramen.

Q. Shortly after leaving the skull, the trunk of the facial nerve gives rise to three branches. They are . . .

A. The nerve to the posterior belly of the digastric muscle, the nerve to the stylohyoid muscle, and the posterior auricular nerve. The posterior auricular nerve supplies the occipital belly of the occipitofrontalis muscle. It also supplies the muscles that "move" the ear. These muscles are derived from the embryonic second pharyngeal arch.

Q. The facial nerve then passes into . . .

A. The parotid gland.

Q. In the substance of the parotid gland, where it lies superficially, the facial nerve divides into its terminal branches to the muscles of the face. These branches are . . .

A. The temporal branches, the zygomatic branches, the buccal branches, the marginal, mandibular branches, and the cervical branches.

Q. The muscles supplied by the temporal branch of the facial nerve are . . .

A. The frontal belly of the occipitofrontalis muscle and the upper part of the orbicularis oculi muscle.

Q. The muscles supplied by the zygomatic branch of the facial nerve are . . .

A. The lower half of the orbicularis oculi muscle, the muscles of the nose, and, of course, the zygomaticus major and the zygomaticus minor muscles.

Q. The buccal branch of the facial nerve supplies the buccinator muscle and the orbicularis oris muscle. It then divides into upper and lower divisions. The most important function of the buccinator muscle is . . .

A. To prevent food from accumulating in the vestibule of the mouth during mastication. The vestibule of the mouth is the space between the teeth and the cheek.

Q. Paralysis of the orbicularis oris causes . . .

A. Saliva and food to dribble from the corner of the mouth on the affected side.

Q. The muscles supplied by the upper division of the buccal branch of the facial nerve are . . .

A. The muscles of the upper lip.

Q. The muscles supplied by the lower division of the buccal branch of the facial nerve are . . .

A. The muscles of the lower lip.

Q. The muscles of the chin are supplied by . . .

A. The marginal mandibular branch of the facial nerve.

Q. The platysma receives its innervation from . . .

A. The cervical branch of the facial nerve.

Q. The most important function of the facial nerve is . . .

A. To protect the eye. Not only do the muscles it supplies close the eye, but, by a circuitous route, it supplies secretomotor fibers to the lacrimal gland. The secretions of the lacrimal gland, tears, lubricate the conjunctiva and the cornea.

Q. The facial artery arises from . . .

A. The external carotid artery.

Q. After curving around the submandibular gland, the facial artery enters the face by crossing the mandible, lying in a shallow notch. It is separated from the skin by . . .

A. The platysma muscle. The facial artery is readily palpable where it runs through this notch.

Q. The facial artery winds a tortuous course, first to the angle of the mouth and then to the inner canthus of the eye. The major branches of the facial artery are . . .

A. The superior and the inferior labial arteries, the lateral nasal artery, and the inferior and the superior medial palpebral arteries.

Q. The labial arteries lie just deep to the mucous membrane of the lips and can be readily palpated by slightly compressing the lip between the thumb and the index finger, with the index finger in the vestibule of the mouth. Therefore, profuse bleeding is most likely from a cut on . . .

A. The inside of the lower or the upper lip.

Q. The three important features of the facial vein are . . .

A. That it is superficial, that it does not have valves, and that it communicates via the ophthalmic veins with the cavernous sinus. This communication is a potential pathway for an infected thrombus to travel, via the inferior ophthalmic veins, to the cavernous sinus, with life-threatening results.

Q. The capsule of the parotid gland is formed from . . .

A. The deep cervical fascia.

Q. The major relations of the parotid gland are . . .

A. The external auditory meatus superiorly, the sternocleidomastoid muscle posteriorly, and the ramus of the mandible anteriorly.

Q. The length of the parotid duct is approximately . . .

A. 5 cm (2 inches).

Q. The parotid duct crosses superficially . . .

A. The masseter muscle.

Q. The parotid duct curves medially around the anterior border of the masseter muscle to penetrate . . .

A. The buccinator muscle.

Q. The parotid duct enters the vestibule of the mouth opposite . . .

A. The second upper molar tooth.

Q. The skin of the scalp differs from that of the face in that . . .

A. The skin of the scalp is much thicker, it is firmly adherent to the underlying aponeurosis of the occipitofrontalis muscle, and it has many more and larger hair follicles.

Q. The scalp consists of five layers. They are . . .

A. The **S**kin, a layer of dense sub**C**utaneous tissue, which binds the skin firmly to the underlying **A**poneurosis, a layer of **L**oose areolar tissue over which the scalp moves freely, and the **P**eriosteum, which is firmly attached to the underlying bone.

Q. In scalping, the now obsolete method of keeping a body count, the layers of scalp removed were . . .

A. The skin, the subcutaneous tissue, and the aponeurosis of the occipitofrontalis muscle.

Q. The function of the periosteum is both to form and to remodel bone. The cells involved are . . .

A. The osteoblasts, which form bone, and the osteoclasts, which absorb bone. Both osteoblasts and osteoclasts are needed in the remodeling of bone.

Q. The arterial supply to the scalp is mainly from . . .

A. The two branches, anterior and posterior, of the superficial temporal artery. The majority of surgical flaps, which include both the skin and the underlying aponeurosis and are designed to give access to the underlying cranium and its contents, are based on these vessels.

Q. The superficial temporal artery is a terminal branch of . . .

A. The external carotid artery.

Q. The arterial supply to the scalp over the frontal bone is derived from . . .

A. The superior orbital branch and the supratrochlear branch of the frontal branch of the ophthalmic artery.

Q. The arterial supply of the scalp over the occipital bone is derived from . . .

A. The posterior auricular branch of the facial artery and the lesser occipital branch of the external carotid artery.

Q. The sensory innervation of the frontal and the parietal region of the scalp is . . .

A. The supraorbital branch of the ophthalmic division of the trigeminal nerve. This reflects the large embryological contribution made to the region by the frontonasal process of the first pharyngeal arch.

Q. The sensory innervation of the temporal region of the scalp is derived from . . .

A. The auriculotemporal branch of the mandibular division of the trigeminal nerve.

Q. The sensory innervation of the occipital region of the scalp is derived from . . .

A. The lesser occipital nerve and the greater occipital nerve.

Q. The lesser occipital nerve, which accompanies the artery of the same name, arises from . . .

A. The cervical plexus. The cervical plexus is formed by the anterior primary rami of the upper four cervical nerves.

Q. The area of the scalp over the occipital bone is supplied with sensory fibers from the greater occipital nerve. These sensory, cutaneous fibers are derived from . . .

A. The posterior primary ramus of the second cervical nerve.

Q. The innervation of the muscles of the scalp and auricle is derived from . . .

A. Branches of the facial nerve.

Q. In Figure 3-1, identify A.

A. The orbicularis oculi muscle. It closes, and hence protects, the eye. It is attached medially to the nasal bone and to the medial palpebral ligament.

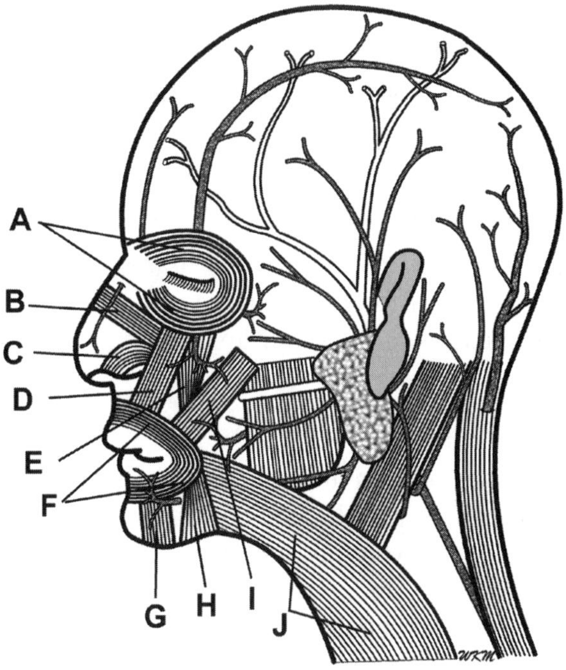

Q. In Figure 3-1, identify B.

A. The compressor naris. It is the transverse part of the nasalis muscle.

Q. In Figure 3-1, identify C.

A. The dilator naris muscle. It is the alar part of the nasalis muscle.

Q. In Figure 3-1, identify D.

A. The levator labii superioris muscle.

Figure 3-1 The Face and Scalp: Muscles of the Eye, Nose, and Mouth

Q. In Figure 3-1, identify E.

A. The levator anguli oris muscle. The levator anguli oris muscle, the levator labii superioris muscle, and the nasalis muscle arise from the maxilla.

Q. In Figure 3-1, identify F.

A. The orbicularis oris muscle. It is a facial muscle that has no attachment to bone.

Q. In Figure 3-1, identify G.

A. The depressor labii inferioris muscle. It arises from the mandible.

Q. In Figure 3-1, identify H.

A. The depressor anguli oris muscle. It arises from the mandible.

Q. In Figure 3-1, identify I.

A. The zygomaticus major muscle. It arises from the zygoma.

Q. In Figure 3-1, identify J.

A. The platysma muscle. Its atrophy in old age is the cause of "chicken neck."

Q. In Figure 3-2, identify A.

A. The cervical branch of the facial nerve. It supplies the platysma muscle.

Q. In Figure 3-2, identify B.

A. The marginal mandibular branch of the facial nerve. It supplies the muscles of the lower lip and chin.

Q. In Figure 3-2, identify C.

A. The buccal branch of the facial nerve. It supplies the buccinator muscle, which is not shown in this diagram, and, via superior and inferior branches, the muscle of the upper and lower lip.

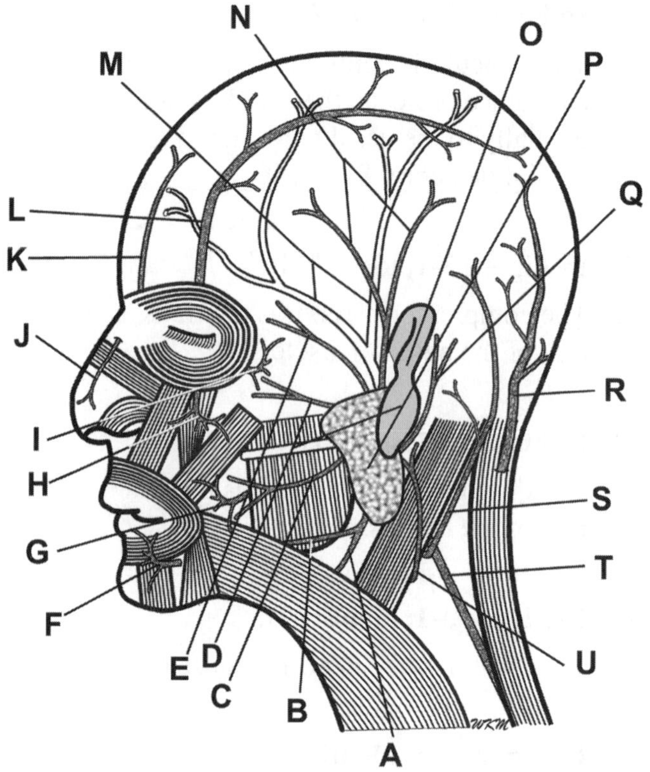

Figure 3-2 The Face and Scalp: Motor and Sensory Nerves

Q. In Figure 3-2, identify D.

A. The zygomatic branch of the facial nerve. It supplies the inferior part of the orbicularis oculi muscle, the nasalis muscle, and the zygomatic muscles.

Q. In Figure 3-2, identify E.

A. The temporal branch of the facial nerve. It supplies the upper part of the orbicularis oculi muscle, the small muscles of the forehead, and the frontal belly of the occipitofrontalis muscle.

Q. In Figure 3-2, identify F.

A. The mental nerve. It is sensory to the chin and is the terminal branch of the inferior alveolar branch of the mandibular division of the trigeminal nerve.

Q. In Figure 3-2, identify G.

A. The buccal branch of the mandibular nerve. It is sensory to the skin of the cheek.

Q. In Figure 3-2, identify H.

A. The infraorbital branch of the maxillary division of the trigeminal nerve. It is sensory to the skin of the upper lip and the upper part of the cheek.

Q. In Figure 3-2, identify I.

A. The zygomaticofacial branch of the maxillary nerve. It supplies the skin over the zygoma.

Q. In Figure 3-2, identify J.

A. The external nasal branch of the anterior ethmoidal nerve. It is a terminal branch of the nasociliary nerve, which is one of the three terminal branches of the ophthalmic division of the trigeminal nerve. It is sensory to the skin of the nose.

Q. In Figure 3-2, identify K.

A. The supratrochlear branch of the frontal nerve. It supplies the skin of the medial part of the forehead. The frontal nerve is a branch of the ophthalmic division of the trigeminal nerve.

Q. In Figure 3-2, identify L.

A. The large supraorbital nerve. It is the larger terminal branch of the frontal nerve and supplies the skin of the scalp as far back as lambda.

Q. In Figure 3-2, identify M.

A. The anterior and the posterior temporal branches of the superficial temporal artery. The superficial temporal artery is the major artery to the scalp. This vessel is commonly used in surgery to supply skin flaps.

Q. In Figure 3-2, identify N.

A. The anterior and the posterior branches of the auriculotemporal nerve. The auriculotemporal nerve is a cutaneous branch of the mandibular division of the trigeminal nerve. It supplies the lateral aspect of the auricle and the temporal region of the scalp.

Q. In Figure 3-2, identify O.

A. The auricle. It has been pulled forward to display the posterior auricular branch of the facial nerve.

Q. In Figure 3-2, identify P.

A. The parotid duct and the parotid gland. The parotid duct runs across the masseter muscle. The parotid gland lies in the space between the ramus of the mandible and the external auditory meatus and the mastoid process. In acute infective parotitis (mumps), the location of the parotid gland makes opening the mouth and jaw painful.

Q. In Figure 3-2, identify Q.

A. The posterior auricular branch of the facial nerve. It supplies the occipital belly of the occipitofrontalis muscle. It also supplies insignificant auricular muscles.

Q. In Figure 3-2, identify R.

A. The greater occipital nerve. It is the cutaneous component of the posterior primary ramus of the second cervical nerve. It emerges through the semispinalis capitis muscle and the trapezius muscle to supply the skin over the occipital bone.

Q. In Figure 3-2, identify S.

A. The lesser occipital nerve. It is the cutaneous component of the anterior primary ramus of the second cervical nerve. It loops around the accessory nerve and ascends under cover of the posterior border of the sternomastoid muscle to supply the skin posterior to the auricle.

Q. In Figure 3-2, identify T.

A. The spinal part of the accessory nerve. It is seen here crossing the posterior triangle of the neck to supply the trapezius muscle.

Q. In Figure 3-2, identify U.

A. The great auricular nerve. It arises from the anterior primary rami of the second and third cervical nerves. It supplies the skin over the medial and over the lower part of the lateral surface of the auricle. It also supplies the skin over the angle of the mandible.

THE SKULL

Q. In Figure 3-3, identify bone A.

A. The frontal bone. In the fetus, right and left frontal bones are present. They fuse in the midline before birth. A remnant of this fusion sometimes remains as a metopic suture.

Q. In Figure 3-3, identify B.

A. The superior orbital fissure. It connects the orbit with the middle cranial fossa.

Q. In Figure 3-3, identify suture C.

A. The zygomaticofrontal suture. It is usually readily palpable.

Q. In Figure 3-3, identify bone D.

A. The zygoma.

Q. In Figure 3-3, identify E.

A. The zygomatic arch.

Q. In Figure 3-3, identify F.

A. The maxilla.

Q. In Figure 3-3, the nerve that emerges through foramen G is . . .

A. The mental nerve. It arises from the inferior alveolar branch of the mandibular division of the trigeminal nerve. It is sensory to the skin of the chin.

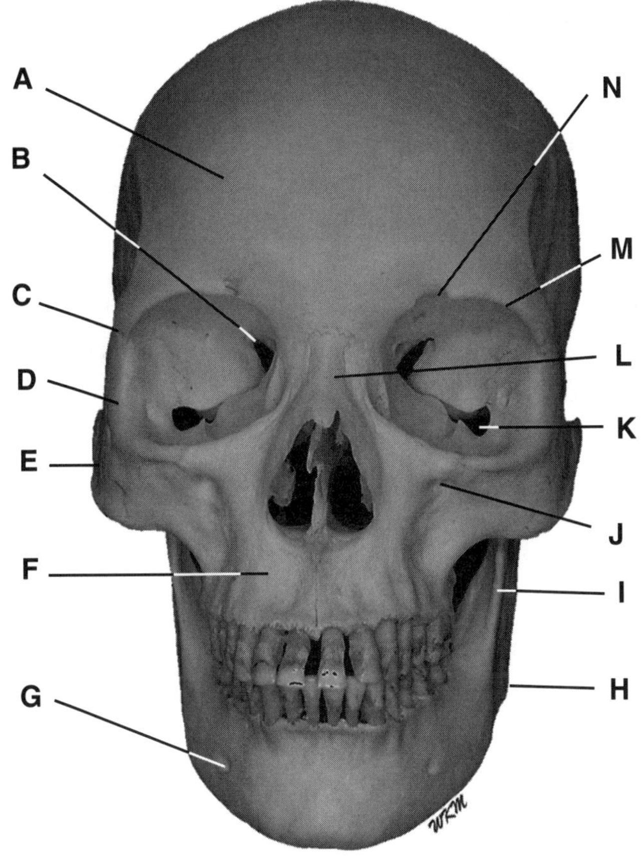

Figure 3-3 The Skull, Frontal Aspect

Q. In Figure 3-3, identify H.

A. The angle of the mandible. It tends to be everted in the male and inverted in the female.

Q. In Figure 3-3, identify I.

A. The coronoid process of the mandible.

Q. In Figure 3-3, identify J.

A. The infraorbital foramen. It transmits the infraorbital branch of the maxillary division of the trigeminal nerve. It is sensory to the skin of the cheek.

Q. In Figure 3-3, identify K.

A. The inferior orbital fissure. It connects the orbit to the pterygopalatine fossa and the infratemporal fossa.

Q. In Figure 3-3, identify L.

A. The left nasal bone. It articulates superiorly with the nasal process of the frontal bone.

Q. In Figure 3-3, identify M.

A. The supraorbital margin of the frontal bone. Laterally sharp, it is rounded medially.

Q. In Figure 3-3, identify N.

A. The supraorbital foramen for the supraorbital branch of the frontal nerve. The margin may be incomplete inferiorly. It then becomes a palpable notch.

Q. In Figure 3-4, identify A.

A. The sagittal suture.

Q. In Figure 3-4, identify B.

A. The frontal air sinus. The right and left sinuses are of unequal size. On occasion, only one frontal air sinus is present.

Q. In Figure 3-4, identify C.

A. The zygoma. It articulates with the zygomatic process of the temporal bone at the zygomaticotemporal suture.

Q. In Figure 3-4, identify D.

A. The coronoid process of the mandible.

Q. In Figure 3-4, identify E.

A. The angle of the mandible. In the male, the mandible is heavier and the mandibular angle is usually more everted.

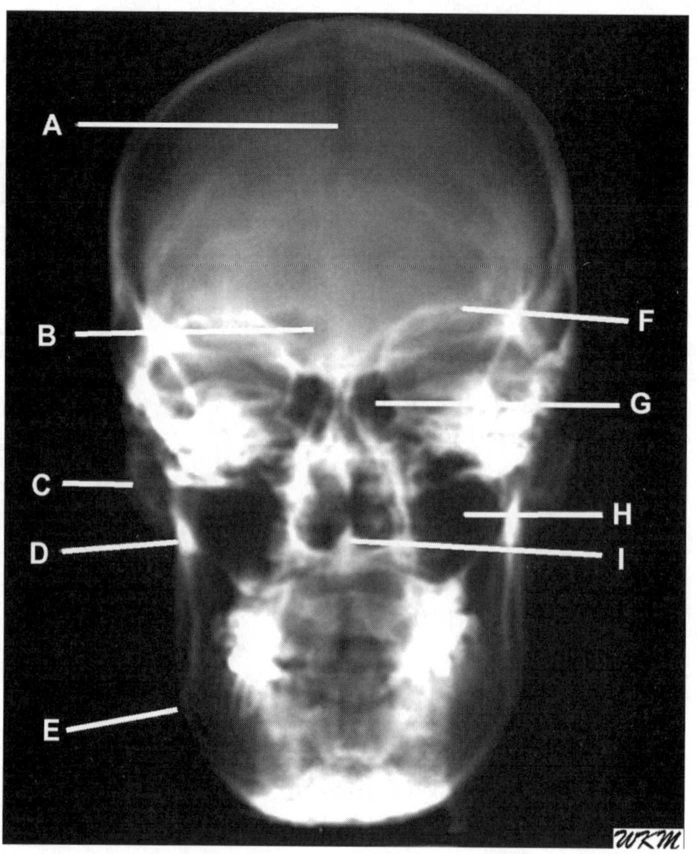

Figure 3-4 PA X-ray of the Skull

Q. In Figure 3-4, identify F.

A. The supraorbital margin.

Q. In Figure 3-4, identify G.

A. The ethmoid sinuses. There are three groups on the lateral side of both right and left nasal cavities anterior, middle, and posterior. In a posteroanterior X-ray, they are, as here, superimposed over one another. The orbital plate of the ethmoid, the lamina papyracea ethmoidale, is very thin, thus infection of the ethmoid sinuses can readily spread to the orbit.

Q. In Figure 3-4, identify H.

A. The maxillary sinus.

Q. In Figure 3-4, identify I.

A. The nasal spine. It is readily palpable.

Q. In Figure 3-5, identify A.

A. The frontal eminence.

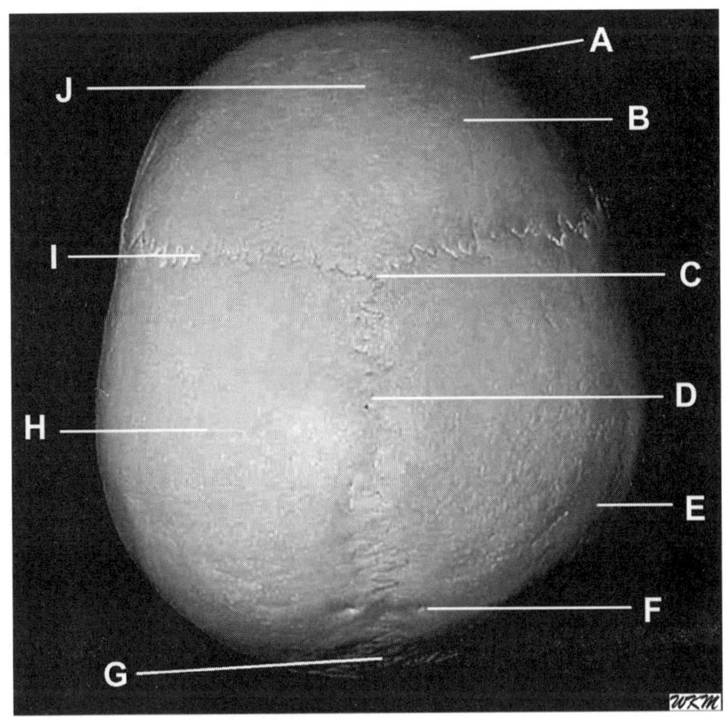

Figure 3-5 The Skull, Superior Aspect: Norma Verticalis

Q. In Figure 3-5, identify B.

A. The frontal bone.

Q. In Figure 3-5, identify C.

A. The bregma, the anterior fontanelle of the neonate.

Q. In Figure 3-5, identify D.

A. The sagittal suture.

Q. In Figure 3-5, identify E.

A. The parietal eminence. In congenital syphilis, the frontal and parietal eminences are exaggerated and give the appearance of a "hot-cross bun."

Q. In Figure 3-5, identify F.

A. An emissary parietal foramen for an emissary vein.

Q. In Figure 3-5, identify G.

A. Lambda. It is the point at which the sagittal sutures and the two lambdoid sutures meet. It is an easily palpable landmark. In the neonate, it is the posterior fontanelle.

Q. In Figure 3-5, identify H.

A. The parietal bone.

Q. In Figure 3-5, identify I.

A. The coronal suture.

Q. In Figure 3-5, identify J.

A. The almost obliterated, metopic suture. The single adult frontal bone originates from two embryonic frontal bones. The metopic suture persists in approximately 5 percent of skulls, depending on their ethnic origin. When the metopic suture persists, it can be palpated for a variable distance toward the bregma, where it joins the coronal and sagittal sutures.

Q. In Figure 3-6, identify A.

A. The mental foramen.

Q. In Figure 3-6, identify B.

A. The anterior nasal spine.

Q. In Figure 3-6, identify C.

A. The nasion.

Q. In Figure 3-6, identify D.

A. The frontozygomatic suture.

Q. In Figure 3-6, identify E.

A. The pterion.

Q. In Figure 3-6, identify F.

A. The coronal suture.

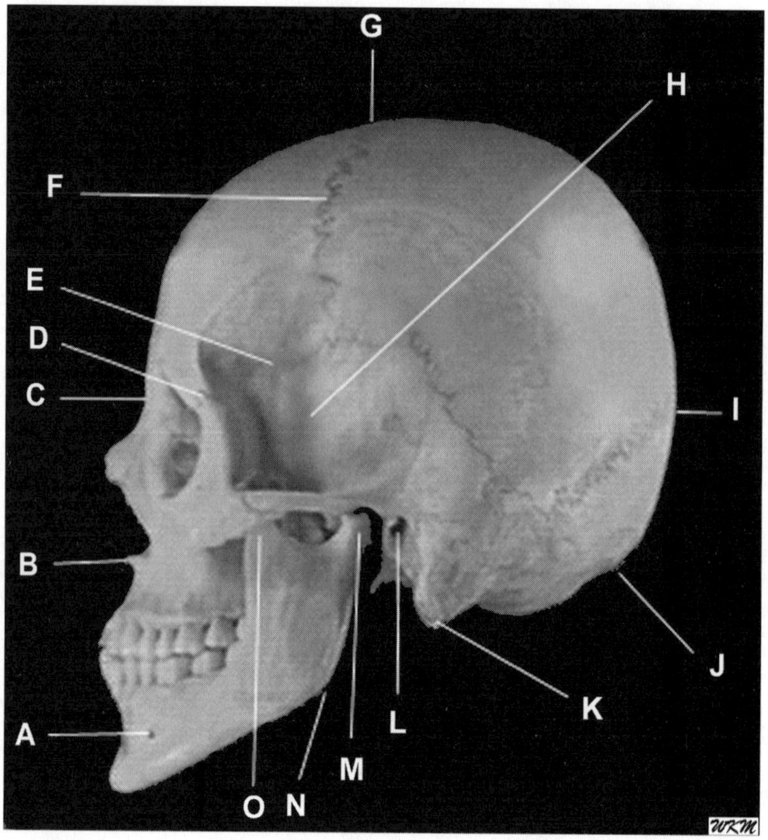

Figure 3-6 The Skull, Lateral Aspect: Norma Lateralis

Q. In Figure 3-6, identify G.

A. The bregma. It is the site of the anterior fontanelle, which is often not closed until approximately 18 months of extrauterine life.

Q. In Figure 3-6, identify area H.

A. The temporal fossa.

Q. In Figure 3-6, identify I.

A. Lambda, the point of union of the lambdoid and the sagittal sutures. It is the site of the posterior fontanelle, which remains open during the first six months of extrauterine life.

Q. In Figure 3-6, identify J.

A. The inion. It is the external occipital protuberance of the occipital bone.

Q. In Figure 3-6, identify K.

A. The mastoid process.

Q. In Figure 3-6, identify L.

A. The external auditory meatus.

Q. In Figure 3-6, identify M.

A. The condyloid process of the mandible.

Q. In Figure 3-6, identify N.

A. The angle of the mandible.

Q. In Figure 3-6, identify O.

A. The coronoid process of the mandible.

Q. In Figure 3-7, identify A.

A. The frontal air sinuses.

Q. In Figure 3-7, identify B.

A. The orbital plate of the frontal bone.

Q. In Figure 3-7, identify C.

A. The hypophyseal (pituitary) fossa. It is bounded by the anterior and the posterior clinoid processes and, anteroinferiorly, by the sphenoidal air sinuses.

Q. In Figure 3-7, identify D.

A. The anterior nasal spine.

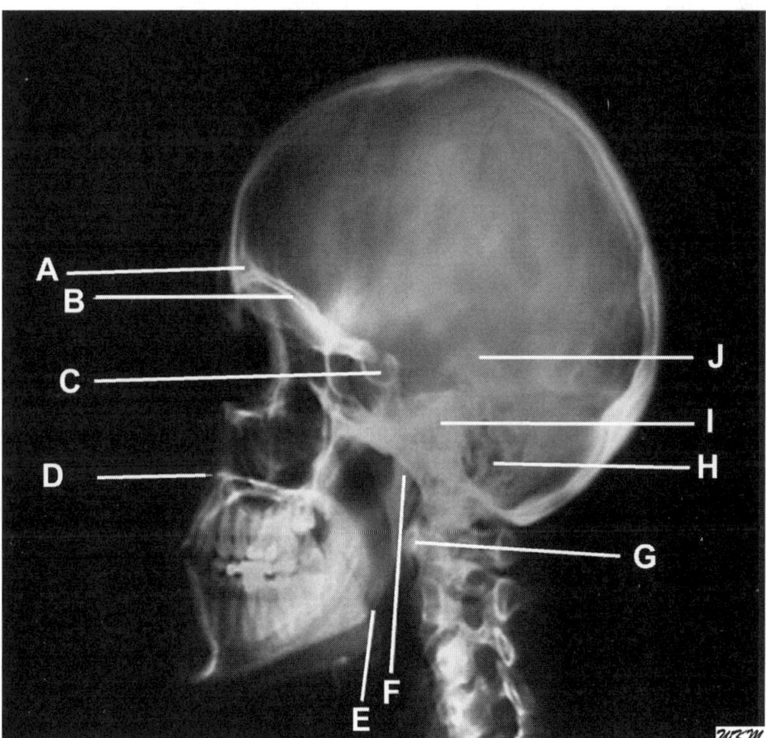

Figure 3-7 Lateral X-ray of the Skull

Q. In Figure 3-7, identify E.

A. The angle of the mandible.

Q. In Figure 3-7, identify F.

A. The condyloid process of the mandible.

Q. In Figure 3-7, identify G.

A. The anterior arch of the atlas.

Q. In Figure 3-7, identify H.

A. The mastoid air cells.

Q. In Figure 3-7, identify I.

A. The petrous temporal bone.

Q. In Figure 3-7, identify J.

A. The curved helix of the ear.

Q. In Figure 3-8, identify A.

A. The frontal crest.

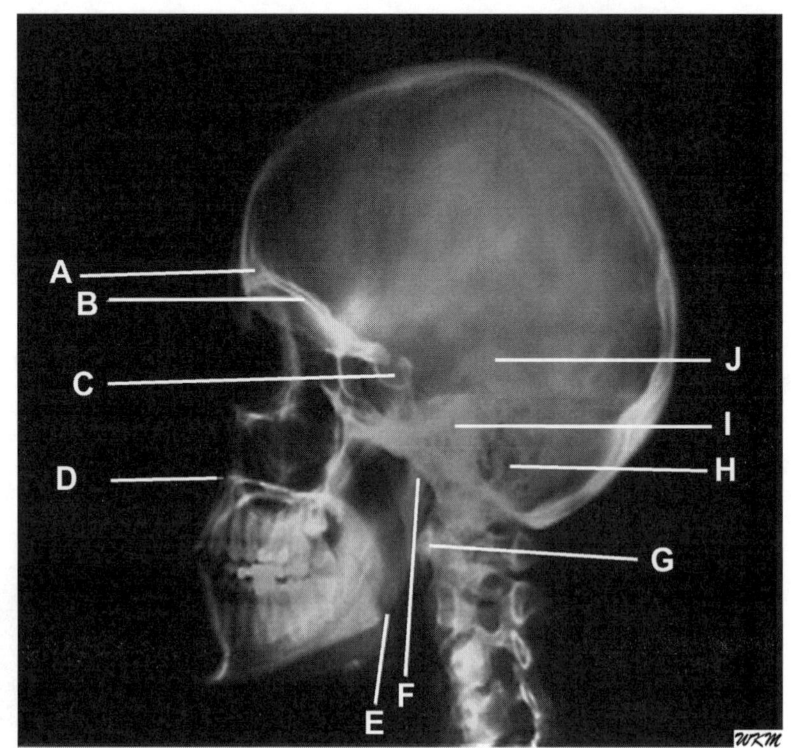

Figure 3-7 Lateral X-ray of the Skull

Q. In Figure 3-8, identify B.

A. Two of the grooves for the branches of the middle meningeal artery.

Q. In Figure 3-8, identify C.

A. A hollow for an arachnoid granulation.

Q. In Figure 3-8, identify D.

A. The parietal emissary foramen.

Q. In Figure 3-8, identify E.

A. The inner table of the skull.

Q. In Figure 3-8, identify F.

A. The diploe of the skull.

Q. In Figure 3-8, identify G.

A. The outer table of the skull.

Q. In Figure 3-8, identify H.

A. The groove for the superior sagittal sinus.

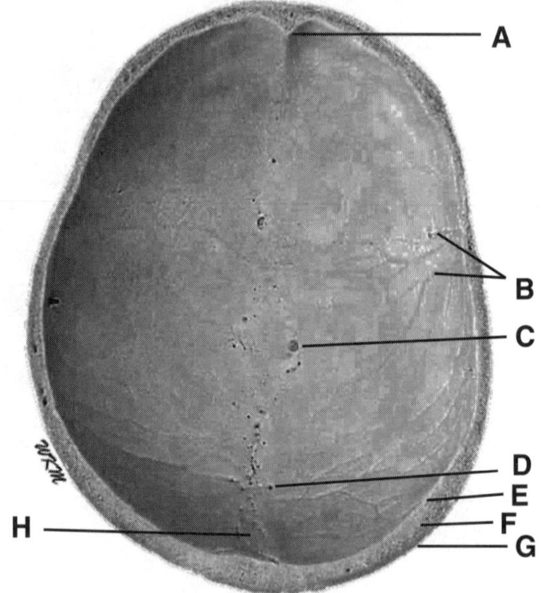

Figure 3-8 The Skull: Inferior Aspect of the Calvaria

Q. In Figure 3-9, identify A.

A. The orbital plate of the frontal bone.

Q. In Figure 3-9, identify B.

A. The lesser wing of the sphenoid bone.

Q. In Figure 3-9, identify C.

A. The greater wing of the sphenoid bone.

Q. In Figure 3-9, identify D.

A. The middle cranial fossa.

Q. In Figure 3-9, identify E.

A. The clivus, the basisphenoid, and the basal part of the occipital bone.

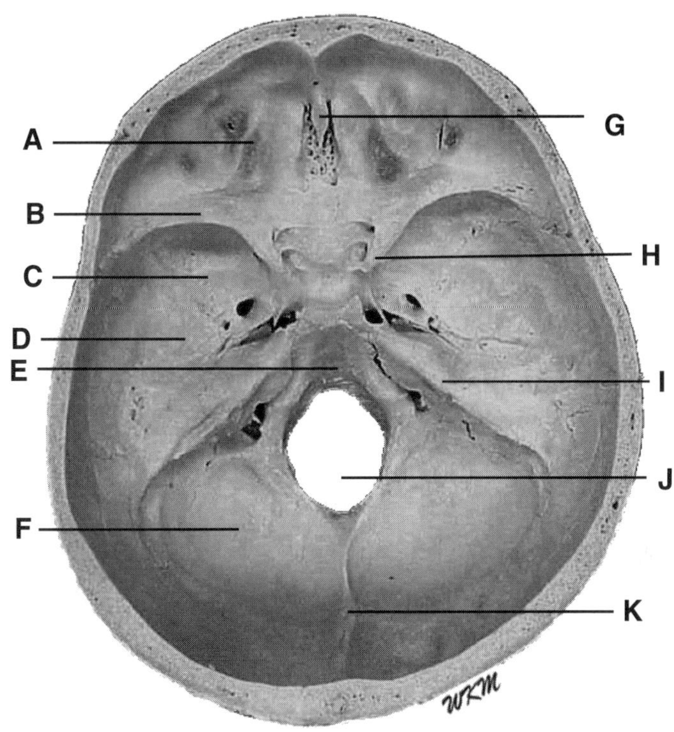

Figure 3-9 The Skull: Superior Aspect of the Base

Q. In Figure 3-9, identify F.

A. The posterior cranial fossa, the squamous plate of the occipital bone.

Q. In Figure 3-9, identify G.

A. The crista galli.

Q. In Figure 3-9, identify H.

A. The anterior clinoid process.

Q. In Figure 3-9, identify I.

A. The petrous temporal bone.

Q. In Figure 3-9, identify J.

A. The foramen magnum.

Q. In Figure 3-9, identify K.

A. The internal occipital protuberance.

Q. In Figure 3-10, identify A.

A. The lamina cribrosa ethmoidale.

Q. The structures that pass through the cribriform plate of the ethmoid bone are . . .

A. The olfactory nerve filaments.

Q. In Figure 3-10, identify B.

A. The optic foramen.

Q. In Figure 3-10, identify C.

A. The superior orbital fissure.

Q. The cranial nerves that pass through the superior orbital fissure are . . .

A. The oculomotor (third cranial) nerve, the trochlear (fourth cranial) nerve, the abducent (sixth cranial) nerve, and the ophthalmic division of the trigeminal (fifth cranial) nerve.

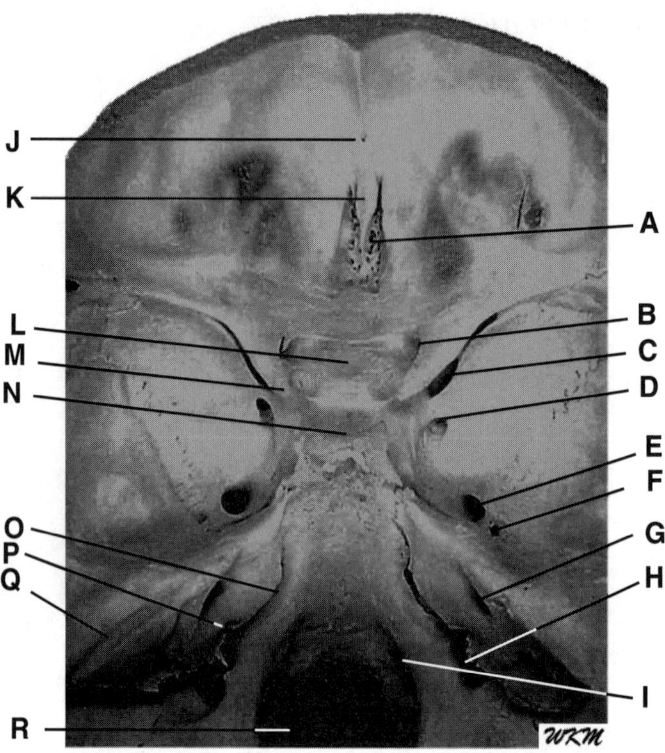

Figure 3-10 The Skull: Foramina of the Base, Superior Aspect

Q. In Figure 3-10, identify D.

A. The foramen rotundum.

Q. The cranial nerve that passes through the foramen rotundum is . . .

A. The maxillary division of the trigeminal (fifth cranial) nerve.

Q. In Figure 3-10, identify E.

A. The foramen ovale.

Q. The structure that passes through the foramen ovale is . . .

A. The mandibular division of the trigeminal (fifth cranial) nerve.

Q. In Figure 3-10, identify F.

A. The foramen spinosum.

Q. The structures that pass through the foramen spinosum are . . .

A. The middle meningeal artery and the nervous spinosum. The nerve is a sensory branch of the mandibular nerve to the dura mater.

Q. In Figure 3-10, identify G.

A. The internal auditory meatus.

Q. The structures that pass through the internal auditory meatus are . . .

A. The facial (seventh cranial) nerve, the vestibulocochlear (eighth cranial) nerve, and the labyrinthine (internal auditory) artery.

Q. In Figure 3-10, identify H.

A. The jugular foramen.

Q. The structures that pass through the jugular foramen are . . .

A. The glossopharyngeal (ninth cranial) nerve, the vagus (tenth cranial) nerve, the accessory (11th cranial) nerve, the inferior petrosal sinus, and the internal jugular vein.

Q. In Figure 3-10, identify I.

A. The anterior condylar canal.

Q. The structure that passes through the anterior condylar canal is . . .

A. The hypoglossal (12th cranial) nerve.

Q. In Figure 3-10, identify J.

A. The foramen cecum. It may transmit a vein from the nasal mucosa to the superior sagittal sinus.

Q. In Figure 3-10, identify K.

A. The crista galli.

Q. In Figure 3-10, the structure that lies in groove L is . . .

A. The optic chiasma.

Q. In Figure 3-10, identify the bony process M.

A. The anterior clinoid process.

Q. In Figure 3-10, identify N.

A. The dorsum sellae, the pituitary fossa.

Q. In Figure 3-10, the structure that lies in groove O is . . .

A. The inferior petrosal sinus.

Q. In Figure 3-10, the structure that lies in notch P is . . .

A. The glossopharyngeal (ninth cranial) nerve. The superior and inferior petrosal ganglia of the glossopharyngeal nerve receive their names from this relationship.

Q. In Figure 3-10, the structure that lies in groove Q is . . .

A. The superior petrosal sinus. It connects the basilar sinus to the transverse sinus.

Q. In Figure 3-10, identify the large foramen R.

A. The foramen magnum.

Q. The structures that pass through the foramen magnum are . . .

A. The spinal meninges and their contents, the medulla oblongata, the accessory nerves, and the vertebral arteries.

Q. The outer layer of the spinal meninges is . . .

A. The dura mater. It fuses with the periosteum of the occipital bone, the so-called periosteal layer of the cranial dura mater, at the margins of the foramen magnum.

Q. Closely applied to the spinal dura mater is . . .

A. The arachnoid mater. It encloses the subarachnoid space, which contains the cerebrospinal fluid that separates the arachnoid mater from the pia mater.

Q. The main contents of the subarachnoid space in the foramen magnum are . . .

A. The vertebral arteries and the spinal roots of the accessory nerves.

Q. The segment of the brainstem that lies in the foramen magnum is . . .

A. The medulla oblongata. The adherent pia mater separates it from the subarachnoid space.

THE CRANIAL MENINGES, THE VENOUS SINUSES, AND THE CRANIAL NERVES

Q. The meninges of the spinal cord can be divided into two functionally separate components: a protective component and a nutritional, or vascular, component. The protective layer is called . . .

A. The pachymeninx, the dura mater, or the hard mother. It extends from the atlas to the sacrum. Unlike the cranial dura mater, it is entirely separate from the periosteum.

Q. The layer containing the blood vessels is known as . . .

A. The leptomeninx.

Q. The leptomeninx is commonly subdivided into . . .

A. The arachnoid mater, or the spider mother, and the pia mater, or the tender mother.

Q. The layer firmly attached to the spinal cord is . . .

A. The pia mater.

Q. The arachnoid mater is much thinner than the pia mater. It is separated from the pia mater by . . .

A. The subarachnoid space.

Q. The subarachnoid space contains . . .

A. The arteries and the veins of the central nervous system and about 150 ml of cerebrospinal fluid.

Q. The arachnoid mater is kept in contact with the dura mater by . . .

A. The pressure of the cerebrospinal fluid.

Q. At the margins of the foramen magnum in the occipital bone, the spinal dura mater fuses with the periosteum of that bone. The cranial dura mater is therefore said to be composed of two layers, which are . . .

A. The inner (meningeal) layer and the outer endosteal (periosteal) layer.

Q. These two layers are firmly adherent except in . . .

A. The areas where there are venous sinuses. They also are separate where the meningeal layer is reflected to form baffles or partitions between the various parts of the brain.

Q. The venous sinuses lie between the outer (periosteal) layer and the inner (meningeal) layer of the dura mater. They are, therefore, kept permanently open by the rigidity of their walls. Their lining consists of . . .

A. Thin vascular endothelium.

Q. The superficial veins of the brain lie . . .

A. In the subarachnoid space, between the arachnoid mater and the pia mater.

Q. The cerebral veins drain into . . .

A. The rigid venous sinuses.

Q. To reach the venous sinuses, the superficial cerebral veins pass through the flimsy arachnoid mater and cross . . .

A. The potential subdural space.

Q. Sudden, usually violent, movements of the cranium, particularly in elderly people, whose brains tend to be diminished in size, can tear the cerebral veins from their attachment to the rigid walls of the venous sinuses. This results in . . .

A. Bleeding into the subdural space, a subdural hematoma.

Q. The longest venous sinus lies at the attachment of the longitudinal falx cerebri, which separates the two cerebral hemispheres. This sinus is . . .

A. The superior sagittal sinus.

Q. The superior sagittal sinus extends from the crista galli anteriorly to . . .

A. The internal occipital protuberance posteriorly. It joins the confluence of the sinuses.

Q. At the confluence of the sinuses, the superior sagittal sinus communicates with the end of the straight sinus and then turns to the left to become . . .

A. The left transverse sinus.

Q. The transverse sinus lies at the posterior attachment of . . .

A. The tentorium cerebelli.

Q. The tentorium cerebelli is a double layer of the meningeal dura mater, which separates the cerebellum from . . .

A. The occipital lobes of the cerebrum.

Q. The free edge of the falx cerebri, a double fold of meningeal dura mater that separates from the periosteal dura mater on either side of the superior sagittal sinus, contains . . .

A. The inferior sagittal sinus.

Q. Posteriorly, the falx cerebri fuses with . . .

A. The superior surface of the tentorium cerebelli.

Q. At this point, the inferior sagittal sinus is joined by . . .

A. The great cerebral vein. During a difficult delivery, this vein may be torn by distortion of the fetal skull as it is forced or pulled through the bony, rigid, pelvis. This results in intrapartum, intracranial bleeding, which may be severe enough to result in a stillbirth or in death in the first few days of extrauterine life.

Q. The continuation of the inferior sagittal sinus posteriorly in the junction of the falx cerebri and the tentorium cerebelli is . . .

A. The straight sinus.

Q. The straight sinus communicates with the end of the superior sagittal sinus at the confluence of the sinuses and becomes . . .

A. The right transverse sinus.

Q. Each right and left transverse sinus ends by becoming . . .

A. The appropriate sigmoid sinus.

Q. As each transverse sinus turns inferiorly to become the sigmoid sinus, each is joined by . . .

A. The appropriate superior petrosal sinus.

Q. Each superior petrosal sinus runs along . . .

A. The ipsilateral superior border of the petrous temporal bone.

Q. Each superior petrosal sinus terminates in the end of the corresponding transverse sinus. They originate from . . .

A. The appropriate posterolateral angle of the cavernous sinus.

Q. In Figure 3-11, identify A.

A. The cavernous sinus. It is lined by endothelium, covered by the meningeal layer of the dura mater, and separated from the sphenoid bone by the endosteal layer of the dura mater.

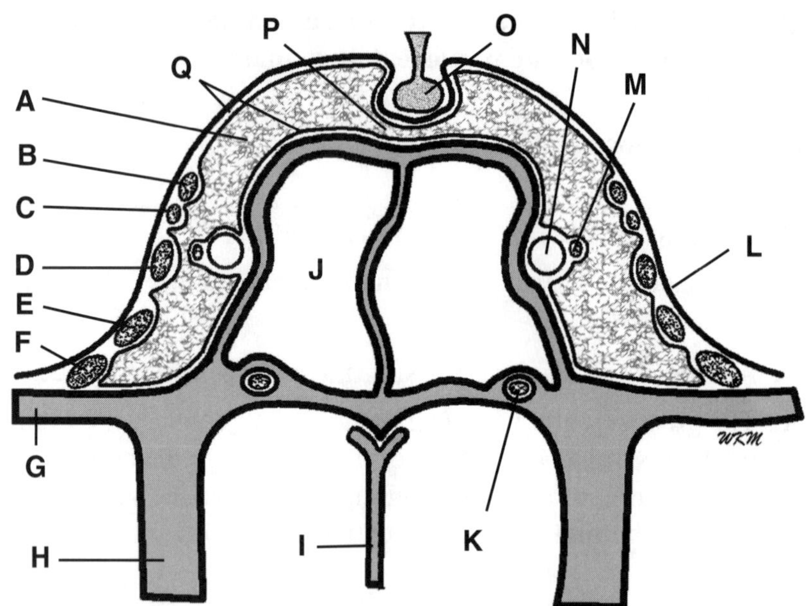

Figure 3-11 The Cavernous Sinus, Coronal Section

Q. In Figure 3-11, identify B.

A. The oculomotor nerve. It penetrates the meningeal dura in the posterior cranial fossa between the free and the attached borders of the tentorium cerebelli.

Q. In Figure 3-11, identify C.

A. The trochlear nerve. It pierces the meningeal dura mater in the posterior cranial fossa, just posterior to the posterior clinoid process.

Q. In Figure 3-11, identify D.

A. The ophthalmic division of the trigeminal nerve. It pierces the meningeal dura mater at the distal end of the cavum trigeminale in the middle cranial fossa. It enters the "cave" at its entrance in the posterior cranial fossa.

Q. In Figure 3-11, identify E.

A. The maxillary division of the trigeminal nerve. Its course, to this point, is identical to that of the ophthalmic division of the trigeminal nerve. It leaves the cranium through the foramen rotundum.

Q. In Figure 3-11, identify F.

A. The mandibular division of the trigeminal nerve. It leaves the cranium through the foramen ovale.

Q. In Figure 3-11, identify G.

A. The greater wing of the sphenoid bone. It forms the superior boundary of the infratemporal fossa.

Q. In Figure 3-11, identify H.

A. The pterygoid process of the sphenoid bone.

Q. In Figure 3-11, identify I.

A. The vomer. It forms the posterior part of the nasal septum.

Q. In Figure 3-11, identify space J.

A. The sphenoidal air sinus.

Q. In Figure 3-11, identify K.

A. The nerve of the pterygoid canal.

Q. In Figure 3-11, identify L.

A. The meningeal layer of the dura mater.

Q. In Figure 3-11, identify M.

A. The abducent nerve. It pierces the meningeal dura mater medial to the apex of the petrous temporal bone and inferior to the petrosphenoidal ligament. Together with the oculomotor nerve, the trochlear nerve, the abducent nerve, and the ophthalmic division of the trigeminal nerve, it enters the orbit through the superior orbital fissure.

Q. In Figure 3-11, identify N.

A. The internal carotid artery. It is surrounded by a plexus of postganglionic sympathetic nerve fibers.

Q. In Figure 3-11, identify O.

A. The adenohypophysis (the pituitary). It is connected to the hypothalamus by its stalk.

Q. In Figure 3-11, identify P.

A. The intercavernous sinus.

Q. In Figure 3-11, identify Q.

A. The endothelium of the cavernous sinus.

Q. Each sigmoid sinus commences at the lateral ends of the ipsilateral transverse sinus and traverses an S shaped groove in . . .

A. The mastoid part of the temporal bone.

Q. Each sigmoid sinus terminates in the ipsilateral jugular vein after passing through the posterior part of . . .

A. The appropriate jugular foramen.

Q. Other structures pass through the jugular foramen. They are . . .

A. The glossopharyngeal (ninth cranial) nerve, the vagus (10th cranial) nerve, the accessory (11th cranial) nerve, and the inferior petrosal sinus.

Q. The inferior petrosal sinus originates at . . .

A. The posterior end of the cavernous sinus.

Q. The inferior petrosal sinus runs in . . .

A. The groove between the petrous temporal bone and the occipital bone.

Q. The olfactory (first cranial) nerve leaves the cranial cavity through . . .

A. The cribriform plate of the ethmoid bone to reach the nasal cavity.

Q. The optic (second cranial) nerves are formed at the optic chiasma. They enter the orbits through . . .

A. The optic foramina.

Q. The oculomotor (third cranial), trochlear (fourth cranial), and abducent (sixth cranial) nerves are the nerves of the embryonic preotic somites. They enter the orbit through . . .

A. The superior orbital fissure.

Q. The sphenoid bone is, therefore, formed from . . .

A. The preotic sclerotomes of the embryo.

Q. The other nerves, which enter the orbit through the superior orbital fissure, are . . .

A. The lacrimal nerve, the frontal nerve, and the nasociliary nerve. They are the three branches of the ophthalmic division of the trigeminal (fifth cranial) nerve.

Q. The maxillary division of the trigeminal (fifth cranial) nerve leaves the cranial cavity through . . .

A. The foramen rotundum in the middle cranial fossa.

Q. The mandibular division of the trigeminal (fifth cranial) nerve leaves the cranial cavity through . . .

A. The foramen ovale in the middle cranial fossa.

Q. The cavum trigeminale is . . .

A. The pouch (recess) of the meningeal layer of the dura mater of the posterior cranial fossa. It is formed by the trigeminal nerve as it evaginates this layer inferior to the medial end of the superior petrosal sinus.

Q. Therefore, the cavum trigeminale will lie between the meningeal and the periosteal layers of the dura mater in the floor of . . .

A. The middle cranial fossa. It is situated on the apex of the petrous temporal bone.

Q. The oculomotor (third cranial), trochlear (fourth cranial), and abducent (sixth cranial) nerves penetrate the meningeal layer of the dura mater of the posterior cranial fossa to traverse . . .

A. The cavernous sinus to reach the superior orbital fissure.

Q. The facial (seventh cranial) nerve and the vestibulocochlear (eighth cranial) nerve run together and enter . . .

A. The internal auditory meatus.

Q. The facial (seventh cranial) nerve ultimately leaves the skull through . . .

A. The stylomastoid foramen.

Q. The glossopharyngeal (9th cranial), vagus (10th cranial), and accessory (11th cranial) nerves all leave the skull through . . .

A. The jugular foramen.

Q. In the jugular foramen, the glossopharyngeal (ninth cranial) nerve lies in a notch in the inferior aspect of . . .

A. The petrous temporal bone.

Q. In the jugular foramen, the glossopharyngeal (9th cranial) nerve is separated from the vagus (10th cranial) nerve and the accessory (11th cranial) nerve by . . .

A. The termination of the inferior petrosal sinus.

Q. The hypoglossal (12th cranial) nerve leaves the skull through . . .

A. The anterior condylar canal.

Q. The anterior condylar canal passes through . . .

A. The occipital bone.

Q. The occipital bone is formed in utero by fusion of several embryonic sclerotomes. The muscles of the tongue, which are supplied by the hypoglossal nerve, are, therefore, derived from . . .

A. The embryonic occipital myotomes.

THE AUDITORY APPARATUS—THE EXTERNAL EAR

Q. The auditory apparatus consists of . . .

A. The external ear, the middle ear, and the inner ear.

Q. The external ear serves to collect and to transmit sound to the tympanic membrane. It consists of two parts. They are . . .

A. The auricle and the external auditory meatus.

Q. In Figure 3-12, identify A.

A. The scaphoid fossa. It is a sulcus, which lies between the helix and the antihelix.

Q. In Figure 3-12, identify B.

A. The helix.

Q. In Figure 3-12, identify C.

A. The antihelix.

Q. In Figure 3-12, identify D.

A. The external auditory meatus. Its external opening is hidden by the tragus.

Q. In Figure 3-12, identify E.

A. The lobule of the ear. It tends to increase in size with advancing age, especially with continued use of heavy earrings. The entire external ear continues to grow throughout life.

Q. In Figure 3-12, identify F.

A. The antitragus.

Q. In Figure 3-12, identify G.

A. The intertragic incisure.

Q. In Figure 3-12, identify H.

A. The concha. The skin here contains numerous sebaceous glands.

Q. In Figure 3-12, identify I.

A. The tragus. Pressure on the tragus closes the external auditory meatus.

Q. In Figure 3-12, identify J.

A. The crura of the antihelix. The triangular fossa lies between the crura.

Q. The skeleton of the auricle is . . .

A. The auricular cartilage. The overlying thin skin is firmly attached to it.

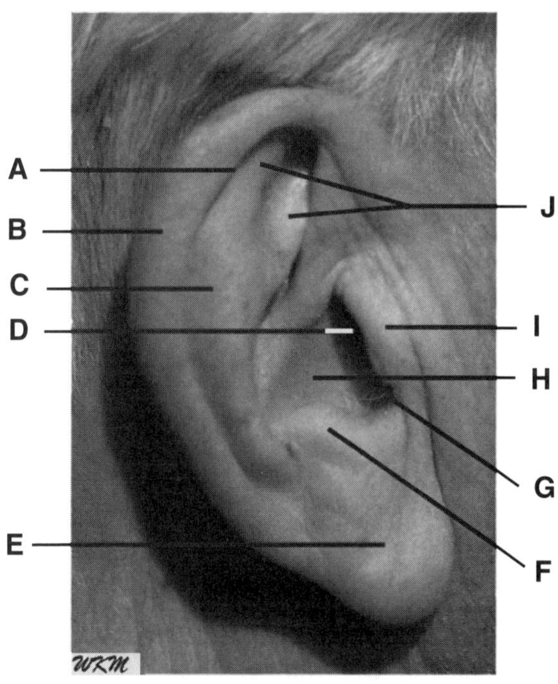

Figure 3-12 The External Ear of an Elderly Male

Q. The sensory innervation of the cranial surface of the auricle is via . . .

A. The great auricular nerve. It is formed by the anterior primary rami of the second and third cervical nerves. The lesser occipital nerve, from the anterior primary ramus of the second cervical nerve, supplies a small area on the upper part of the cranial surface of the auricle.

Q. The sensory innervation of the lateral surface of the auricle is provided by . . .

A. The auriculotemporal branch of the mandibular division of the trigeminal nerve and the great auricular nerve. The auriculotemporal nerve supplies the upper anterior region of the lateral surface. The great auricular nerve supplies the greater part of the posterior part of the lateral surface. The skin of the concha is supplied by the auricular branch of the vagus nerve and sensory twigs from the facial nerve. The major function of the facial nerve is, of course, to supply motor fibers to the muscles of facial expression.

Q. The lymphatics of the auricle drain to . . .

A. The parotid lymph nodes, the mastoid lymph nodes, and the upper deep cervical lymph nodes.

Q. The external auditory meatus extends from the concha to the tympanic membrane. In the adult, this is a distance of . . .

A. 25 to 30 mm (just over 1 inch).

Q. The lymphatics of the external auditory meatus drain to . . .

A. The parotid lymph nodes, the mastoid lymph nodes, and the upper deep cervical lymph nodes. These are the same groups of nodes that drain the auricle.

Q. The skeleton of the external auditory meatus, in its lateral one-third, is . . .

A. Cartilage. It is continuous with the cartilage of the auricle.

Q. The skeleton of the medial two-thirds of the external auditory meatus is osseous. It is formed by . . .

A. The tympanic part of the temporal bone.

Q. The bony segment of the external auditory meatus is much shorter in the first year of life. It does not reach adult length until the teen years. At birth it is only . . .

A. 2 mm long. It is therefore necessary to exercise extreme care when carrying out an otoscopic examination on babies and young children.

Q. In the adult, the narrowest point of the external auditory meatus is situated at the junction of the lateral cartilaginous one-third and . . .

A. The medial bony two-thirds of the meatus.

Q. The adult external auditory meatus is not straight, but S-shaped. It can be straightened during otoscopic examination by pulling the auricle . . .

A. Upward and backward.

Q. The skin of the external auditory meatus is replete with hair follicles and their associated specialized sebaceous glands, the ceruminous glands. The skin is firmly attached to . . .

A. The underlying cartilaginous and bony segments of the external auditory meatus. The density and thickness of the hairs diminishes in the bony part of the meatus. Both increase with age.

Q. Anterior to the external auditory meatus lies . . .

A. The temporomandibular joint.

Q. Posterior to the external auditory meatus lie . . .

A. The mastoid process and its air cells.

Q. Inferior to the cartilaginous part of the external auditory meatus lies . . .

A. The parotid gland.

Q. Superior to the osseous part of the external auditory meatus lie . . .

A. The middle cranial fossa, laterally, and the epitympanic recess, medially.

Q. The sensory innervation of the external auditory meatus is via . . .

A. The auricular branch of the vagus nerve and the auriculotemporal branch of the mandibular division of the trigeminal nerve.

Q. The medial end of the external auditory meatus is closed by the tympanic membrane, which is set obliquely, so that the lateral surface of the membrane faces . . .

A. Downward and forward. The downward inclination is even more pronounced in the infant. To get a good view of the tympanic membrane in infants, the auricle should be pulled downward rather than upward and backward, as in adults. It is essential to remember the shortness of the infant external auditory meatus to prevent damaging the tympanic membrane.

Q. The approximate diameter of the tympanic membrane is . . .

A. 10 mm (just less than half an inch).

Q. The tympanic membrane is composed of three layers. They are . . .

A. Skin, fibrous tissue, and mucous membrane. The latter is continuous with the lining of the middle ear and the pharyngotympanic tube.

Q. Two structures lie under the mucous membrane on the medial surface of the tympanic membrane. They are . . .

A. The chorda tympani nerve and the handle of the malleus.

Q. In Figure 3-13, identify A.

A. The pars flaccida of the tympanic membrane.

Q. In Figure 3-13, identify B.

A. The anterior malleolar fold.

Q. In Figure 3-13, identify C.

A. The handle of the malleus as seen through the tympanic membrane. It is attached to the medial surface of the membrane by connective tissue.

Q. In Figure 3-13, identify D.

A. The umbo. It is the inverted center of the tympanic membrane at the end of the handle of the malleus.

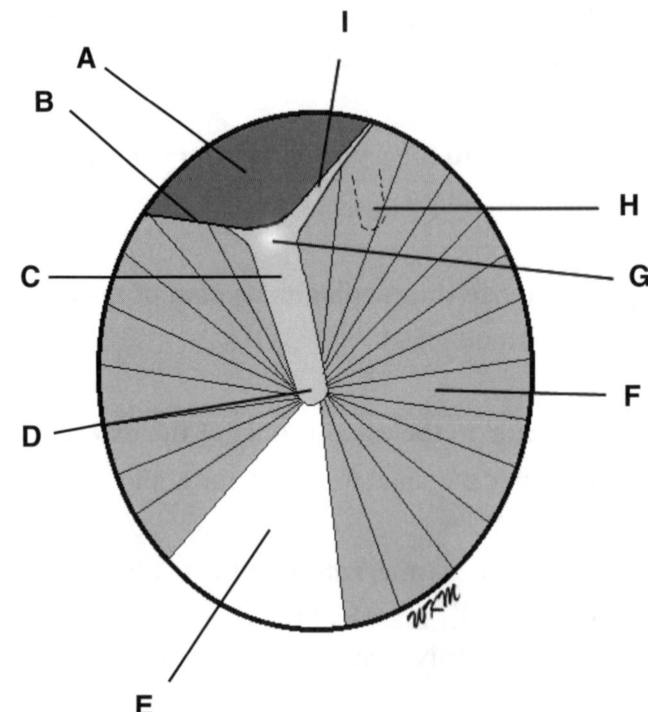

Figure 3-13 The Left Tympanic Membrane

Q. In Figure 3-13, identify E.

A. The cone of light seen on otoscopic examination. This bright area results from the reflection of the light from the otoscope by the curvature of a segment of the pars tensa of the tympanic membrane.

Q. In Figure 3-13, identify F.

A. The pars tensa of the tympanic membrane.

Q. In Figure 3-13, identify G.

A. The lateral process of the malleus. At this point, it is firmly attached to the medial surface of the tympanic membrane.

Q. In Figure 3-13, identify H.

A. The vague outline of the long process of the incus as seen through the tympanic membrane.

Q. In Figure 3-13, identify I.

A. The posterior malleolar fold.

THE AUDITORY APPARATUS—THE MIDDLE EAR

Q. The middle ear serves to . . .

A. Transmit and diminish in amplitude and increase in force the rapid air pressure variations (sound) to the inner ear.

Q. The cavity of the middle ear occupies . . .

A. The petrous part of the temporal bone.

Q. The cavity of the middle ear is a narrow rectangular space, varying in width from 2 to 6 mm. The vertical and horizontal dimensions are both approximately . . .

A. 15 mm (just over half an inch).

Q. The plane of this cavity is approximately anteroposterior. The lateral wall of the cavity is largely formed by . . .

A. The tympanic membrane. It closes the medial end of the external auditory meatus.

Q. The medial wall of the middle ear cavity is formed by . . .

A. The petrous part of the temporal bone. It encloses the labyrinths of the inner ear.

Q. The part of the membranous labyrinth that lies immediately lateral to the middle ear is . . .

A. The cochlear apparatus. The first turn of the cochlea, in fact, bulges into the medial wall of the middle ear, forming the promontory.

Q. The roof of the middle ear cavity is formed by . . .

A. The tegmen tympani. It forms part of the floor of the middle cranial fossa.

Q. The anterior wall of the middle ear cavity has opening into it superiorly . . .

A. The canal for the tensor tympani muscle, and, below that, the pharyngotympanic tube.

Q. The anterior wall of the middle ear cavity is formed inferiorly by . . .

A. A thin plate of bone, which separates it from the internal carotid artery.

Q. Embedded in the posterior wall of the middle ear cavity is . . .

A. The canal for the facial nerve.

Q. Posteriorly, the middle ear cavity is related to . . .

A. The sigmoid sinus, medially, and the mastoid air cells, laterally. The middle ear cavity communicates with the mastoid air cells via the tympanic aditus. This opening lies high on the posterior wall of the cavity.

Q. In Figure 3-14, identify A.

A. The mastoid air cells. They are prone to infection in untreated otitis media (infection of the middle ear).

Q. In Figure 3-14, identify B.

A. The mastoid antrum.

Q. In Figure 3-14, identify C.

A. The tympanic aditus to the mastoid antrum.

Q. In Figure 3-14, identify D.

A. The incus. Note that it has a short and a long process.

Q. In Figure 3-14, identify E.

A. The head of the malleus. Note that it has a long handle, which is attached to the tympanic membrane at the umbo.

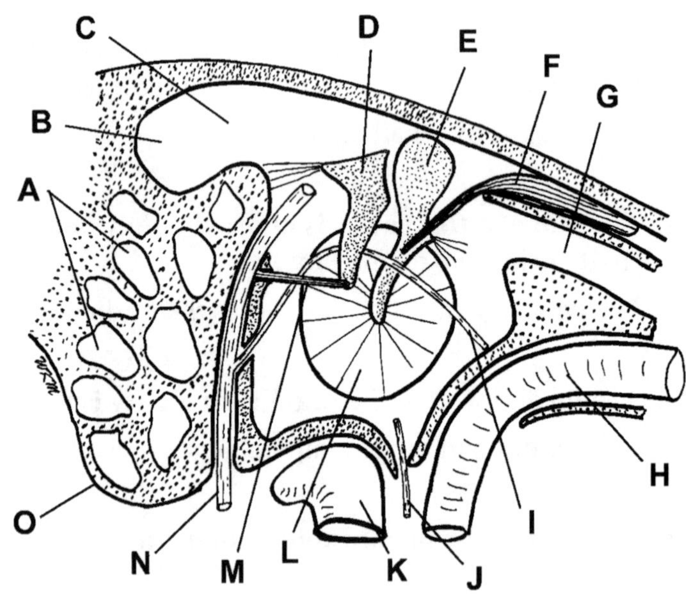

Figure 3-14 The Middle Ear, Lateral Wall

Q. In Figure 3-14, identify F.

A. The tensor tympani muscle. It is attached to the base of the long handle of the malleus. Its nerve supply is from the mandibular division of the trigeminal nerve.

Q. In Figure 3-14, identify G.

A. The pharyngotympanic (Eustachian) tube.

Q. In Figure 3-14, identify H.

A. The carotid artery in the carotid canal. The wall of this canal is very thin and may even be fenestrated where it lies in close proximity to the middle ear cavity. In the case of untreated otitis media, these canal wall features can result in the spread of infection to the internal carotid artery.

Q. In Figure 3-14, identify I.

A. The chorda tympani nerve. It supplies taste to the anterior two-thirds of the tongue and secretomotor fibers to the submandibular salivary gland and to the sublingual salivary gland.

Q. The secretomotor and taste fibers in the chorda tympani nerve reach their final destinations via . . .

A. The lingual nerve.

Q. The chorda tympani nerve is separated from the middle ear cavity only by . . .

A. Mucous membrane.

Q. In Figure 3-14, identify J.

A. The tympanic branch of the glossopharyngeal nerve. It supplies secretomotor fibers to the parotid gland via the otic ganglion.

Q. In Figure 3-14, identify K.

A. The bulb of the internal jugular vein.

Q. In Figure 3-14, identify L.

A. The tympanic membrane.

Q. In Figure 3-14, identify M.

A. The stapedius muscle. It is attached to the neck of the stapes, which is also derived from the second pharyngeal arch; therefore the nerve supply is the facial nerve. The stapedius muscle serves to dampen movement of the stapes. Its paralysis results in hyperacusis (increased sensitivity to loud noises).

Q. In Figure 3-14, identify N.

A. The facial nerve emerging from the stylomastoid foramen.

Q. In Figure 3-14, identify O.

A. The mastoid process of the petrous temporal bone.

Q. The space above the tympanic cavity in which the head of the malleus and most of the incus lie is . . .

A. The epitympanic recess.

Q. The thin layer of bone covering the epitympanic recess is . . .

A. The tegmen tympani, the roof of the middle ear.

Q. Immediately above the meninges, which cover the superior surface of the tegmen tympani, lies . . .

A. The temporal lobe of the brain. Hence, meningitis and a temporal lobe abscess are both possible complications of otitis media. Otitis media is particularly common in children. It is estimated that about 50 percent of children suffer from this complaint.

Q. In Figure 3-15, identify A.

A. The aditus to the mastoid antrum.

Q. In Figure 3-15, identify B.

A. The bulge of the lateral semicircular canal.

Q. In Figure 3-15, identify C.

A. The canal for the facial nerve.

Q. In Figure 3-15, identify D.

A. The fenestra ovale, fenestra vestibuli. It is closed by the foot piece of the stapes.

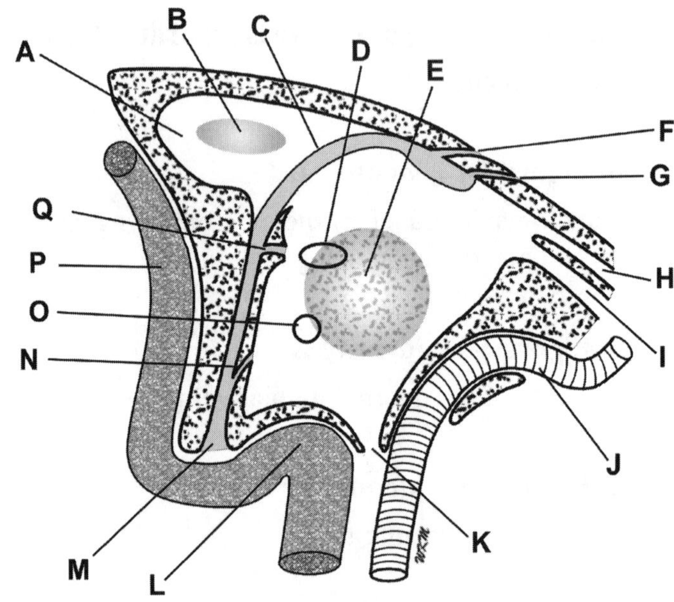

Figure 3-15 The Middle Ear, Medial Wall

Q. In Figure 3-15, identify E.

A. The promontory. It overlies the first turn of the cochlea and is covered by a nerve plexus that is largely formed from the tympanic branch of the glossopharyngeal nerve.

Q. In Figure 3-15, identify F.

A. The foramen for the greater petrosal nerve. It joins the facial nerve at the geniculate ganglion. It carries sensory fibers from the soft palate and preganglionic, secretomotor fibers to the lacrimal gland and the nasal glands.

Q. In Figure 3-15, identify G.

A. The foramen for the lesser petrosal nerve. It carries preganglionic, secretomotor fibers to the parotid gland. They originate from the glossopharyngeal nerve via its tympanic branch and the tympanic plexus on the promontory of the middle ear. They synapse in the otic ganglion.

Q. In Figure 3-15, identify H.

A. The bony canal for the tensor tympani muscle.

Q. In Figure 3-15, identify I.

A. The bony canal for the pharyngotympanic tube.

Q. In Figure 3-15, identify J.

A. The internal carotid artery.

Q. In Figure 3-15, identify K.

A. The foramen for the tympanic branch of the glossopharyngeal nerve.

Q. In Figure 3-15, identify L.

A. The bulb of the jugular vein.

Q. In Figure 3-15, identify M.

A. The stylomastoid foramen. The facial nerve emerges through it from the skull.

Q. The facial nerve exits the cranial cavity through . . .

A. The internal auditory meatus.

Q. In Figure 3-15, identify N.

A. The foramen for the chorda tympani branch of the facial nerve.

Q. In Figure 3-15, identify O.

A. The fenestra rotundum, fenestra cochleae. It is closed by the secondary tympanic membrane.

Q. In Figure 3-15, identify P.

A. The sigmoid sinus.

Q. In Figure 3-15, identify Q.

A. The aperture in the base of the pyramidal eminence. It transmits the nerve to the minute stapedius muscle, whose tendon emerges from the bony aperture in the pyramidal eminence to be inserted into the neck of the stapes bone.

THE AUDITORY APPARATUS—THE INNER EAR

Q. The inner ear serves . . .

A. To transduce (convert) the fluid vibrations transmitted to the perilymph by the vibrations of the ossicles of the middle ear into nerve impulses. These nerve impulses are then carried to the brain via the cochlear part of the vestibulocochlear (eighth cranial) nerve.

Q. The inner ear has two additional functions. They are . . .

A. To determine the posture of the head and to detect any movements thereof.

Q. In Figure 3-16, identify A.

A. The canal for the tensor tympani muscle. It is separated by a bony shelf from the osseous segment of the pharyngotympanic tube.

Q. The nerve supply of the tensor tympani muscle is from . . .

A. The mandibular division of the trigeminal nerve. The tensor tympani muscle develops in the mesenchyme of the embryonic first pharyngeal arch. Therefore, it receives its nerve supply from the nerve supplying that arch.

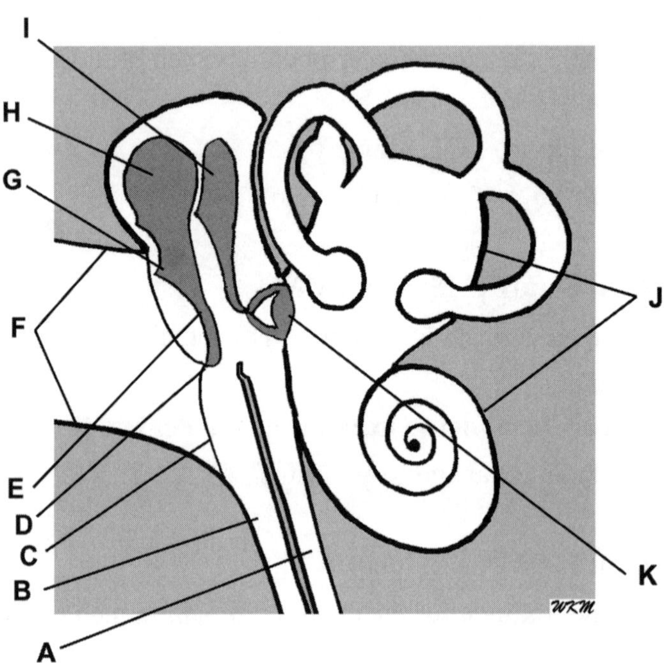

Figure 3-16 The Auditory Apparatus, Schematic Anterosuperior View

Q. In Figure 3-16, identify B.

A. The osseous segment of the pharyngotympanic tube. It is formed by the squamous and the petrous parts of the temporal bone.

Q. In Figure 3-16, identify C.

A. The pars tensa of the tympanic membrane.

Q. The middle ear serves . . .

A. To transmit and to diminish in amplitude and increase in force the rapid air pressure variations, which constitute sound, to the inner ear.

Q. In Figure 3-16, identify D.

A. The umbo, the boss of a shield, of the tympanic membrane. At this point, the free end of the manubrium mallei is attached to the tympanic membrane.

Q. In Figure 3-16, identify E.

A. The manubrium mallei, the handle of the malleus.

Q. In Figure 3-16, identify F.

A. The osseous segment of the external auditory meatus. It is the tympanic part of the temporal bone.

Q. In Figure 3-16, identify G.

A. The lateral process of the malleus. It is attached to the apex of the pars flaccida of the tympanic membrane.

Q. In Figure 3-16, identify H.

A. The head of the malleus. It articulates with the body of the incus.

Q. In Figure 3-16, identify I.

A. The body of the incus. The incus has two crura (legs). Here, the crus longum incudis can be seen articulating with the head of the stapes.

Q. In Figure 3-16, identify J.

A. The bony labyrinth. It is lined by periosteum. That part of the petrous temporal bone immediately surrounding it is considerably denser and harder than the remainder of the petrous temporal bone, of which it is a part.

Q. In Figure 3-16, identify K.

A. The foot piece of the stapes. It occupies the oval fenestra vestibuli. The vibrations of the tympanic membrane are transmitted to it by the chain of ossicles in the middle ear. These rapid movements are themselves transmitted to the perilymph in the cochlear, and hence to the organ of Corti, which converts them to nerve impulses.

Q. The bony labyrinth is a complex cavity in the petrous temporal bone. It is lined by periosteum, which covers a particularly dense layer of compact bone. In the cavity of the bony labyrinth lies . . .

A. The membranous labyrinth. It contains endolymph and is separated by perilymph from the walls of the bony labyrinth.

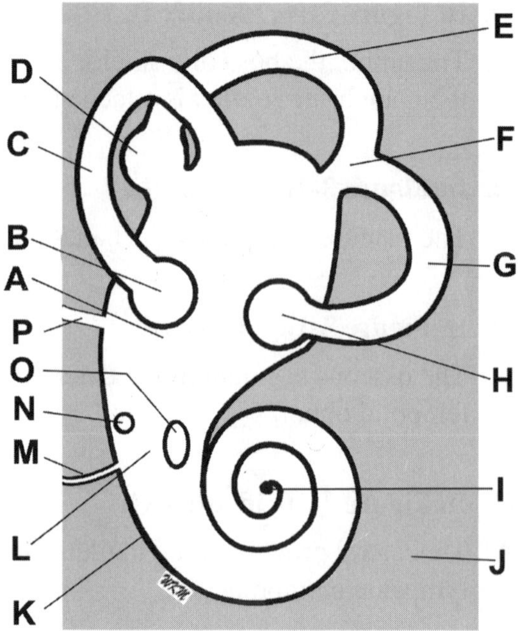

Figure 3-17 The Right Bony Labyrinth, Superolateral Aspect

Q. In Figure 3-17, identify A.

A. The vestibule of the bony labyrinth. It contains the utricle and the saccule of the membranous labyrinth. A small canal, the aqueduct of the vestibule, runs from it to the posterior surface of the petrous temporal bone. It contains the ductus endolymphaticus and the saccus endolymphaticus. Both are parts of the membranous labyrinth.

Q. In Figure 3-17, identify B.

A. The ampulla of the lateral semicircular canal.

Q. In Figure 3-17, identify C.

A. The lateral semicircular canal. As can be seen in Figures 3-15 and 3-16, it bulges into the medial wall of the mastoid antrum immediately posterior to the facial canal. It is the only semicircular canal that lies in a horizontal plane. Thus, it is sometimes called the horizontal canal.

Q. In Figure 3-17, identify D.

A. The ampulla of the posterior semicircular canal.

Q. In Figure 3-17, identify E.

A. The posterior semicircular canal. It is set vertically, and its plane almost coincides with the long axis of the petrous temporal bone.

Q. In Figure 3-17, identify F.

A. The crus commune of the posterior and the anterior semicircular canals.

Q. In Figure 3-17, identify G.

A. The anterior semicircular canal. It is set in a vertical plane at right angles to the plane of the posterior semicircular canal, and hence to the long axis of the petrous temporal bone. It forms a small bulge on the anterior part of the arcuate eminence, which is situated on the superior surface of the petrous temporal bone.

Q. In Figure 3-17, identify H.

A. The ampulla of the anterior semicircular canal.

Q. In Figure 3-17, identify I.

A. The modiolus of the cochlear. The osseospiral lamina, which is a major attachment of the cochlear duct, winds around it.

Q. In Figure 3-17, identify J.

A. The compact petrous part of the temporal bone.

Q. In Figure 3-17, identify K.

A. The dense layer of compact bone, which is covered by an internal layer of periosteum, that forms the walls of the bony labyrinth.

Q. In Figure 3-17, identify L.

A. The first turn of the cochlea. It communicates with the subarachnoid space via the cochlear aqueduct, which lies in the cochlear canaliculus.

Q. In Figure 3-17, identify M.

A. The cochlear canaliculus. It runs to a notch on the inferior surface of the petrous temporal bone. It serves as a direct connection between the perilymph and the subarachnoid space round the inferior ganglion of the glossopharyngeal nerve.

Q. In Figure 3-17, identify N.

A. The fenestra cochleae, the round window. It is closed by the secondary tympanic membrane.

Q. In Figure 3-17, identify O.

A. The fenestra vestibuli. It opens into the osseous cochlear canal at its junction with the vestibule and is closed by the foot piece of the stapes. Both the fenestra vestibule and the fenestra cochleae lie in the lateral wall of the bony labyrinth and can be identified in the medial wall of the middle ear.

Q. In Figure 3-17, identify P.

A. The aqueduct of the vestibule. It contains the endolymphatic duct, which leads to the endolymphatic sac.

Q. The wall of the membranous labyrinth, although thin, consists of three distinct layers. They are . . .

A. An outer fibrous vascular layer; an intermediate, more delicate, connective tissue layer containing capillaries; and an inner layer of epithelial cells resting on a basal lamina.

Q. In Figure 3-18, identify A.

A. The utricle of the membranous labyrinth.

Q. The sensory organ in the wall of the utricle is . . .

A. The macula of the utricle. This is a horizontally oriented area of sensory hair cells that detect variations in the gravitational pull of the otoliths on their surface.

Q. In Figure 3-18, identify B.

A. The saccule of the membranous labyrinth.

Q. The sensory organ in the wall of the saccule is . . .

A. The macula of the saccule. This is a vertically oriented area of sensory hair cells that detect variations in the gravitational pull of the otoliths on their surface.

Q. The two maculae in the inner ear lie at right angles to one another, and therefore provide information concerning . . .

A. The posture of the head. They are sometimes called the static labyrinth.

Q. In Figure 3-18, identify C.

A. The cochlear duct.

Q. The sensory organ in the cochlear duct is . . .

A. The spiral organ of Corti.

Q. The organ of Corti is a complex structure whose function is to . . .

A. Translate vibrations in the perilymph, and hence in the endolymph, into nerve impulses that convey the sense of hearing.

Q. In Figure 3-18, identify D.

A. The ductus reuniens. It connects the saccule to the base of the cochlear duct.

Q. In Figure 3-18, identify E.

A. The ductus endolymphaticus. It lies in the aqueduct of the vestibule.

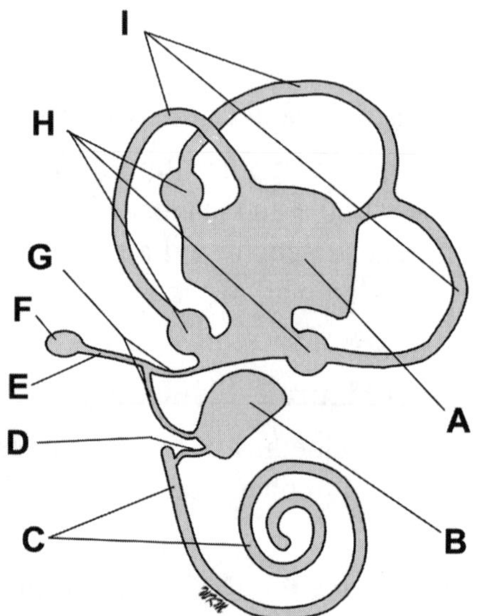

Figure 3-18 Right Membranous Labyrinth, Superior Aspect

Q. In Figure 3-18, identify F.

A. The saccus endolymphaticus.

Q. The function of the saccus endolymphaticus is . . .

A. The absorption of endolymph. Blockage of the ductus endolymphaticus causes increased pressure in both the vestibular and the cochlear apparatuses and impairs their function.

Q. In Figure 3-18, identify G.

A. The utriculosaccular duct.

Q. In Figure 3-18, identify H.

A. The ampullae of the three semicircular ducts. Each ampulla contains a crista whose hair cells respond to movements of the endolymph, which are caused by movements of the head.

Q. The semicircular canals and their contained ducts together form . . .

A. The kinetic labyrinth.

Q. In Figure 3-18, identify I.

A. The three semicircular ducts of the membranous labyrinth. In cross-section they are only about one-quarter the diameter of the osseous semicircular canals that they occupy.

Q. The three layers of the wall of the membranous labyrinth are . . .

A. An outer, vascular, fibrous periosteal layer; a middle, delicate, vascular layer; and an inner layer of simple epithelial cells.

Q. In Figure 3-19, identify A.

A. The layer of dense compact bone that forms the wall of the bony labyrinth.

Q. In Figure 3-19, identify B.

A. The compact bone of the petrous temporal bone.

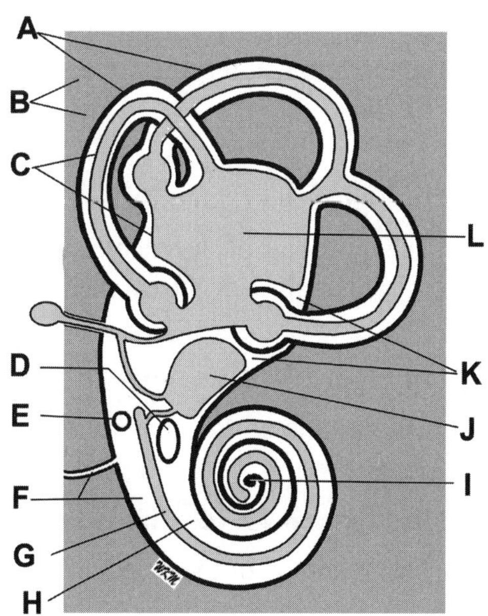

Figure 3-19 The Labyrinths of the Internal Ear

Q. In Figure 3-19, identify C.

A. The thin three-layered wall of the membranous labyrinth.

Q. In Figure 3-19, identify D.

A. The fenestra vestibuli. It is closed by the foot piece of the stapes. The stapes transmits vibrations to the perilymph of the scala vestibuli.

Q. In Figure 3-19, identify E.

A. The fenestra cochleae. It is closed by the secondary tympanic membrane to permit the vibration of the perilymph in the scala tympani. These vibrations originate with the stapes and are transmitted through the perilymph of the scala vestibuli.

Q. In Figure 3-19, identify F.

A. The scala tympani. It contains perilymph. It is closed at the fenestra cochlea, the round window, by the secondary tympanic membrane. It can be seen communicating with the subarachnoid space via the cochlear aqueduct, which traverses the cochlear canaliculus.

Q. In Figure 3-19, identify G.

A. The cochlear duct. It spirals around the modiolus of the cochlea between the scala tympani and the scala vestibuli. It contains the organ of Corti, which detects the vibrations of its two walls and translates them into nerve impulses.

Q. In Figure 3-19, identify H.

A. The scala vestibuli. It communicates with the scala cochleae by a small opening, the helicotrema, at the apex of the modiolus of the cochlea.

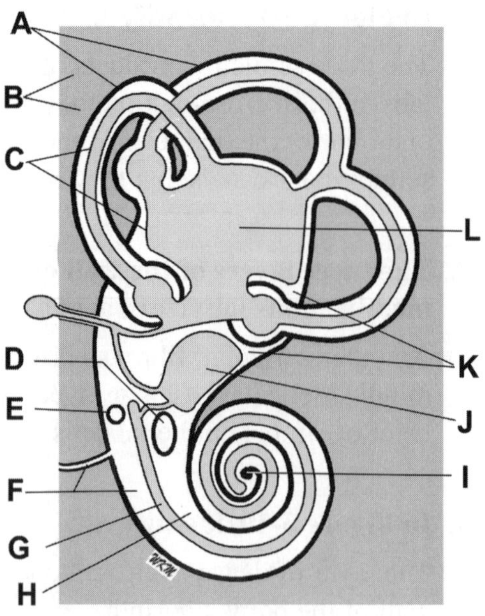

Figure 3-19 The Labyrinths of the Internal Ear

Q. In Figure 3-19, identify I.

A. The modiolus of the cochlea. It contains the spiral ganglion of the cochlea.

Q. In Figure 3-19, identify J.

A. The saccule of the membranous labyrinth.

Q. In Figure 3-19, identify K.

A. The vestibule of the osseous labyrinth.

Q. In Figure 3-19, identify L.

A. The utricle of the membranous labyrinth.

THE ORBIT

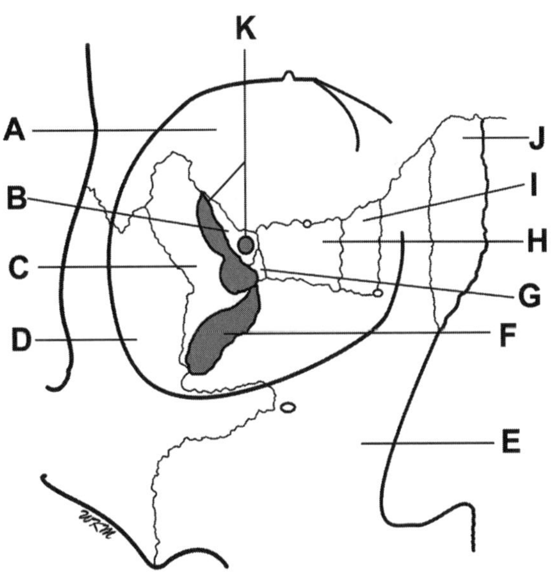

Figure 3-20 The Bones of the Right Orbit

Q. In Figure 3-20, identify A.

A. The orbital plate of the frontal bone.

Q. In Figure 3-20, identify B.

A. The lesser wing of the sphenoid bone.

Q. In Figure 3-20, identify C.

A. The greater wing of the sphenoid bone.

Q. In Figure 3-20, identify D.

A. The orbital plate of the zygoma.

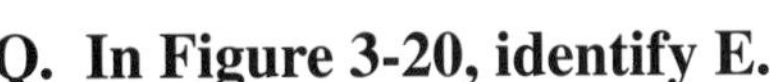

Q. In Figure 3-20, identify E.

A. The maxilla.

Q. In Figure 3-20, identify F.

A. The inferior orbital fissure.

Q. In Figure 3-20, identify G.

A. The orbital plate of the palatine bone.

Q. In Figure 3-20, identify H.

A. The orbital plate of the ethmoid bone, the lamina papyracea ethmoidale.

Q. In Figure 3-20, identify I.

A. The lacrimal bone.

Q. In Figure 3-20, identify J.

A. The nasal bone.

Q. In Figure 3-20, identify K.

A. The superior orbital fissure and the optic foramen. The superior orbital fissure separates the greater and lesser wings of the sphenoid bone. The optic foramen lies between the two roots of the lesser wing of the sphenoid bone.

Q. In Figure 3-21, identify A.

A. The optic foramen. It transmits the optic nerve and the ophthalmic artery.

Q. In Figure 3-21, identify B.

A. The superior orbital fissure.

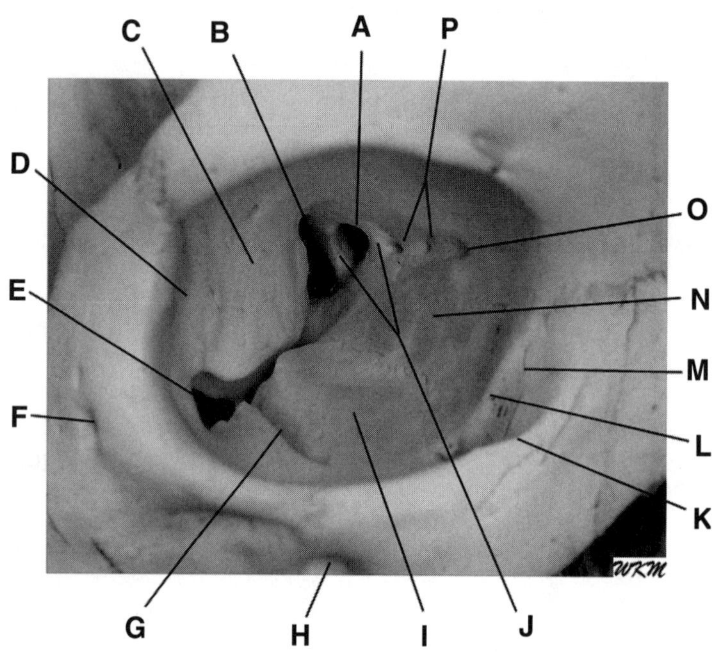

Figure 3-21 The Right Orbit

Q. The bony boundaries of the superior orbital fissure are . . .

A. The greater and the lesser wings of the sphenoid bone.

Q. In Figure 3-21, identify C.

A. The greater wing of the sphenoid bone.

Q. In Figure 3-21, identify D.

A. The orbital plate of the zygoma.

Q. In Figure 3-21, identify E.

A. The inferior orbital fissure.

Q. The three bones that form the boundaries of the inferior orbital fissure are . . .

A. The greater wing of the sphenoid bone, the orbital plate of the zygoma, and the orbital plate of the maxillary bone.

Q. In Figure 3-21, identify F.

A. The opening of the zygomaticofacial foramen.

Q. The zygomaticofacial foramen is traversed by the zygomaticofacial nerve. This nerve is a branch of . . .

A. The zygomatic nerve, which is, itself, a branch of the maxillary division of the trigeminal nerve.

Q. In Figure 3-21, identify G.

A. The infraorbital groove in the maxilla.

Q. In Figure 3-21, identify H.

A. The infraorbital foramen.

Q. The infraorbital branch of the maxillary nerve that emerges from the infraorbital foramen is . . .

A. The sensory nerve to the cheek.

Q. In Figure 3-21, identify I.

A. The thin orbital plate of the maxilla. A blow to the eye can easily cause the plate to fracture. The inferior rectus muscle may then become trapped, causing inability to elevate the affected eye.

Q. In Figure 3-21, identify J.

A. The two roots of the lesser wing of the sphenoid bone. They form the boundaries of the optic foramen, the optic canal.

Q. In Figure 3-21, identify K.

A. The anterior lacrimal crest on the frontal process of the maxilla.

Q. In Figure 3-21, identify L.

A. The posterior lacrimal crest on the lacrimal bone.

Q. The structure that lies between the anterior and posterior lacrimal crests is . . .

A. The junction between the lacrimal sac and the upper end of the nasolacrimal duct.

Q. In Figure 3-21, identify suture M.

A. The lacrimomaxillary suture.

Q. In Figure 3-21, identify N.

A. The lamina papyracea ethmoidale, the thin orbital plate of the ethmoid bone.

Q. In Figure 3-21, identify O.

A. The anterior ethmoidal foramen. It transmits the anterior ethmoidal nerve and its accompanying vessels. The anterior ethmoidal nerve is a terminal branch of the nasociliary branch of the ophthalmic nerve. The other terminal branch is the infratrochlear nerve.

Q. In Figure 3-21, identify P.

A. The middle and posterior ethmoidal foramina. They transmit similarly named nerves and vessels.

Q. The ethmoidal nerves are branches of the nasociliary branch of the trigeminal nerve. The ethmoidal arteries are branches of . . .

A. The ophthalmic artery.

Q. In Figure 3-22, identify A.

A. The optic foramen.

Q. In Figure 3-22, identify B.

A. The inferior orbital fissure.

Q. In Figure 3-22, identify C.

A. The superior orbital fissure.

Q. In Figure 3-22, identify D.

A. The lateral rectus muscle.

Q. In Figure 3-22, identify E.

A. The zygomaticofrontal suture.

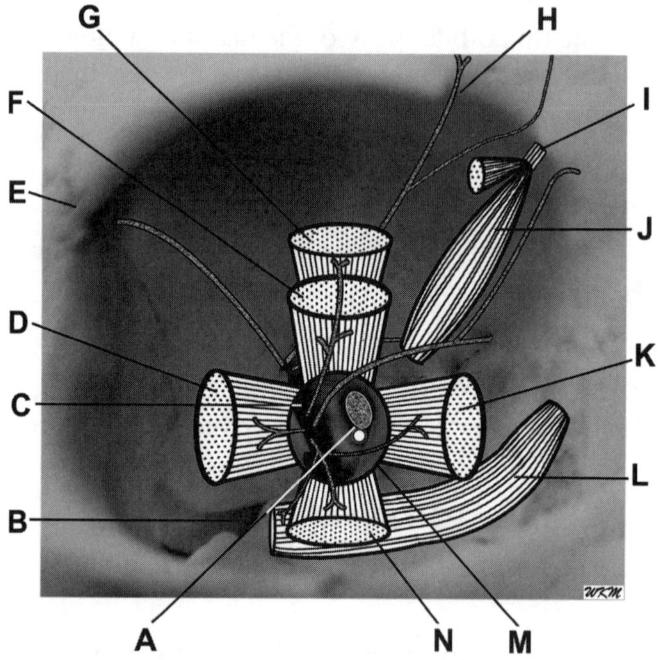

Figure 3-22 The Right Orbit: Muscles and Bones

Q. In Figure 3-22, identify F.

A. The superior rectus muscle.

Q. In Figure 3-22, identify G.

A. The levator palpebrae superioris muscle.

Q. In Figure 3-22, identify H.

A. The supraorbital notch. Sometimes, the notch converts into a foramen.

Q. In Figure 3-22, identify I.

A. The trochlea. This "pulley" changes the direction of pull of the superior oblique muscle.

Q. In Figure 3-22, identify J.

A. The superior oblique muscle.

Q. In Figure 3-22, identify K.

A. The medial rectus muscle.

Q. In Figure 3-22, identify L.

A. The inferior oblique muscle.

Q. In Figure 3-22, identify M.

A. The annulus fibrosus, the common annular tendon.

Q. In Figure 3-22, identify N.

A. The inferior rectus muscle.

Q. Three nerves enter the orbit through the superior orbital fissure outside the annulus tendineus. From the lateral to the medial side, they are . . .

A. The lacrimal nerve, the frontal nerve, and the trochlear nerve.

Q. The most important fibers in the lacrimal nerve are . . .

A. The secretomotor fibers to the lacrimal gland. The lacrimal nerve also carries sensory fibers to the conjunctiva and to the upper eyelid.

Q. The secretomotor fibers to the lacrimal gland synapse in . . .

A. The pterygopalatine ganglion.

Q. These parasympathetic fibers originate in . . .

A. The pons. They leave in the facial nerve and pass via the greater petrosal nerve to the nerve of the pterygoid canal, and hence to the pterygopalatine ganglion.

Q. These secretomotor fibers reach the lacrimal nerve from the pterygopalatine ganglion via . . .

A. The zygomatic branch of the maxillary nerve. The zygomatic nerve enters the orbit through the inferior orbital fissure and communicates with the lacrimal nerve.

Q. In Figure 3-23, identify A.

A. The lacrimal nerve. It is one of the three terminal branches of the ophthalmic division of the trigeminal nerve. It supplies sensory branches to the upper eyelid and secretomotor branches to the lacrimal gland. These secretomotor fibers originate in the facial nerve, synapse in the pterygopalatine ganglion, and join the lacrimal nerve via the zygomatic branch of the maxillary division of the trigeminal nerve.

Q. In Figure 3-23, identify B.

A. The frontal nerve. It is one of the three terminal branches of the ophthalmic division of the trigeminal nerve. It supplies sensory branches to the forehead and scalp as far back as lambda via its terminal branches, which are the supratrochlear and supraorbital nerves.

Q. In Figure 3-23, identify C.

A. The superior ophthalmic vein. Both it and the inferior ophthalmic vein communicate with the facial veins. Thus, they are possible routes of infection to the cavernous sinus.

Q. In Figure 3-23, identify D.

A. The trochlear nerve. It supplies the superior oblique muscle of the eye.

Q. In Figure 3-23, identify E.

A. The superior division of the oculomotor nerve. It supplies the superior rectus muscle and the levator palpebrae superioris muscle.

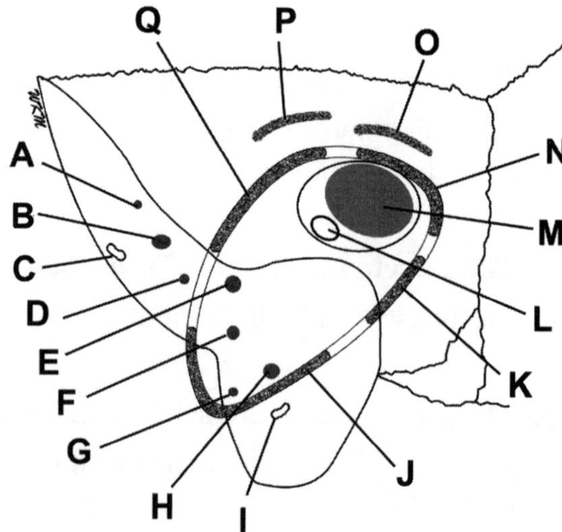

Figure 3-23 The Nerves Entering the Right Orbit

Q. In Figure 3-23, identify F.

A. The nasociliary nerve. It carries sensory fibers to the eyeball and the nose. Most importantly, it is sensory to the conjunctiva.

Q. In Figure 3-23, identify G.

A. The abducent nerve. It supplies the lateral rectus muscle.

Q. In Figure 3-23, identify H.

A. The inferior division of the oculomotor nerve. It supplies the medial rectus muscle, the inferior oblique muscle, and the inferior rectus muscle.

Q. In Figure 3-23, identify I.

A. The inferior ophthalmic vein.

Q. In Figure 3-23, identify J.

A. The origin of the lateral rectus muscle from the tendinous ring.

Q. In Figure 3-23, identify K.

A. The origin of the inferior rectus muscle from the tendinous ring.

Q. In Figure 3-23, identify L.

A. The ophthalmic artery.

Q. In Figure 3-23, identify M.

A. The optic nerve. The optic nerve and the ophthalmic artery enter the orbit through the optic canal. The optic nerve is surrounded by a dural sheath, which contains an extension of the subarachnoid space. Increased intracranial pressure may obstruct the vein, causing retinal hemorrhages and papilledema (edema of the optic disk).

Q. In Figure 3-23, identify N.

A. The origin of the medial rectus muscle from the tendinous ring. Note its proximity to the optic nerve. The proximity of the muscle to the optic nerve may cause pain on medial deviation of the eye when optic neuritis is present.

Q. In Figure 3-23, identify O.

A. The origin of the superior oblique muscle from the lesser wing of the sphenoid bone.

Q. In Figure 3-23, identify P.

A. The origin of the levator palpebrae superioris muscle from the lesser wing of the sphenoid bone.

Q. In Figure 3-23, identify Q.

A. The origin of the superior rectus muscle from the tendinous ring.

Q. The frontal nerve is one of the three terminal branches of . . .

A. The ophthalmic division of the trigeminal nerve. The other two branches are the lacrimal nerve and the nasociliary nerves.

Q. The frontal nerve terminates by dividing into . . .

A. The small, medial, supratrochlear nerve, and the larger, lateral, supraorbital nerve. Before dividing, the frontal nerve runs forward immediately below the roof of the orbit, lying on the superior surface of the levator palpebrae superioris muscle.

Q. The supraorbital nerve and the supratrochlear nerve supply . . .

A. The skin of the forehead, the scalp, the root of the nose, and the upper eyelid.

Q. The area of the scalp supplied by the medial and the lateral branches of the supraorbital nerve is . . .

A. The forehead and the vertex, extending back almost to the lambdoid suture.

Q. The trochlear nerve supplies . . .

A. The superior oblique muscle.

Q. The superior oblique muscle turns . . .

A. The cornea downward and laterally.

Q. To test the superior oblique muscle, and hence the trochlear nerve, the patient is asked to . . .

A. Adduct the eye and then look down. When the eye is adducted, the inferior rectus can no longer act as a depressor; hence the superior oblique muscle is now acting alone.

Q. Immediately inferior to the frontal nerve lie two muscles. They are . . .

A. The levator palpebrae superioris muscle and the superior rectus muscle.

Q. The nerve supply of the levator palpebrae superioris muscle and of the superior rectus muscle is . . .

A. The superior division of the oculomotor nerve, which enters their inferior surface.

Q. In addition to the optic nerve, three other nerves can be seen inferior to the levator palpebrae superioris muscle and superior rectus muscle. They are . . .

A. The laterally situated abducent nerve; the more medially situated nasociliary nerve; and finally, situated more inferiorly on the lateral side of the optic nerve lies the inferior division of the oculomotor nerve.

Q. In the same plane as the superior rectus and on its medial side lies . . .

A. The superior oblique muscle.

Q. The superior oblique muscle is inserted into . . .

A. The sclera. It passes forward along the medial side of the roof of the orbit. Now tendinous, it passes around the trochlea, a small pulley-like sling of fascia attached to the orbital plate of the zygomatic bone. It then turns posterolaterally to reach its insertion.

Q. The ciliary ganglion lies between the nasociliary nerve and the inferior division of the oculomotor nerve. Parasympathetic fibers synapse in it. These parasympathetic fibers are from . . .

A. The inferior division of the oculomotor nerve.

Q. The ciliary ganglion also receives a branch from the nasociliary nerve. These nerve fibers traverse, but do not synapse in, the ciliary ganglion. They are . . .

A. Sensory fibers to the globe and sympathetic motor fibers to the dilator pupillae muscle.

Q. The sympathetic fibers to the ciliary ganglion have already synapsed in . . .

A. The superior cervical sympathetic ganglion of the sympathetic chain. The sympathetic fibers are, therefore, postganglionic.

Q. The fibers from the ciliary ganglion reach the globe via . . .

A. The short ciliary nerves. They consist of both sympathetic and parasympathetic postganglionic fibers to the sphincter pupillae muscle and the ciliaris muscle. They also carry afferent sensory fibers from the globe.

Q. The long ciliary nerves also enter the globe of the eye. They originate from . . .

A. The nasociliary nerve. They carry postganglionic sympathetic fibers to the dilator pupillae muscle and sensory fibers from the cornea.

Q. The nasal branch of the nasociliary nerve crosses to the medial side of the orbit, superior to the optic nerve. It terminates by dividing into . . .

A. The anterior ethmoidal nerve and the infratrochlear nerves.

Q. The anterior ethmoidal nerve enters the nose via . . .

A. The anterior ethmoidal foramen.

Q. The anterior ethmoidal nerve supplies . . .

A. The lateral wall of the nose, the ethmoidal sinuses, and the anterior part of the nasal septum.

Q. The anterior ethmoidal nerve leaves the nose between the nasal bone and the nasal cartilages to become . . .

A. The external nasal nerve. It supplies the skin over the cartilages of the nose.

Q. The skin over the nasal bones is supplied by . . .

A. The infratrochlear branch of the nasociliary nerve.

Q. The inferior division of the oculomotor nerve continues forward to supply . . .

A. The inferior oblique muscle, the inferior rectus muscle, and the medial rectus muscle.

Q. The branch from the inferior division of the oculomotor nerve reaches the medial rectus muscle by crossing the optic nerve . . .

A. Inferiorly.

Q. The action of the inferior oblique muscle is to . . .

A. Turn the eye upward and laterally.

Q. To test the inferior oblique muscle, the patient is asked . . .

A. To adduct the eye and then look upwards. Adducting the eye prevents the superior rectus muscle from elevating the eye, leaving only the inferior oblique muscle as an elevator.

Q. To test the inferior rectus muscle, the patient is asked . . .

A. To look laterally and then downward. With the eye abducted, the superior oblique muscle can no longer depress the pupil, leaving only the inferior rectus muscle to act as a depressor.

Q. The subarachnoid space surrounding the optic nerve ends at the point where . . .

A. The dural covering of the optic nerve fuses with the sclera. This is important clinically because increased pressure of the cerebrospinal fluid can obstruct venous return from the retina.

Q. The ophthalmic artery enters the orbit accompanied by . . .

A. The optic nerve. They both enter the orbit through the optic foramen.

Q. At first, the ophthalmic artery lies lateral to the optic nerve, but then it crosses to its medial side by passing . . .

A. Superior to the optic nerve. It is accompanied by the nasociliary nerve.

Q. The most important branch of the ophthalmic artery is . . .

A. The central artery of the retina. Its other branches, which are numerous, follow the nerves already described.

Q. The lacrimal branch of the ophthalmic artery supplies the lacrimal gland, but it may also give a recurrent meningeal branch, which anastomoses with . . .

A. The anterior branch of the middle meningeal artery. It may replace the lacrimal artery proper.

Q. In Figure 3-24, identify A.

A. The inferior division of the oculomotor nerve.

Q. In Figure 3-24, identify B.

A. The abducent nerve.

Q. In Figure 3-24, identify C.

A. The superior division of the oculomotor nerve.

Q. In Figure 3-24, identify D.

A. The lacrimal nerve.

Q. In Figure 3-24, identify E.

A. The frontal nerve.

Q. In Figure 3-24, identify F.

A. The supraorbital nerve.

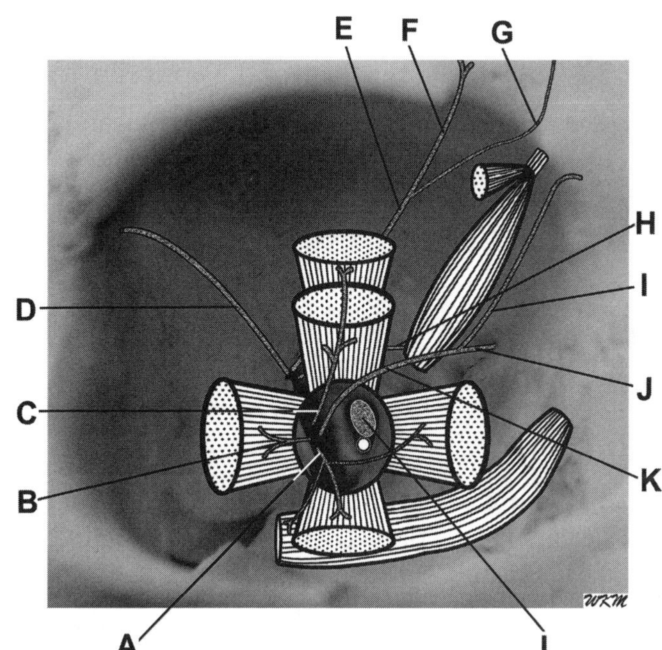

Figure 3-24 The Right Orbit: Nerves

Q. In Figure 3-24, identify G.

A. The supratrochlear nerve. As can be seen, it is the smaller branch of the frontal nerve.

Q. In Figure 3-24, identify H.

A. The trochlear nerve. It runs through the superior orbital fissure outside the tendinous ring.

Q. In Figure 3-24, identify I.

A. The infratrochlear nerve. It is a branch of the nasociliary nerve.

Q. In Figure 3-24, identify J.

A. The anterior ethmoidal nerve. It traverses the nose to emerge as the external nasal nerve.

Q. In Figure 3-24, identify K.

A. The nasociliary nerve.

Q. In Figure 3-24, identify L.

A. The optic nerve.

THE POSTERIOR TRIANGLE

Q. The boundaries of the posterior triangle are . . .

A. The posterior border of the sternocleidomastoid muscle, the anterior border of the trapezius muscle, and the superior border of the clavicle.

Q. The muscles in the floor of the posterior triangle, starting superiorly, are . . .

A. The edge of the semispinalis capitis muscle; the splenius capitis muscle; the two bellies of the levator scapulae muscle, which is often mistaken for two muscles; the edge of the scalenus posterior muscle, which is often insignificant; the scalenus medius muscle; and the lateral edge of the scalenus anterior muscle.

Q. The posterior triangle is divided into a superior, occipital triangle and an inferior, supraclavicular triangle by . . .

A. The inferior (posterior) belly of the omohyoid muscle.

Q. The muscles in the floor of the posterior triangle are covered by a thick layer of fascia. This is the lateral extension of . . .

A. The prevertebral fascia. This thick layer of fascia separates the anterior visceral and the vascular compartments of the neck from the posterior musculoskeletal compartment.

Q. Emerging into the floor of the posterior triangle from between the scalenus medius muscle and the scalenus anterior muscle are the roots of . . .

A. The cervical plexus and the brachial plexus.

Q. The roof of the posterior triangle is formed by . . .

A. The investing layer of the cervical fascia.

Q. The important nerve that crosses in the fascial roof of the posterior triangle is . . .

A. The spinal accessory nerve. It leaves the sternocleidomastoid muscle in the upper part of the triangle and enters the anterior border of the trapezius muscle in its lower part.

Q. The structures supplied by the spinal accessory nerve are . . .

A. The sternocleidomastoid muscle and the trapezius muscle.

Q. Lying in the superficial fascia and, therefore, superficial to the investing layer of the cervical fascia is . . .

A. The platysma muscle.

Q. The nerve supply of the platysma muscle is . . .

A. The cervical branch of the facial nerve.

Q. The structure that lies deep to the platysma muscle and is superficial to the investing layer of the cervical fascia is . . .

A. The external jugular vein.

Q. The veins that unite to form the external jugular vein are . . .

A. The posterior branch of the retromandibular vein and the posterior auricular vein.

Q. The retromandibular vein is formed by the union of . . .

A. The superficial temporal vein and the maxillary vein.

Q. The external jugular vein runs inferiorly on the surface of . . .

A. The sternocleidomastoid muscle.

Q. The external jugular vein ends by piercing . . .

A. The investing layer of the cervical fascia at the posterior border of the lower part of the sternocleidomastoid muscle. In the supraclavicular triangle, it terminates in the subclavian vein.

Q. The anterior branch of the retromandibular vein joins . . .

A. The facial vein. The facial vein is, itself, also joined by a vein or veins, sometimes known as the deep facial veins, which drain the pterygoid venous plexus.

Q. The facial vein, which is sometimes called the common facial vein, terminates in . . .

A. The internal jugular vein at the superior angle of the carotid triangle.

Q. The cervical plexus lies in . . .

A. The occipital triangle.

Q. The major structure in the anteroinferior angle of the occipital triangle is . . .

A. The proximal (superior) part of the brachial plexus.

Q. In Figure 3-25, identify A.

A. The semispinalis capitis muscle.

Q. In Figure 3-25, identify B.

A. The splenius capitis muscle.

Q. In Figure 3-25, identify C.

A. The levator scapulae muscle.

Q. In Figure 3-25, identify D.

A. The scalenus medius muscle. The roots of the brachial plexus emerge between it and the scalenus anterior muscle.

Q. In Figure 3-25, identify E.

A. The trapezius muscle. It forms the posterior border of the posterior triangle.

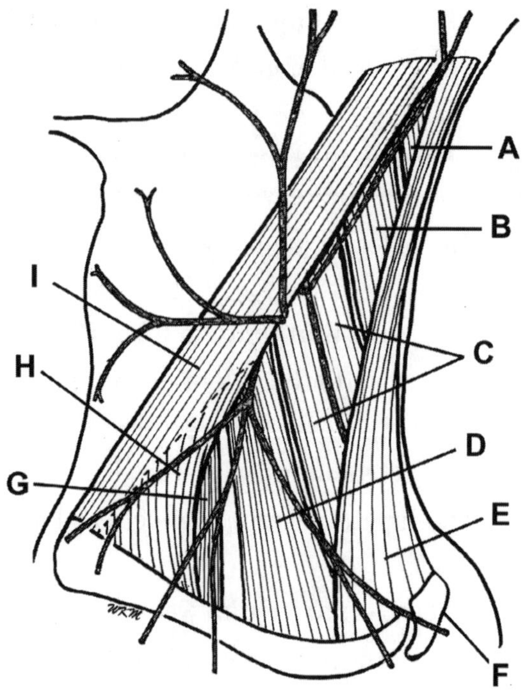

Figure 3-25 The Left Posterior of the Neck: Muscles

Q. In Figure 3-25, identify F.

A. The acromial process of the scapula. It forms the point of the shoulder.

Q. In Figure 3-25, identify G.

A. The edge of the scalenus anterior muscle, deep to the clavicular head of the sternocleidomastoid muscle.

Q. In Figure 3-25, identify muscle H.

A. The clavicular head of the sternocleidomastoid muscle.

Q. In Figure 3-25, identify muscle I.

A. The sternal head of the sternocleidomastoid muscle. The sternocleidomastoid muscle forms the anterior border of the posterior triangle.

Q. In Figure 3-26, identify A.

A. The lateral branch of the supraclavicular nerve. It supplies the skin as far medially as the medial border of the scapula.

Q. In Figure 3-26, identify B.

A. The intermediate branch of the supraclavicular nerve.

Q. In Figure 3-26, identify C.

A. The medial branch of the supraclavicular nerve. The supraclavicular nerves arise from the anterior primary rami of C3 and C4.

Q. Figure 3-26, identify D.

A. The anterior cutaneous nerve of the neck, the transverse cervical nerve, C2 and C3.

Q. In Figure 3-26, identify E.

A. The great auricular nerve, C2 and C3. It supplies the skin over the angle of the mandible and the lateral surface of the auricle.

Q. In Figure 3-26, identify F.

A. The lesser occipital nerve. It winds around the accessory nerve as that nerve leaves the sternocleidomastoid muscle. It then ascends, along the posterior border of that muscle, to the skin of the lateral part of the occipital region and the medial surface of the auricle.

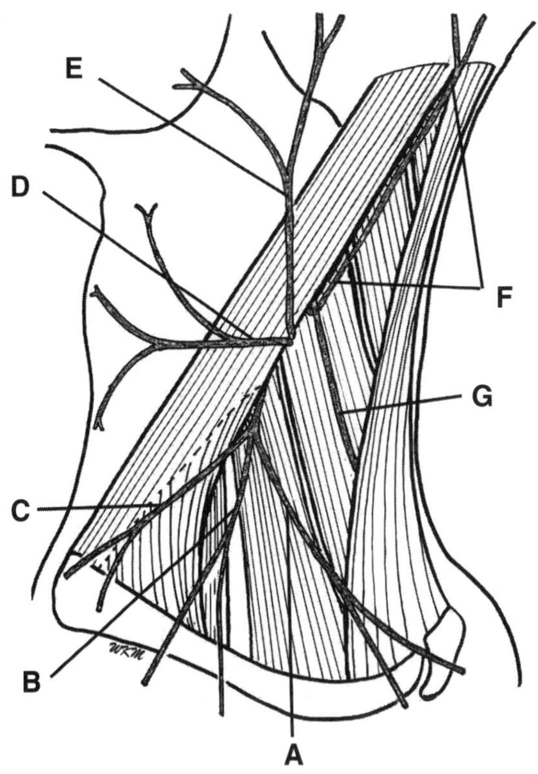

Figure 3-26 The Left Posterior Triangle of the Neck: Nerves

Q. In Figure 3-26, identify G.

A. The accessory nerve, which is supplying the trapezius muscle. It lies in the investing layer of the cervical fascia.

Q. The major neural structure located in the supraclavicular triangle, colloquially called "the salt cellar," is . . .

A. The distal, inferior, but still supraclavicular, part of the brachial plexus. The brachial plexus is crossed by the inferior belly of the omohyoid muscle.

Q. The largest, and therefore most important, vessels in the supraclavicular triangle are . . .

A. The third part of the subclavian artery and the subclavian vein. These vessels can be obstructed by firm pressure directed inferiorly on this triangle. This triangle is sometimes called the "subclavian triangle." However, this term is misleading, because the triangle is above the clavicle, not below it.

Q. The cutaneous branches of the cervical plexus are . . .

A. The lesser occipital nerve, C2; the great auricular nerve, C2 and C3; the transverse cervical nerve, C2 and C3; and the supraclavicular nerves, C3 and C4.

Q. The muscular branches of the cervical plexus are deeply situated. They are divided into a medial and a lateral group. The lateral group supplies . . .

A. The levator scapulae muscle and the scalenus medius muscle. They also assist in supplying the sternocleidomastoid muscle and the trapezius muscles. These latter muscles are, however, supplied mainly by the spinal part of the accessory (11th cranial) nerve.

Q. The medial group supplies the prevertebral muscles and . . .

A. The strap muscles via the inferior root, C2 and C3, of the ansa cervicalis, and the diaphragm via the phrenic nerve, C3, C4, and C5.

Q. The supraclavicular triangle is clearly a "vascular" triangle. Name the vessels that are located in it.

A. The subclavian artery and subclavian vein, the transverse cervical artery and vein, and the suprascapular artery and vein. The subclavian vein is often used for the placement of a central venous line.

Q. In Figure 3-27, identify A.

A. The hypoglossal nerve. It is joined by the anterior primary ramus of the first cervical nerve. Some of the first cervical nerve fibers soon leave the hypoglossal nerve to supply the geniohyoid muscle and the thyrohyoid muscle; others form the superior ramus of the cervical plexus.

Q. In Figure 3-27, identify B.

A. The superior ramus of the ansa cervicalis. It supplies the superior belly of the omohyoid muscle.

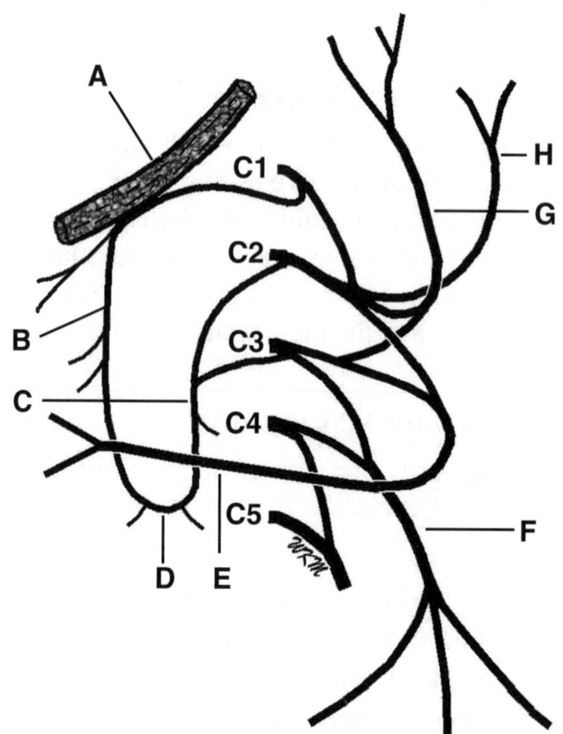

Figure 3-27 The Left Cervical Plexus

Q. In Figure 3-27, identify C.

A. The inferior ramus of the ansa cervicalis. It supplies the inferior belly of the omohyoid muscle.

Q. In Figure 3-27, identify D.

A. The ansa cervicalis. It supplies the sternothyroid muscle and the sternohyoid muscle.

Q. The superior and inferior rami of the ansa cervicalis and the ansa itself supply . . .

A. The cervical strap muscles: the sternohyoid muscle, the sternothyroid muscle, and the two bellies of the omohyoid muscle.

Q. The thyrohyoid muscle and the geniohyoid muscle are supplied by . . .

A. Branches from the hypoglossal nerve. These nerve fibers have, however, joined the hypoglossal nerve from the anterior primary ramus of the first cervical nerve.

Q. In Figure 3-27, identify E.

A. The transverse cervical nerve, C2 and C3.

Q. The transverse cervical nerve supplies . . .

A. The skin of the front and side of the neck.

Q. In Figure 3-27, identify F.

A. The supraclavicular nerve, C3 and C4.

Q. The supraclavicular nerve divides into three major branches. They are . . .

A. The medial supraclavicular nerve, the intermediate supraclavicular nerve, and the lateral supraclavicular nerve.

Q. The supraclavicular nerves supply . . .

A. The skin of the root of the neck, the skin over the clavicle, and the skin over the spine of the scapula.

Q. In Figure 3-27, identify G.

A. The great auricular nerve, C2 and C3.

Q. The great auricular nerve supplies . . .

A. The skin over the medial and lateral surfaces of the lower part of the auricle and the skin over the parotid gland and the angle of the mandible.

Q. In Figure 3-27, identify H.

A. The lesser occipital nerve, C2.

THE ANTERIOR TRIANGLE

Q. The boundaries of the anterior triangle of the neck are . . .

A. The line of the body of the mandible superiorly, the midline of the neck anteriorly, and the anterior border of the sternocleidomastoid muscle posteriorly.

Q. The anterior triangle is divided into four triangles. They are . . .

A. The submandibular digastric triangle, the unpaired submental triangle, the carotid triangle, and the muscular triangle.

Q. The boundaries of the submandibular triangle are . . .

A. The anterior and the posterior bellies of the digastric muscle and the body of the mandible.

Q. The boundaries of the submental triangle are . . .

A. The anterior bellies of the right and the left digastric muscles and the body of the hyoid bone. The apex of the triangle is at the chin, and the base is the body of the hyoid bone. It is, therefore, an unpaired triangle.

Q. The boundaries of the carotid triangle are . . .

A. The posterior belly of the digastric muscle, the superior belly of the omohyoid muscle, and the anterior border of the sternocleidomastoid muscle.

Q. The boundaries of the muscular triangle are . . .

A. The superior belly of the omohyoid muscle, the anterior border of the sternocleidomastoid muscle, and the midline of the neck.

Q. In Figure 3-28, identify muscle A.

A. The mylohyoid muscle. The left and the right mylohyoid muscles together form the floor of the submental triangle.

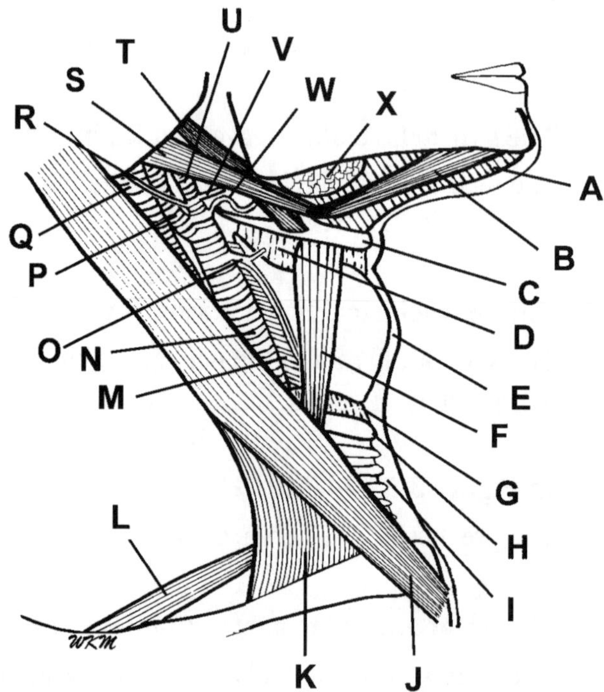

Figure 3-28 The Right Anterior Triangle of the Neck

Q. In Figure 3-28, identify muscle B.

A. The anterior belly of the digastric muscle. The anterior bellies of the right and the left digastric muscles form the two superior boundaries of the submental triangle.

Q. In Figure 3-28, identify bone C.

A. The body of the hyoid bone. It forms the base of the submental triangle.

Q. In Figure 3-28, identify D.

A. The thyrohyoid membrane. An emergency surgical airway cannot be established by an incision at this point. It would penetrate the epiglottis above the larynx.

Q. In Figure 3-28, identify E.

A. The thyroid cartilage, the laryngeal prominence. It becomes much more prominent in the male at puberty.

Q. In Figure 3-28, identify muscle F.

A. The superior belly of the omohyoid muscle.

Q. In Figure 3-28, identify G.

A. The cricothyroid membrane. This area is used for establishing an emergency surgical airway.

Q. In Figure 3-28, identify H.

A. The cricoid cartilage. Upward movement of the anterior ring of the cricoid cartilage can be felt while singing a high note. This pivoting movement around the cricothyroid articulation serves to tighten the vocal cords.

Q. In Figure 3-28, identify I.

A. The trachea. The first four cartilaginous rings are clearly depicted. In life, the second and the third tracheal rings are covered by the isthmus of the thyroid gland.

Q. In Figure 3-28, identify muscle J.

A. The sternal head of the sternocleidomastoid muscle. This muscle forms the posterior boundary of the anterior triangle.

Q. In Figure 3-28, identify muscle K.

A. The clavicular head of the sternocleidomastoid muscle.

Q. In Figure 3-28, identify muscle L.

A. The inferior belly of the omohyoid muscle. This muscle divides the posterior triangle into an occipital triangle and a supraclavicular triangle.

Q. In Figure 3-28, identify muscle M.

A. The inferior constrictor muscle of the pharynx. It forms part of the floor of the carotid triangle.

Q. In Figure 3-28, identify artery N.

A. The common carotid artery.

Q. In Figure 3-28, identify artery O.

A. The superior thyroid artery. In this individual, it is arising from the common carotid artery. Usually, it is the first branch of the external carotid artery. The superior thyroid artery gives off the internal laryngeal artery, which pierces the thyrohyoid membrane to enter the larynx with the internal laryngeal branch of the superior laryngeal nerve.

Q. The superior thyroid artery continues down the neck to the upper pole of the thyroid gland. It is accompanied by . . .

A. The external laryngeal branch of the superior laryngeal nerve.

Q. The external laryngeal nerve supplies . . .

A. The cricothyroid muscle. The cricothyroid muscle serves to tighten the ipsilateral vocal cord when a person sings a high note. It is the only muscle supplied by the external laryngeal nerve.

Q. In Figure 3-28, identify artery P.

A. The internal carotid artery. It has no branches in the neck.

Q. Applying pressure to or massaging the internal carotid artery at this point causes . . .

A. Slowing of the heart and a fall in blood pressure.

Q. The bradycardia and fall in blood pressure is due to . . .

A. The presence of baroceptors in the carotid sinus.

Q. This reflex is mediated through . . .

A. The vagus nerve and the glossopharyngeal nerve.

Q. **In Figure 3-28, identify vein Q.**

A. The internal jugular vein.

Q. **In Figure 3-28, identify artery R.**

A. The occipital branch of the external carotid artery.

Q. **In Figure 3-28, identify muscle S.**

A. The posterior belly of the digastric muscle. It forms the superior border of the carotid triangle.

Q. **The nerve supply of the posterior belly of the digastric muscle is . . .**

A. The facial nerve. The anterior belly of the digastric is supplied by the nerve to the mylohyoid muscle.

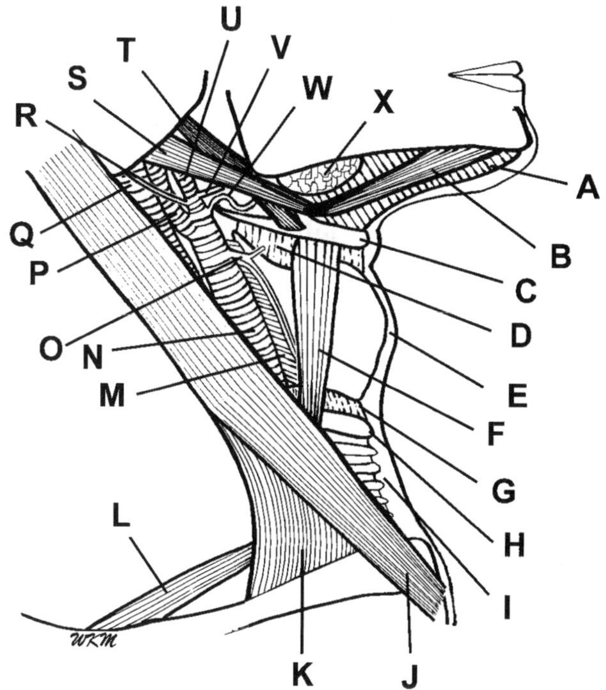

Figure 3-28 The Right Anterior Triangle of the Neck

Q. **In Figure 3-28, identify muscle T.**

A. The stylohyoid muscle and the closely related stylohyoid ligament. The stylohyoid muscle is supplied by the facial nerve, as are the posterior belly of the digastric muscle and the muscles of facial expression. They are all derived from the second pharyngeal arch of the embryo.

Q. **In Figure 3-28, identify artery U.**

A. The external carotid artery.

Q. **In Figure 3-28, identify artery V.**

A. The facial artery. It arises from the external carotid artery. On its way to the face, the facial artery supplies the submandibular salivary gland.

Q. **In Figure 3-28, identify artery W.**

A. The lingual artery. It also arises from the external carotid artery. The upward loop of the lingual artery is characteristic. It is crossed by the hypoglossal nerve, as can be seen in Figure 3-29.

Q. **In Figure 3-28, identify structure X.**

A. The submandibular salivary gland.

Q. The submandibar salivary gland can easily be palpated between the thumb, pressed upwards deep and slightly anterior to the angle of the mandible, and a finger in . . .

A. The linguogingival sulcus.

Q. In Figure 3-29, identify nerve A. Both ends of the nerve are labelled.

A. The hypoglossal (12th cranial) nerve. It supplies the muscles of the tongue.

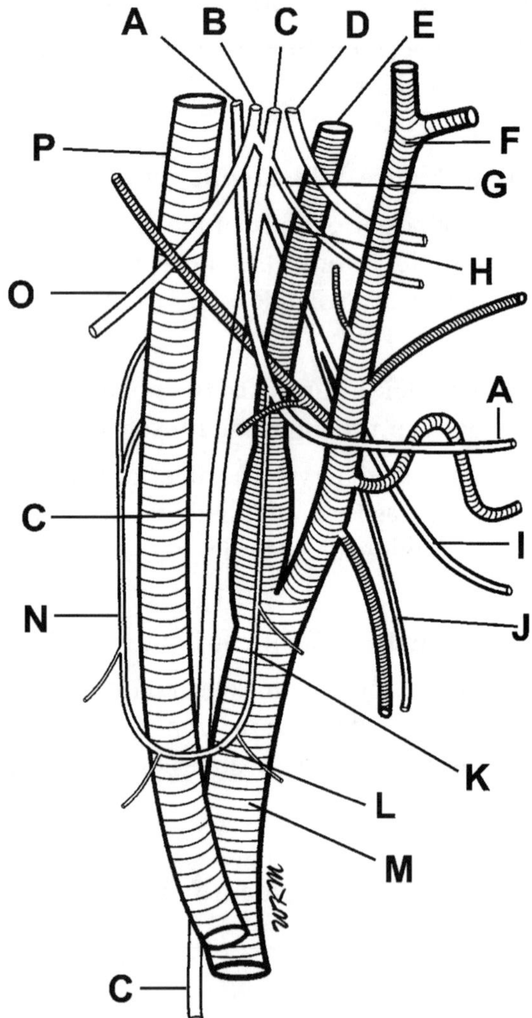

Figure 3-29 The Last Four Cranial Nerves Emerging From the Skull, Right Side, Anterolateral Aspect

Q. In Figure 3-29, identify nerve B.

A. The accessory nerve (11th cranial) nerve. It has both cranial and spinal components. The cranial component joins the vagus nerve; the spinal component supplies the sternocleidomastoid muscle and the trapezius muscle.

Q. In Figure 3-29, identify nerve C. It is labelled three times.

A. The vagus (10th cranial) nerve.

Q. In Figure 3-29, identify nerve D.

A. The glossopharyngeal (ninth cranial) nerve. It supplies the posterior one-third of the tongue and the oropharynx with both general sensory and taste fibers. It also supplies the stylopharyngeus muscle.

Q. In Figure 3-29, identify artery E.

A. The internal carotid artery. It normally does not have branches in the neck.

Q. In Figure 3-29, identify artery F.

A. The external carotid artery.

Q. In Figure 3-29, identify nerve G.

A. The pharyngeal branch of the vagus nerve.

Q. In Figure 3-29, identify nerve H.

A. The superior laryngeal branch of the vagus.

Q. In Figure 3-29, identify nerve I.

A. The internal laryngeal branch of the superior laryngeal nerve. It enters the larynx through the thyrohyoid membrane to supply the mucous membrane above the glottis.

Q. In Figure 3-29, identify nerve J.

A. The external laryngeal branch of the superior laryngeal nerve. It supplies the cricothyroid muscle, which tightens the vocal cords when a high note is sung.

Q. In Figure 3-29, identify nerve K.

A. The superior ramus to the ansa cervicalis. Although its fibers come from the anterior primary ramus of the first cervical nerve, they travel for part of their course with the hypoglossal nerve.

Q. In Figure 3-29, identify nerve L.

A. The ansa cervicalis. The ansa and its two roots supply the strap muscles of the larynx.

Q. In Figure 3-29, identify artery M.

A. The common carotid artery. At the level of the hyoid bone, it divides into internal and external branches. The internal carotid artery does not have branches in the neck. It supplies most of the brain, the orbit and the globe of the eye, and part of the nose.

Q. In Figure 3-29, identify nerve N.

A. The inferior ramus to the ansa cervicalis. It arises from the anterior primary rami of the second and third cervical nerves.

Q. In Figure 3-29, identify nerve O.

A. The spinal accessory nerve. It supplies the sternocleidomastoid muscle and the trapezius muscle.

Q. In Figure 3-29, identify vein P.

A. The internal jugular vein. It is enclosed in the carotid sheath together with the carotid artery and the vagus nerve.

Q. The external carotid artery has two groups of branches, superficial branches and deep branches. The superficial branches are . . .

A. The facial artery, the superficial temporal artery, and the occipital artery. They supply the superficial structures of the face and scalp.

Q. The deep branches of the external carotid artery are . . .

A. The superior thyroid artery, the lingual artery, the ascending pharyngeal artery, and the maxillary artery.

Q. The structures supplied by the deep branches of the external carotid artery are all part of . . .

A. The mechanisms of the upper alimentary tract or the respiratory tract.

Q. In Figure 3-30, identify A.

A. The internal carotid artery.

Q. In Figure 3-30, identify B.

A. The superficial temporal artery. It accompanies the auricular temporal nerve to supply the upper part of the auricle and the temporal region of the scalp.

Q. In Figure 3-30, identify C.

A. The maxillary artery. It supplies all of the structures in the infratemporal fossa, the maxillary region of the face, and the posterior part of the nasal cavity.

Q. In Figure 3-30, identify D.

A. The ascending pharyngeal artery. It supplies the upper part of the pharynx. It also gives off the inferior tympanic artery, branches to the last four cranial nerves, and, via its posterior meningeal branch, the meninges of the posterior cranial fossa.

Q. In Figure 3-30, identify E.

A. The facial artery. It winds around the submandibular gland, which it supplies, and then grooves the lower border of the mandible to reach the face. It can be easily palpated where it lies in a groove in the mandible.

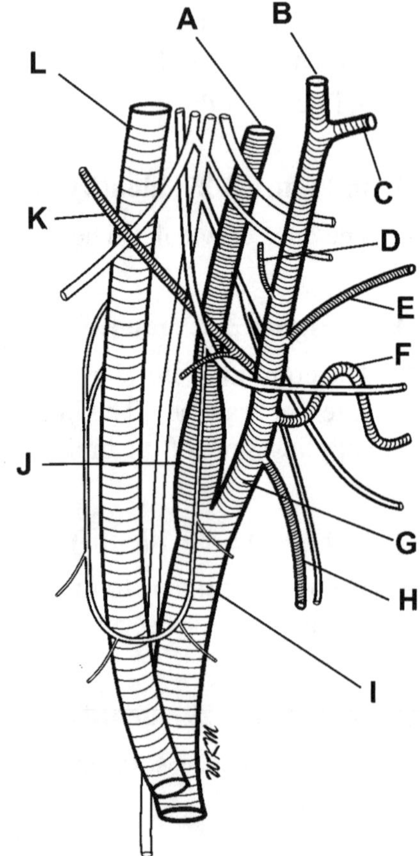

Figure 3-30 The Branches of the Right External Carotid Artery

Q. In Figure 3-30, identify F.

A. The lingual artery. It forms a characteristic loop, where it is crossed by the hypoglossal nerve. It then runs forward, deep to the hyoglossus muscle, which separates it from the hypoglossal nerve and its venae comitantes. Finally, it turns upward and forward to end as the arteria profunda linguae on the undersurface of the tongue.

Q. In Figure 3-30, identify G.

A. The stem of the external carotid artery.

Q. In Figure 3-30, identify H.

A. The superior thyroid artery. In addition to branches to the thyroid gland, it supplies the larynx above the glottis.

Q. In Figure 3-30, identify I.

A. The common carotid artery. This artery, together with the internal jugular vein and the vagus nerve, is enclosed in the carotid sheath of connective tissue.

Q. In Figure 3-30, identify J.

A. The carotid bulb. It contains baroceptors in its wall. They control the pressure of arterial blood to the brain via feedback carried by the glossopharyngeal and vagus nerves.

Q. In Figure 3-30, identify K.

A. The occipital artery. One of its branches to the sternomastoid muscle hooks around the hypoglossal nerve. This is a useful surgical landmark. The occipital artery is the major blood supply to the occipital region of the scalp.

Q. In Figure 3-30, identify L.

A. The internal jugular vein. It leaves the skull through the jugular foramen, together with the glossopharyngeal nerve, the vagus nerve, and the accessory nerve.

Q. In the jugular foramen, the glossopharyngeal nerve is separated from the vagus and accessory nerves by . . .

A. The inferior petrosal sinus.

Q. The inferior petrosal sinus connects the cavernous sinus to . . .

A. The internal jugular vein.

Q. The hypoglossal nerve leaves the skull through . . .

A. The anterior condylar canal in the occipital bone.

Q. The hypoglossal nerve is the motor nerve to . . .

A. The muscles of the tongue.

THE INFRATEMPORAL FOSSA

Q. In Figure 3-31, identify A.

A. The maxilla.

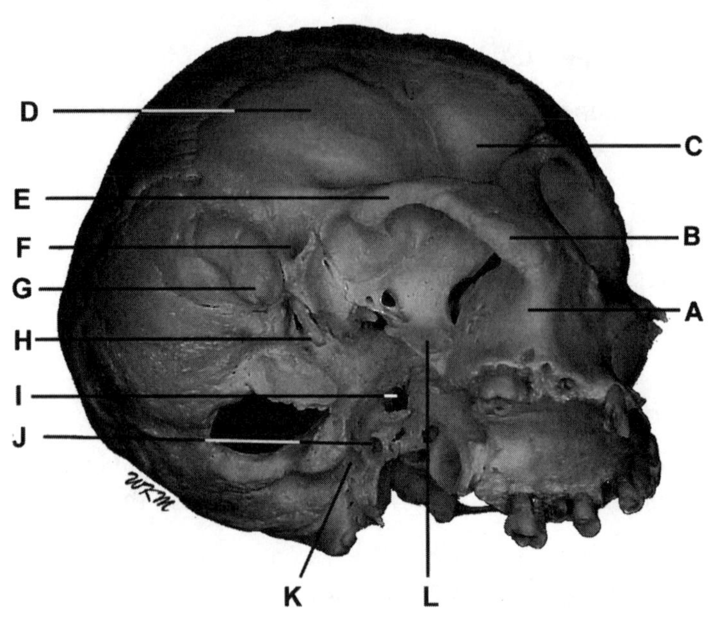

Figure 3-31 Orientation of the Right Infratemporal Fossa

Q. In Figure 3-31, identify B.

A. The zygoma.

Q. In Figure 3-31, identify C.

A. The greater wing of the sphenoid bone.

Q. In Figure 3-31, identify D.

A. The squamous temporal bone.

Q. In Figure 3-31, identify E.

A. The zygomatic process of the temporal bone.

Q. In Figure 3-31, identify F.

A. The external auditory meatus.

Q. In Figure 3-31, identify G.

A. The mastoid process of the temporal bone.

Q. In Figure 3-31, identify H.

A. The styloid process of the temporal bone. It represents part of the skeleton of the embryonic second pharyngeal arch.

Q. In Figure 3-31, identify I.

A. The foramen lacerum. The deep petrosal nerve passes through the lower half of this foramen; the greater superficial petrosal nerve passes through the upper half. These two nerves join to form the nerve of the pterygoid canal, which opens onto the anterior wall of the foramen lacerum.

Q. In Figure 3-31, identify J.

A. The carotid canal.

Q. In Figure 3-31, identify K.

A. The jugular foramen.

Q. In Figure 3-31, identify L.

A. The pterygoid process of the sphenoid bone.

Q. The bony roof of the infratemporal fossa is . . .

A. The infratemporal surface of the greater wing of the sphenoid bone. It is covered by the superior head of the lateral pterygoid muscle.

Q. The bony medial wall of the infratemporal fossa is composed of . . .

A. The lateral surface of the lateral pterygoid plate. It is covered by the inferior head of the lateral pterygoid muscle, which arises from it.

Q. The bony anterior wall of the infratemporal fossa is formed by . . .

A. The posterior surface of the maxilla.

Q. The bony lateral wall of the infratemporal fossa is formed by . . .

A. The medial surface of the angle and of the ramus of the mandible.

Q. The muscle that is attached to the medial surface of the angle of the mandible is . . .

A. The medial pterygoid muscle.

Q. The superior attachment of the medial pterygoid muscle is to . . .

A. The medial surface of the lateral pterygoid plate and the tubercle of the maxilla.

Q. The medial pterygoid muscle, descending from its upper attachment, at first lies medial to . . .

A. The inferior head of the lateral pterygoid muscle.

Q. The medial pterygoid muscle then passes downward and laterally, leaving a narrow angle between its fibers and the ramus of the mandible. This space is sometimes called . . .

A. The pterygomandibular space or interval.

Q. The three nerves that pass through the pterygomandibular space are . . .

A. The buccal nerve, the lingual nerve, and the inferior alveolar nerve. Consequently, dentists frequently inject local anesthetic into this space to anesthetize the lower teeth and jaw. They call such an injection "a mandibular nerve block," although, of course, only these three nerves are paralyzed.

Q. A needle inserted too deeply into the pterygomandibular space would penetrate . . .

A. The parotid gland.

Q. Injection of local anesthetic into the parotid salivary gland would result in paralysis of . . .

A. The facial nerve as it traverses this gland.

Q. An important nerve enters the infratemporal fossa through a foramen in its roof. This foramen is . . .

A. The foramen ovale.

Q. The nerve that passes through the foramen ovale is . . .

A. The mandibular division of the trigeminal nerve.

Q. As it leaves the foramen ovale, the mandibular nerve lies on . . .

A. The tensor palati muscle.

Q. Between the tensor palati muscle and the trunk of the mandibular nerve lies . . .

A. The otic ganglion.

Q. The otic ganglion is . . .

A. A parasympathetic ganglion. Parasympathetic preganglionic fibers synapse in the otic ganglion on their way to the parotid gland.

Q. The preganglionic fibers to the otic ganglion originate from . . .

A. The glossopharyngeal nerve.

Q. Preganglionic fibers in the glossopharyngeal nerve reach the otic ganglion via . . .

A. The tympanic branch of the glossopharyngeal nerve to the tympanic plexus in the middle ear. They then leave the tympanic plexus via the lesser petrosal nerve, traversing the foramen ovale to reach the otic ganglion.

Q. The secretomotor fibers from the otic ganglion travel to the parotid gland via . . .

A. The auriculotemporal branch of the trigeminal nerve.

Q. Where the mandibular nerve lies on the tensor palati muscle, it is covered by . . .

A. The superior head of the lateral pterygoid muscle.

Q. The main trunk of the mandibular nerve gives off two branches. One branch is sensory, the other is motor. The sensory branch is . . .

A. The nervus spinosum. It reenters the skull through the foramen spinosum to supply the meninges of the middle cranial fossa.

Q. The motor branch of the main trunk of the mandibular nerve is . . .

A. The nerve to the medial pterygoid muscle. It supplies motor fibers to the tensor palati muscle and to the tensor tympani muscle.

Q. Shortly after the exit of the mandibular nerve from the foramen ovale, it is divided into two trunks by the pterygospinous ligament. These trunks are . . .

A. The anterior trunk and the larger posterior trunk. The anterior trunk is situated anterolaterally to the ligament, and the posterior trunk is situated posteromedially to the ligament. This occurs because the pterygospinous ligament passes obliquely, medially and anteriorly, from the spine of the sphenoid bone to the upper part of the posterior edge of the lateral pterygoid plate of the sphenoid bone.

Q. The smaller anterior trunk of the mandibular nerve can be said to have four motor branches and one sensory branch. The sensory branch of the anterior trunk of the mandibular nerve is . . .

A. The buccal nerve. It is sensory to the cheek and to the buccal gingivae of the molar teeth and the premolar teeth of the lower jaw.

Q. The anterior trunk is motor to the remaining muscles of mastication. These muscles are . . .

A. The lateral pterygoid muscle, the masseter muscle, and the temporalis muscle. The last-named muscle is supplied by two branches, the anterior and the posterior deep temporal nerves. As their names imply, they lie on the deep surface of the temporalis muscle and are in contact with the skull.

Q. The posterior trunk can be said to have four sensory branches and one motor branch. The sensory branches of the posterior trunk are . . .

A. The inferior alveolar nerve, the lingual nerve, and the two roots of the auriculotemporal nerve.

Q. The two roots of the auriculotemporal nerve encircle . . .

A. The middle meningeal branch of the maxillary artery. It ascends to the foramen spinosum.

Q. The motor fibers in the posterior trunk of the mandibular division of the trigeminal nerve supply . . .

A. The mylohyoid muscle and the anterior belly of thc digastric muscle. The nerve to the mylohyoid is a branch of the inferior alveolar branch of the posterior mandibular trunk.

Q. The branch of the facial nerve that traverses the infratemporal fossa is . . .

A. The chorda tympani nerve. It leaves the facial nerve in the facial canal, crosses the tympanic membrane, and then emerges into the infratemporal fossa through the squamotympanic fissure. Finally, it traverses the infratemporal fossa to reach the lingual nerve.

Q. The motor nerve fibers carried in the chorda tympani nerve are . . .

A. Preganglionic parasympathetic nerve fibers. They travel to the submandibular ganglion, where they synapse. The postganglionic secretomotor fibers, which originate in the ganglion, are secretomotor to the submandibular and the sublingual glands.

Q. The sensory fibers carried in the chorda tympani nerve are . . .

A. Sensory fibers for taste from the anterior two-thirds of the tongue. Their cell bodies are in the sensory geniculate ganglion of the facial nerve. Sensory fibers do not, of course, synapse in peripheral ganglia.

Q. The three muscles in the infratemporal fossa responsible for biting are . . .

A. The temporalis muscle, the medial pterygoid muscle, and the masseter muscle. The masseter muscle is incorporated into the lateral wall of the fossa.

Q. The muscle responsible for retracting the jaw is . . .

A. The posterior part of the temporalis muscle. This part of the temporalis muscle is innervated by the posterior deep temporal nerve.

Q. The muscle responsible for protracting the jaw is . . .

A. The lateral pterygoid muscle. The mechanism of chewing involves the sequential action of all of the muscles of mastication.

Q. The only significant artery in the infratemporal fossa is the maxillary artery. It originates from . . .

A. The external carotid artery. It is one of the two terminal branches of this vessel; the other is the superficial temporal artery.

Q. The maxillary artery enters the infratemporal fossa by passing between . . .

A. The sphenomandibular ligament and the ramus of the mandible.

Q. The maxillary artery crosses the infratemporal fossa by passing superficial to, through the substance of, or deep to . . .

A. The lateral pterygoid muscle.

Q. In the infratemporal fossa, the maxillary artery gives off . . .

A. The branches that accompany each of the branches of the mandibular nerve.

Q. The most significant branch of the maxillary artery in the infratemporal fossa is . . .

A. The middle meningeal artery.

Q. The middle meningeal artery ascends from its origin from the maxillary artery. Then, after being encircled by the auriculotemporal nerve, it immediately enters the skull through . . .

A. The foramen spinosum of the sphenoid bone. It is accompanied by the nervus spinosum.

Q. The middle meningeal artery supplies . . .

A. The dura mater and the bones of most of the neurocranium.

Q. Within the skull, the middle meningeal artery lies between . . .

A. The meningeal and the endosteal layers of the dura mater. Its path can be traced by grooves in the inner table of the skull.

Q. Fractures of the skull frequently rupture the middle meningeal artery. The subsequent hemorrhage occurs in . . .

A. The epidural space. It results in an epidural hematoma.

Q. The maxillary artery leaves the infratemporal fossa by passing through . . .

A. The pterygomaxillary fissure into the pterygopalatine fossa.

Q. In Figure 3-32, identify A.

A. The lateral surface of the lateral pterygoid plate.

Q. The muscle that arises from the lateral surface of the lateral pterygoid plate is . . .

A. The lateral pterygoid muscle.

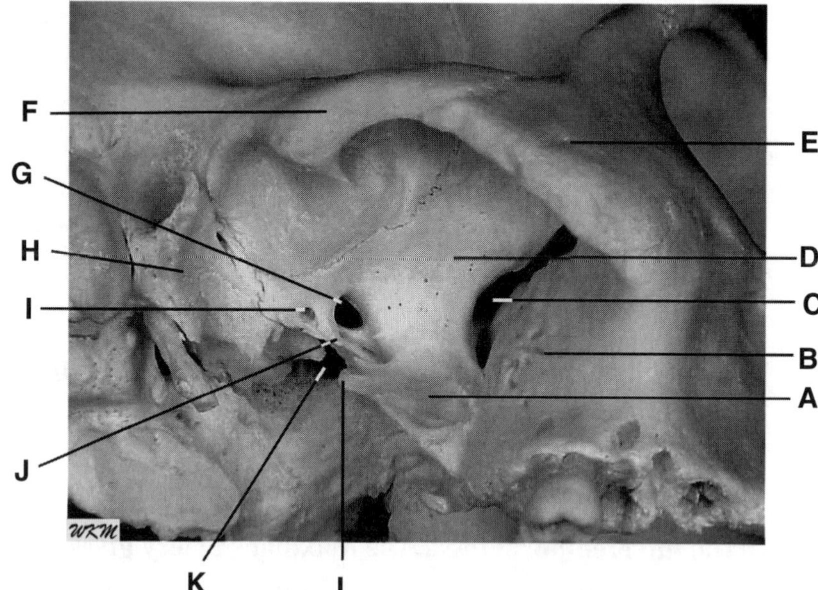

Figure 3-32 Features of the Right Infratemporal Fossa

Q. A second origin of the lateral pterygoid muscle is . . .

A. The infratemporal surface and the infratemporal crest of the greater wing of the sphenoid bone.

Q. In Figure 3-32, identify B.

A. The groove for the posterior superior alveolar nerve on the posterior surface of the maxilla.

Q. The posterior superior alveolar nerve is a branch of . . .

A. The maxillary nerve.

Q. In Figure 3-32, identify C.

A. The pterygomaxillary fissure.

Q. The structures that pass through the pterygomaxillary fissure are . . .

A. The maxillary artery and its accompanying venous plexus and the posterior superior alveolar nerve.

Q. The maxillary artery is one of the two terminal branches of . . .

A. The external carotid artery.

Q. The other terminal branch of the external carotid artery is . . .

A. The superficial temporal artery.

Q. In Figure 3-32, identify D.

A. The infratemporal surface of the greater wing of the sphenoid bone.

Q. In Figure 3-32, identify E.

A. The zygomaticofacial foramen in the zygoma. It is traversed by the nerve of the same name, which is one of the two terminal branches of the zygomatic branch of the maxillary nerve.

Q. In Figure 3-32, identify F.

A. The zygomatic process of the temporal bone.

Q. In Figure 3-32, identify G.

A. The foramen ovale.

Q. The most important structure passing through the foramen ovale is . . .

A. The mandibular division of the trigeminal nerve.

Q. In Figure 3-32, identify H.

A. The tympanic part of the temporal bone. It is the posterior wall of the mandibular fossa.

Q. In Figure 3-32, identify I.

A. The foramen spinosum. It transmits the middle meningeal artery and the nervus spinosum. This branch of the mandibular division of the trigeminal nerve supplies the dura mater of the middle cranial fossa, as does the middle meningeal artery, which is a branch of the maxillary artery.

Q. In Figure 3-32, identify J.

A. The spine of the sphenoid bone. In this specimen, the pterygospinous ligament, which separates the anterior and posterior parts of the mandibular nerve, has become ossified.

Q. In Figure 3-32, identify K.

A. The foramen lacerum.

Q. In Figure 3-32, identify L.

A. The pterygoid hamulus.

THE PREOCCIPITAL REGION

Q. In Figure 3-33, identify A.

A. The apex of the petrous temporal bone.

Q. In Figure 3-33, identify B.

A. The carotid canal.

Q. In Figure 3-33, identify C.

A. The jugular foramen.

Q. In Figure 3-33, identify D.

A. The pharyngeal tubercle. It provides attachment for the median raphe of the pharynx.

Q. In Figure 3-33, identify E.

A. The foramen magnum.

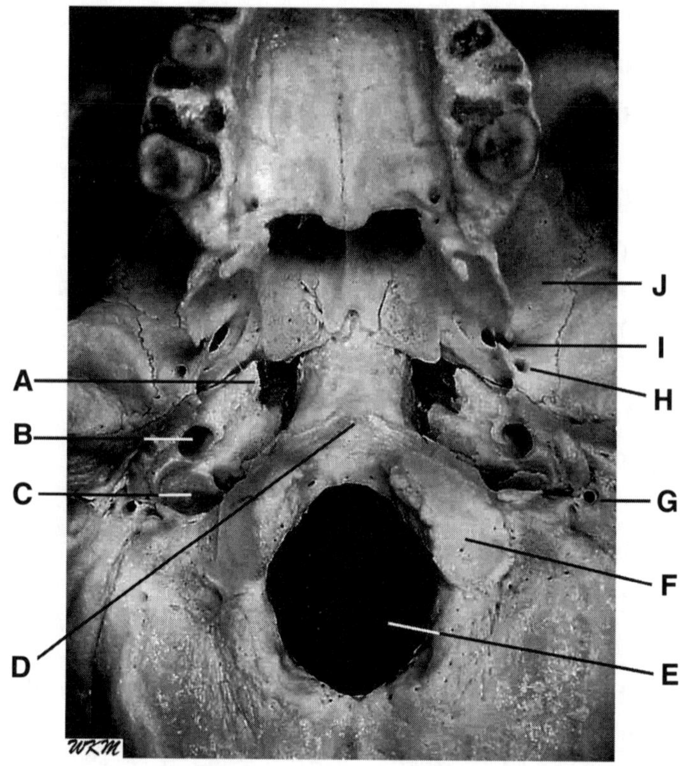

Figure 3-33 Foramina of the Base of the Skull, Inferior Aspect

Q. In Figure 3-33, identify F.

A. The occipital condyle. It articulates with the superior articular facet of the atlas.

Q. In Figure 3-33, identify G.

A. The stylomastoid foramen. The facial nerve emerges from the skull through this foramen.

Q. In Figure 3-33, identify H.

A. The foramen spinosum. The middle meningeal artery passes through it.

Q. In Figure 3-33, identify I.

A. The foramen ovale. It transmits the mandibular division of the trigeminal nerve.

Q. In Figure 3-33, identify fossa J.

A. The infratemporal fossa. The roof of the fossa is the greater wing of the sphenoid bone.

Q. In Figure 3-34, identify A.

A. The carotid canal.

Q. In Figure 3-34, identify B.

A. The stylomastoid foramen. It transmits the facial nerve.

Q. In Figure 3-34, identify C.

A. The part of the jugular foramen occupied by the internal jugular vein.

Q. In Figure 3-34, identify D.

A. The notch for the accessory nerve.

Q. In Figure 3-34, identify E.

A. The notch in the petrous temporal bone for the glossopharyngeal nerve.

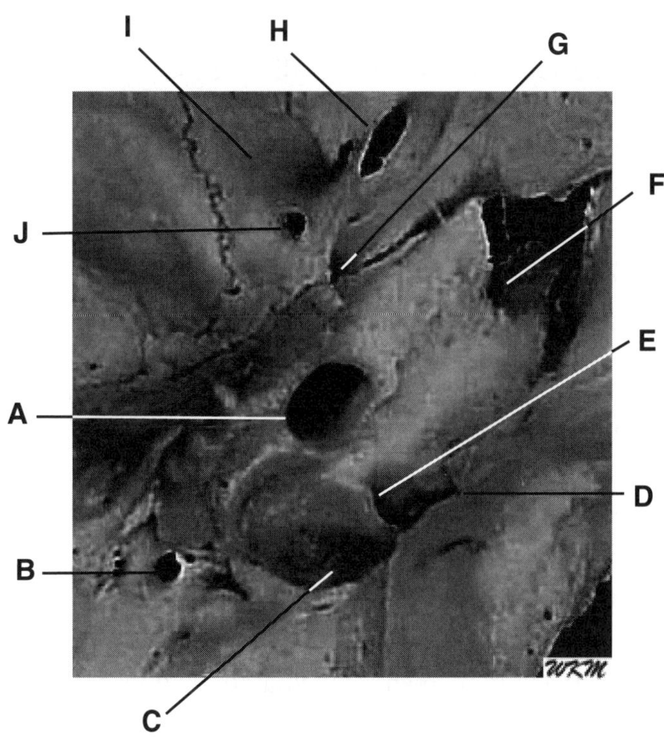

Figure 3-34 Preoccipital Region of the Skull Base, Inferior Aspect

Q. In Figure 3-34, identify F.

A. The opening of the carotid canal. It opens into the posterolateral wall of the foramen lacerum.

Q. In Figure 3-34, identify G.

A. The opening of the osseous pharyngotympanic tube.

Q. In Figure 3-34, identify H.

A. The foramen ovale.

Q. In Figure 3-34, identify I.

A. The infratemporal surface of the greater wing of the sphenoid bone.

Q. In Figure 3-34, identify J.

A. The foramen spinosum. It transmits the middle meningeal artery.

Q. In Figure 3-35, identify A.

A. The superior cervical ganglion of the sympathetic chain. It enters the cranium as a plexus on the internal carotid artery. This plexus is named the carotid nerves.

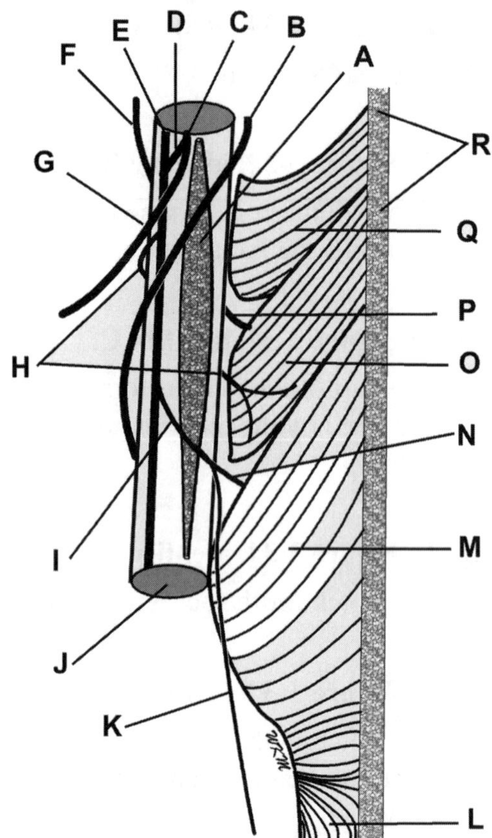

Figure 3-35 The Internal Carotid Artery and the Cranial Nerves, Left Side, Posterior Aspect

Q. In Figure 3-35, identify B.

A. The hypoglossal nerve. It has emerged from the anterior condylar canal. It crosses posterior to the superior cervical sympathetic ganglion, to the internal carotid artery, and then to the vagus nerve. It is closely adherent to the vagus nerve for a short distance.

Q. In Figure 3-35, identify C.

A. The accessory nerve. It has emerged from the jugular foramen anteromedial to the internal jugular vein. Almost immediately, it divides into cranial and spinal divisions. Its cranial division joins the vagus nerve. It is distributed to the pharyngeal plexus by the pharyngeal branch of the vagus nerve.

Q. In Figure 3-35, identify D.

A. The short cranial division of the accessory nerve. It joins the vagus nerve.

Q. In Figure 3-35, identify E.

A. The vagus nerve. It has emerged from the jugular foramen, lateral to the accessory nerve, and anterior to the internal jugular vein.

Q. In Figure 3-35, identify F.

A. The glossopharyngeal nerve. It emerges from the anteromedial part of the jugular foramen in a groove in the petrous temporal bone. In the jugular foramen, it is separated from the vagus nerve by the termination of the inferior petrosal sinus as it enters the bulb of the internal jugular vein.

Q. In Figure 3-35, identify G.

A. The spinal accessory nerve. It supplies the sternocleidomastoid muscle and the trapezius muscle.

Q. In Figure 3-35, identify H.

A. The pharyngeal branch of the vagus nerve. It is the major component of the pharyngeal plexus, which is motor to the constrictor muscles of the pharynx.

Q. In Figure 3-35, identify I.

A. The superior laryngeal branch of the vagus nerve.

Q. In Figure 3-35, identify J.

A. The internal carotid artery.

Q. In Figure 3-35, identify K.

A. The external laryngeal branch of the superior laryngeal nerve. It supplies the cricothyroid muscle.

Q. In Figure 3-35, identify L.

A. The esophagus.

Q. In Figure 3-35, identify M.

A. The inferior constrictor of the pharynx.

Q. In Figure 3-35, identify N.

A. The internal laryngeal branch of the superior laryngeal nerve. It enters the larynx between the inferior constrictor muscle and the middle constrictor muscle of the pharynx. It is sensory to the mucous membrane between the epiglottis and the glottis.

Q. In Figure 3-35, identify O.

A. The middle constrictor muscle of the pharynx.

Q. In Figure 3-35, identify P.

A. The glossopharyngeal nerve. It is labeled for the second time. Here it is seen entering the pharynx, passing between the superior and middle constrictor muscles of the pharynx.

Q. In Figure 3-35, identify Q.

A. The superior constrictor muscle of the pharynx.

Q. In Figure 3-35, identify R.

A. The midline pharyngeal raphe. It is attached to the pharyngeal tubercle of the skull.

THE PTERYGOPALATINE FOSSA

Q. In Figure 3-36, identify A.

A. The superior orbital fissure.

Q. In Figure 3-36, identify B.

A. The lesser wing of the sphenoid bone.

Q. In Figure 3-36, identify C.

A. The greater wing of the sphenoid bone.

Q. In Figure 3-36, identify D.

A. The orbital plate of the sphenoid bone.

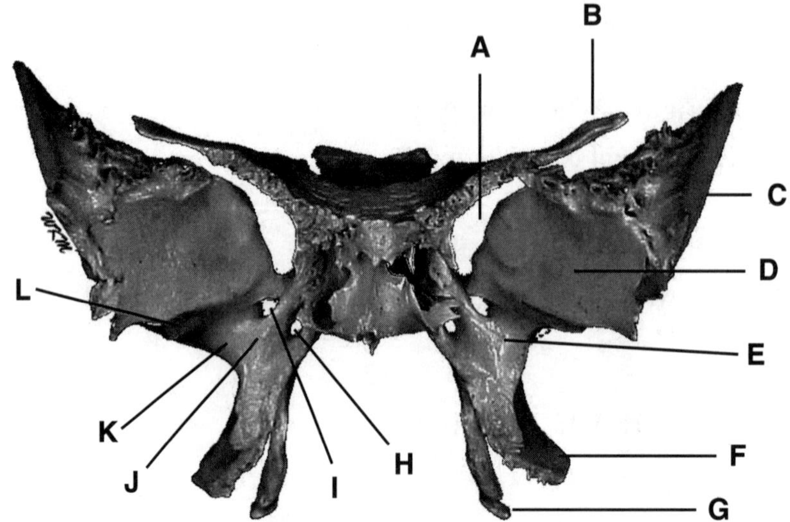

Figure 3-36 The Sphenoid Bone, Anterior Aspect

Q. In Figure 3-36, identify E.

A. The pterygoid process of the sphenoid bone.

Q. In Figure 3-36, identify F.

A. The lateral pterygoid plate of the sphenoid bone.

Q. In Figure 3-36, identify G.

A. The medial pterygoid plate of the sphenoid bone.

Q. In Figure 3-36, identify H.

A. The opening of the pterygoid canal. The nerve of the pterygoid canal is formed in the foramen lacerum by the union of the deep petrosal nerve and the greater petrosal nerve. It carries postganglionic sympathetic fibers from the superior cervical sympathetic ganglion via the deep petrosal nerve and preganglionic parasympathetic fibers from the facial nerve via the greater petrosal nerve. The parasympathetic fibers synapse in the pterygopalatine ganglion for onward transmission to the lacrimal gland and to the mucous glands of the nose.

Q. In Figure 3-36, identify I.

A. The foramen rotundum. It transmits the maxillary division of the trigeminal nerve.

Q. In Figure 3-36, identify J.

A. The posterior wall of the pterygopalatine fossa.

Q. In Figure 3-36, identify K.

A. The posterior boundary of the pterygomaxillary fissure. The pterygomaxillary fissure leads into the pterygopalatine fossa.

Q. In Figure 3-36, identify L.

A. The roof of the infratemporal fossa.

Q. The pterygopalatine fossa is bounded by . . .

A. The perpendicular plate of the palatine bone, medially; the posterior surface of the maxilla, anteriorly; and the body and the pterygoid process of the sphenoid bone, posteriorly.

Q. The two openings in the posterior wall of the pterygopalatine fossa are . . .

A. The foramen rotundum, laterally, and the pterygoid canal, medially.

Q. Through the foramen rotundum passes . . .

A. The maxillary division of the trigeminal nerve.

Q. The maxillary division of the trigeminal nerve conveys sensory fibers to . . .

A. The skin of the face, the interior of the nose, and both surfaces of the palate.

Q. The pterygoid canal is occupied by . . .

A. The nerve of the pterygoid canal and a small branch from the maxillary artery.

Q. The nerve of the pterygoid canal carries . . .

A. The preganglionic parasympathetic fibers from the facial nerve via its greater petrosal branch and the post-ganglionic sympathetic fibers from the superior cervical sympathetic ganglion via the carotid plexus and the deep petrosal nerve.

Q. The preganglionic parasympathetic fibers terminate in . . .

A. The pterygopalatine ganglion.

Q. The postganglionic fibers that result from synapses of the parasympathetic fibers in the pterygopalatine ganglion supply . . .

A. The nasal glands, the palatine glands, some pharyngeal mucous glands, and, most importantly, the lacrimal glands. Hence, the ganglion is sometimes called the "ganglion of hay fever."

Q. The secretomotor fibers reach the lacrimal glands from the pterygopalatine ganglion via . . .

A. The zygomatic branch of the maxillary nerve. The zygomatic nerve enters the orbit through the inferior orbital fissure. In the orbit, the secretomotor fibers leave the zygomatic nerve to join the lacrimal branch of the ophthalmic division of the trigeminal nerve, and hence reach and supply the lacrimal gland.

Q. The zygomatic branch of the maxillary nerve enters a canal in . . .

A. The zygomatic bone, the zygoma.

Q. In the zygomatic bone, the zygomatic nerve divides into two branches. They are . . .

A. The zygomaticotemporal nerve and the zygomaticofacial nerve. They supply the appropriate cutaneous areas.

Q. The maxillary nerve continues through the fossa and leaves it through . . .

A. The infraorbital groove. It emerges on the face through the infraorbital foramen as the infraorbital nerve. It supplies sensory fibers to the skin of the face between the eye and the mouth.

Q. In the infraorbital groove, the infraorbital nerve gives off . . .

A. The middle superior alveolar nerves and the anterior superior alveolar nerves. These nerves supply the premolars, canines, and incisors of the upper jaw.

Q. The posterior superior alveolar nerve, which is a branch of the maxillary nerve, leaves the pterygopalatine fossa via . . .

A. The pterygomaxillary fissure. This constitutes the lateral wall of the fossa. The posterior superior alveolar nerve runs in a groove or canal on the posterior surface of the maxilla before penetrating the bone and dividing to supply the upper molars.

Q. The pterygopalatine ganglion receives fibers from both the nerve of the pterygoid canal and the maxillary nerve. The fibers that synapse in the ganglion are . . .

A. The secretomotor parasympathetic fibers. The sympathetic fibers are already postganglionic, having synapsed in the superior cervical sympathetic ganglion. The sensory fibers have their cell bodies in the trigeminal ganglion. They do not synapse until they reach the trigeminal nucleus in the pons in the central nervous system.

Q. The majority of the fibers leaving the pterygopalatine ganglion are . . .

A. The sensory branches of distribution from the maxillary nerve. They are not true branches of the ganglion.

Q. The branches of the pterygopalatine ganglion are distributed to . . .

A. The palate, the nose, and the pharynx. In addition, the ganglion supplies the branch to the lacrimal gland, as already described.

Q. The smallest named branch of the pterygopalatine ganglion is . . .

A. The pharyngeal nerve. It traverses the palatinovaginal canal to supply the nasopharynx.

Q. The largest branch of the pterygopalatine ganglion is . . .

A. The greater palatine nerve.

Q. The greater palatine nerve descends through the greater palatine canal to terminate by supplying . . .

A. The greater part of the inferior surface of the hard palate. To extract molar or premolar teeth from the upper jaw painlessly, it is necessary to inject local anesthetic close to this nerve. The incisive branch of the nasopalatine nerve supplies a smaller anterior area of the hard palate.

Q. The branches of the greater palatine nerve are . . .

A. The lesser palatine nerves and the nasal branches of the greater palatine nerve.

Q. The lesser palatine nerves supply . . .

A. The mucosa of the soft palate.

Q. The nerve fibers conveyed to the inferior surface of the palate by the palatine nerves carry . . .

A. General sensation and taste from the mucous membrane. They are also secretomotor to the mucous glands.

Q. The tensor palati muscle tenses the soft palate. It is supplied by . . .

A. The mandibular division of the trigeminal nerve.

Q. The levator palati muscle raises the soft palate. It is supplied by . . .

A. The pharyngeal plexus. The motor fibers involved are derived, most probably, from the cranial part of the accessory nerve.

Q. The nasal branches of the pterygopalatine ganglion enter the nose through . . .

A. The sphenopalatine foramen.

Q. The boundaries of the sphenopalatine foramen are . . .

A. The body of the sphenoid bone and the orbital and the sphenoidal processes of the perpendicular plate of the palatine bone.

Q. The largest of the nasal branches of the pterygopalatine ganglion is . . .

A. The nasopalatine nerve. This nerve, accompanied by the sphenopalatine artery, which is the termination of the maxillary artery, runs down the septum of the nose to the incisive foramen.

Q. Smaller nasal branches supply the posterosuperior parts of the medial and the lateral walls of the nose. They are . . .

A. The medial posterior superior nasal branches and the lateral posterior superior nasal branches, respectively.

Q. The maxillary artery enters the pterygopalatine fossa from the infratemporal fossa through . . .

A. The pterygomaxillary fissure.

Q. The maxillary artery leaves the pterygopalatine fossa through . . .

A. The sphenopalatine foramen. It is now named the sphenopalatine artery.

Q. The branches given off by the maxillary artery in the pterygopalatine fossa are . . .

A. The branches that accompany all of the branches of the maxillary nerve and of the pterygopalatine ganglion. They are named appropriately.

THE NOSE AND THE NASAL CAVITY

Q. The upper end of the respiratory tract opens to the exterior at . . .

A. The external nares (nostrils) on the inferior surface of the external nose.

Q. The external nares are bounded on either side by . . .

A. The alae of the nose.

Q. The mobile alae can be flared to permit greater intake of air by . . .

A. The levator labii superioris alaeque nasi muscles and the alar part of the nasalis muscles. Flaring of the nostrils during inspiration at rest is a useful indication of respiratory distress in infants or of anger or fury in adults.

Q. The nerve supply of the nasalis muscle and the levator labii superioris alaeque nasi muscle is . . .

A. The buccal branch of the facial nerve.

Q. The skin over the dorsum of the nose is supplied by branches of . . .

A. The ophthalmic division of the trigeminal nerve via its nasociliary branch.

Q. The cutaneous nerves involved laterally, around the nasofacial crease, are . . .

A. The nasal branches from the infraorbital branch of the maxillary nerve.

Q. The nasociliary nerve supplies two branches to the skin of the nose. They are . . .

A. The infratrochlear nerve and the external nasal nerve. The former supplies the root of the nose. The external nasal nerve emerges between the bony and the cartilaginous parts of the nasal skeleton to supply the remainder of the nasal skin.

Q. The arterial supply to the external nose originates from three sources. They are . . .

A. The dorsal nasal branch of the ophthalmic artery, the nasal branches of the infraorbital branch of the maxillary artery, and the alar and the septal branches of the facial artery.

Q. The lymphatics of the external nose drain to . . .

A. The parotid and the submandibular lymphatic glands.

Q. The skin over the dorsum of the nose is thin and loosely attached to the underlying nasal skeleton. The skin over the alae and tip of the nose is . . .

A. Thick. It contains large sebaceous glands and is firmly attached to the deeper tissues.

Q. The function of the nasal skeleton is to . . .

A. Maintain the patency of the nasal passages.

Q. In Figure 3-37, identify A.

A. The nasion. It is the junction of the nasal process of the frontal bone and the nasal bones. It is readily palpable and is frequently used in craniometry.

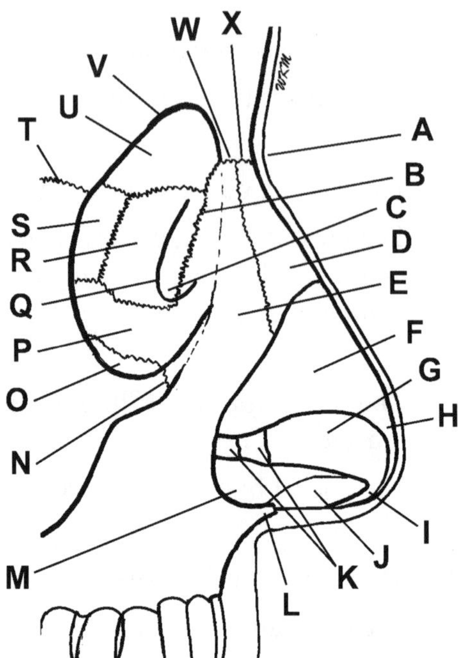

Figure 3-37 The Skeleton of the External Nose and Orbit

Q. In Figure 3-37, identify B.

A. The maxillolacrimal suture. It lies in the floor of the lacrimal groove.

Q. In Figure 3-37, identify C.

A. The superior opening of the nasolacrimal canal.

Q. In Figure 3-37, identify D.

A. The nasal bone. It is often fractured by direct violence.

Q. In Figure 3-37, identify E.

A. The frontal process of the maxilla.

Q. In Figure 3-37, identify F.

A. The right lateral nasal cartilage. Superiorly, it is continuous with the septal cartilage, but anteroinferiorly, the lateral nasal cartilages deviate slightly laterally and are only partially separated from the septal cartilage by a narrow fissure. The fusion of the lateral nasal cartilages with the septal cartilage has led to their alternative joint name of "septodorsal cartilage." Superiorly, both lateral nasal cartilages are firmly attached to the nasal bones.

Q. In Figure 3-37, identify G.

A. The right major alar cartilage.

Q. In Figure 3-37, identify H.

A. The anteroinferior border of the septal (septodorsal) cartilage.

Q. In Figure 3-37, identify I.

A. The septal process of the major alar cartilage. This part of the nasal septum is freely moveable and is called the septum mobile nasi.

Q. In Figure 3-37, identify J.

A. The right external naris. A little more posteriorly, the septum becomes ridged.

Q. In Figure 3-37, identify K.

A. The minor alar cartilages.

Q. In Figure 3-37, identify L.

A. The anterior nasal spine.

Q. In Figure 3-37, identify M.

A. The fibro-adipose part of the ala nasi.

Q. In Figure 3-37, identify N.

A. The zygomaticomaxillary suture on the inferior orbital rim.

Q. In Figure 3-37, identify O.

A. The orbital plate of the zygomatic bone.

Q. In Figure 3-37, identify P.

A. The orbital plate of the maxilla. It forms the thin floor of the orbit. A severe blow to the globe of the eye may drive the globe backward and downward, fracturing this plate. The inferior rectus may get trapped in this fracture, causing fixation of the eye.

Q. In Figure 3-37, identify Q.

A. The nasal crest on the lacrimal bone.

Q. In Figure 3-37, identify R.

A. The lacrimal bone. It is the smallest of the cranial bones.

Q. In Figure 3-37, identify S.

A. The thin orbital plate of the ethmoid bone, the lamina papyracea ethmoidale.

Q. In Figure 3-37, identify T.

A. The zygomaticofrontal suture. It is readily palpable and makes a convenient reference point.

Q. In Figure 3-37, identify U.

A. The orbital plate of the frontal bone.

Q. In Figure 3-37, identify V.

A. The thick superior orbital rim of the frontal bone.

Q. In Figure 3-37, identify W.

A. The frontomaxillary suture.

Q. In Figure 3-37, identify X.

A. The frontonasal suture.

Q. In Figure 3-38, identify A.

A. The frontal sinus. These air sinuses are usually, but not always, bilateral cavities. They are never absolutely symmetrical.

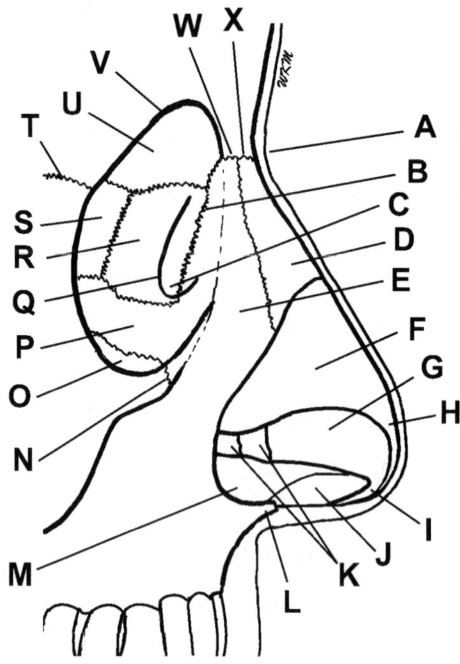

Figure 3-37 The Skeleton of the External Nose and Orbit

Q. In Figure 3-38, identify B.

A. The nasion. It is the location of the frontonasal and frontomaxillary sutures.

Q. In Figure 3-38, identify C.

A. The suture between the two nasal bones.

Q. In Figure 3-38, identify D.

A. The perpendicular plate of the ethmoid bone.

Q. In Figure 3-38, identify E.

A. The septal cartilage. It forms the medial wall of the vestibule and the atrium of the nasal cavity. Note its pointed posterior sphenoidal process.

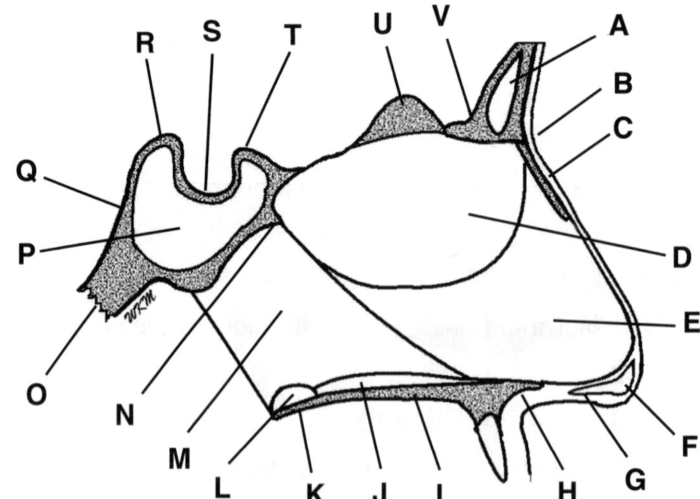

Figure 3-38 The Right Nasal Cavity, Medial (Septal) Wall

Q. In Figure 3-38, identify F.

A. The septal process of the right major alar cartilage. The two septal processes do not join.

Q. In Figure 3-38, identify G.

A. The mobile part of the nasal septum, the septum mobile nasi. It consists of the septal processes (the medial cruri) of the left and right major alar cartilages.

Q. In Figure 3-38, identify H.

A. The anterior nasal spine.

Q. In Figure 3-38, identify I.

A. The palatal process of the maxilla. Together, the right and the left palatal processes of the maxilla form most of the hard palate.

Q. In Figure 3-38, identify J.

A. The nasal crest of the maxilla. With its fellow nasal crest of the opposite side, it forms a groove for the vomer.

Q. In Figure 3-38, identify K.

A. The horizontal palatine process of the palatine bone.

Q. In Figure 3-38, identify L.

A. The nasal crest of the palatine bone.

Q. In Figure 3-38, identify M.

A. The vomer.

Q. In Figure 3-38, identify N.

A. The sphenoidal crest.

Q. In Figure 3-38, identify O.

A. The occipitosphenoidal suture.

Q. In Figure 3-38, identify P.

A. The sphenoidal air sinus. These are paired sinuses, which each open into their respective sphenoethmoidal recess. Inflammation of these sinuses is reputed to impair concentration, an excuse sometimes futilely invoked at examination times or oral examinations.

Q. In Figure 3-38, identify Q.

A. The upper part of the clivus. It is formed by the basisphenoid and the basioccipital bones.

Q. In Figure 3-38, identify R.

A. The dorsum sellae.

Q. In Figure 3-38, identify S.

A. The hypophyseal fossa. Its size is determined by the size of the contained pituitary gland. It tends to be shallower in the elderly.

Q. In Figure 3-38, identify T.

A. The tuberculum sellae. Collectively, the tuberculum sellae, the hypophyseal fossa, and the dorsum sellae are named the sella turcica, the "Turkish saddle."

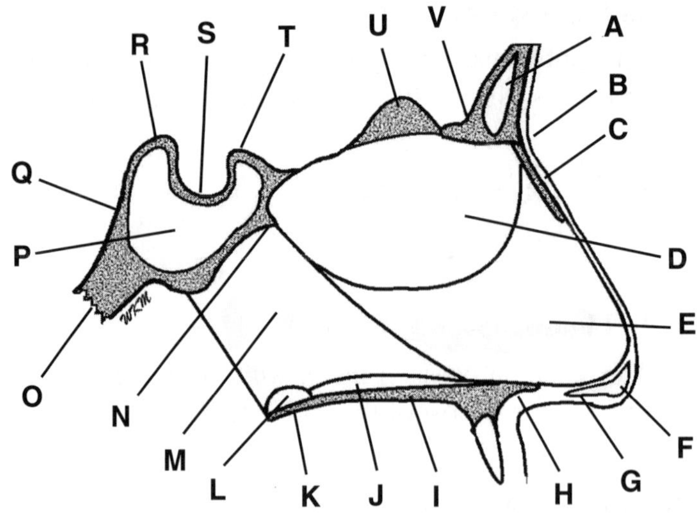

Figure 3-38 The Right Nasal Cavity, Medial (Septal) Wall

Q. In Figure 3-38, identify U.

A. The crista galli of the ethmoid bone. The crista galli serves as an anterior attachment for the falx cerebri.

Q. In Figure 3-38, identify V.

A. The nasal spine of the frontal bone.

Q. In Figure 3-39, identify A.

A. The frontal air sinus.

Q. In Figure 3-39, identify B.

A. The orbital plate of the frontal bone.

Q. In Figure 3-39, identify C.

A. The frontal process of the maxilla.

Q. In Figure 3-39, identify D.

A. The left nasal bone.

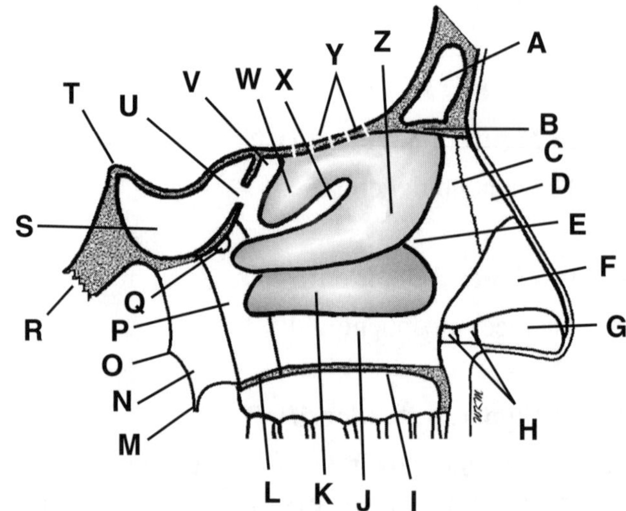

Figure 3-39 The Left Nasal Cavity, Lateral Wall

Q. In Figure 3-39, identify E.

A. The middle meatus of the nose. It lies under the middle concha. The frontal air sinus, the maxillary air sinus, and the anterior and the middle ethmoidal air sinuses open into it.

Q. In Figure 3-39, identify F.

A. The lateral nasal cartilage.

Q. In Figure 3-39, identify G.

A. The left major alar cartilage. The superior border of the major alar cartilage is the limen nasi, the threshold of the nose. The epithelium here changes from skin to respiratory mucosa.

Q. In Figure 3-39, identify H.

A. The minor alar cartilages.

Q. In Figure 3-39, identify I.

A. The palatal process of the maxilla.

Q. In Figure 3-39, identify J.

A. The inferior meatus. The nasolacrimal duct opens into it anteriorly. At its posterior end, the pharyngotympanic tube opens into the nasopharynx.

Q. In Figure 3-39, identify K.

A. The inferior concha. It is the largest of the three nasal conchae, and the only one of the three that is an independent bone.

Q. In Figure 3-39, identify L.

A. The horizontal plate of the palatine bone.

Q. In Figure 3-39, identify M.

A. The pterygoid hamulus. The tensor tympani runs around it to reach the lateral margin of the palatine aponeurosis.

Q. In Figure 3-39, identify N.

A. The medial surface of the medial pterygoid plate.

Q. In Figure 3-39, identify O.

A. The processus tubarius. It is the attachment for the cartilage of the pharyngotympanic tube.

Q. In Figure 3-39, identify P.

A. The perpendicular plate of the palatine bone.

Q. In Figure 3-39, identify Q.

A. The sphenopalatine foramen. It transmits the sphenopalatine branch of the maxillary artery to the nasal cavity and the nasopalatine branch of the maxillary nerve.

Q. In Figure 3-39, identify R.

A. The sphenooccipital suture.

Q. In Figure 3-39, identify S.

A. The sphenoidal air sinus. The pterygoid canal, with its nerve, lies in its floor.

Q. In Figure 3-39, identify T.

A. The dorsum sellae.

Q. In Figure 3-39, identify U.

A. The opening of the sphenoidal sinus into the sphenoethmoidal recess.

Q. In Figure 3-39, identify V.

A. The sphenoethmoidal recess.

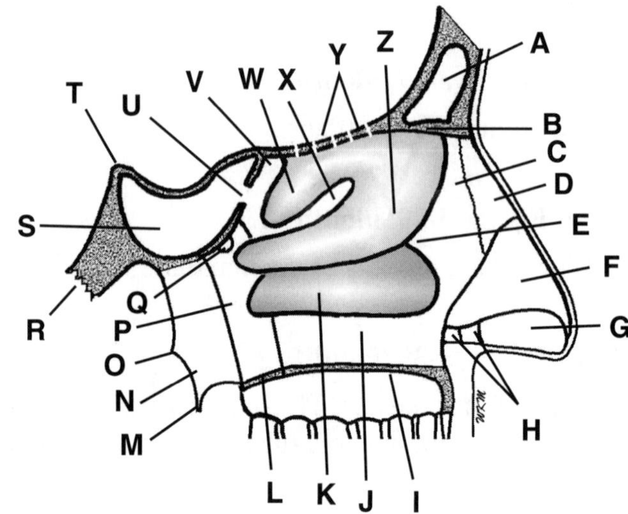

Figure 3-39 The Left Nasal Cavity, Lateral Wall

Q. In Figure 3-39, identify W.

A. The superior nasal concha.

Q. In Figure 3-39, identify X.

A. The superior meatus. The posterior ethmoidal sinuses drain into this meatus.

Q. In Figure 3-39, identify Y.

A. The cribriform plate of the ethmoid bone. The olfactory fibers from the underlying olfactory mucosa exit the nasal cavity through these foramina. They will synapse in the olfactory bulb.

Q. In Figure 3-39, identify Z.

A. The middle concha. It and the middle concha form part of the ethmoid bone. Beneath the middle concha lies the middle meatus, which contains the hiatus semilunaris; the openings of the frontal sinus; the anterior and middle ethmoidal sinuses; and the maxillary sinus.

Q. The external nares open into the nasal cavity, the superior end of the respiratory tract. The cavity of the nose can be divided into three distinct regions. These are . . .

A. The vestibule, which is lined by skin (stratified epithelium); the respiratory region, the nasal cavity proper, which is lined by nasal mucosa (ciliated columnar epithelium); and the olfactory region.

Q. The vestibule has medial and lateral walls composed of . . .

A. The septal and alar cartilages, respectively.

Q. The external opening of the vestibule is, of course, the naris. Posteriorly, its junction with the main nasal cavity is marked by a ridge known as . . .

A. The limen nasi, the threshold of the nose.

Q. The nasal cavity proper has a medial wall, a lateral wall, a roof, and a floor. The roof of the nasal cavity is subdivided into three regions that correspond to the bones involved. The three regions, anteroposteriorly, are . . .

A. The frontal region, the ethmoidal region, and the sphenoidal region.

Q. The floor of the nasal cavity is composed of the palate. The three regions of the palate, anteroposteriorly, are . . .

A. The maxilla, the horizontal plate of the palatine bone, the muscles and aponeurosis of the soft palate, and the uvula.

Q. The medial wall of the nasal cavity, the nasal septum, is rarely flat or strictly in the midline. It is composed of . . .

A. The perpendicular plate of the ethmoid bone and the vomer. The posterior part of the septal cartilage contributes a small area anteroinferiorly.

Q. The lateral wall of the nasal cavity is much more complicated. It is marked by three, anteroposteriorly oriented, prominent elevations. They are . . .

A. The superior nasal concha, which is the smallest; the middle nasal concha; and the inferior nasal concha, which is the largest of the three.

Q. The nasal conchae divide the medial wall into four recesses or passages. They are, from above down and in ascending order of size . . .

A. The sphenoethmoidal recess, the superior meatus, the middle meatus, and the inferior meatus.

Q. The olfactory mucosa is situated in the roof of the sphenoethmoidal recess. This recess has a nasal sinus opening into it. This opening is that of . . .

A. The sphenoidal sinus.

Q. The superior meatus is small and has only one group of sinuses draining into it. They are . . .

A. The posterior ethmoidal sinuses.

Q. The middle meatus commences anteriorly at a dilated area, the atrium. Posterior to the atrium is a semilunar depression known as . . .

A. The hiatus semilunaris.

Q. Posterior to the hiatus semilunaris, the middle ethmoidal sinuses cause a swelling in the middle meatus. This is . . .

A. The bulla ethmoidalis. The openings of the middle ethmoidal sinuses can be found on its surface.

Q. The anterosuperior end of the hiatus semilunaris is usually joined, from the frontal sinus, by the frontonasal duct, together with the openings of the anterior ethmoidal sinuses. Draining into the posterior end of the hiatus semilunaris is . . .

A. The opening of the maxillary sinus. This opening is high on the medial wall of the maxillary sinus. This position clearly hinders the drainage of the maxillary sinus.

Q. Opening into the anterior end of the inferior meatus is . . .

A. The nasolacrimal duct. Just beyond the junction of the nasal cavity with the oropharynx, the pharyngotympanic (Eustachian) tube opens into the lateral wall of the oropharyngeal isthmus.

Q. The nerve supply of the vestibule of the nose is . . .

A. The infraorbital branch of the maxillary nerve.

Q. The anterior ethmoidal branch of the ophthalmic nerve supplies . . .

A. The anterior and superior parts of both the septal and the lateral walls of the nasal cavity.

Q. The remainder of the nasal cavity, the posterior and the inferior parts of both the medial and the lateral walls, and, of course, the floor, are supplied by appropriately named branches from . . .

A. The maxillary nerve and the pterygopalatine ganglion.

Q. The arterial blood supply to the nasal cavity is derived from branches of both . . .

A. The ophthalmic and the maxillary arteries. They correspond in their distribution and, in general, with their names, to the branches of the ophthalmic nerve and the maxillary nerve.

Q. The branch of the ophthalmic artery that contributes to the blood supply of the nose is . . .

A. The nasociliary artery.

Q. The nasociliary artery divides into two terminal branches. They are . . .

A. The anterior ethmoidal artery and the infratrochlear artery.

Q. The anterior ethmoidal artery supplies . . .

A. The upper and anterior part of the nasal septum and the adjacent lateral wall of the nasal cavity.

Q. The branches of the maxillary artery that supply the nasal cavity are . . .

A. The sphenopalatine artery and branches of the descending palatine artery.

Q. The sphenopalatine artery supplies most of . . .

A. The nasal septum.

Q. The descending palatine artery mainly supplies the inferior surface of the palate, but it also supplies . . .

A. The posterior part of the lateral wall of the nasal cavity.

Q. One additional, and important, artery that contributes to the blood supply of the septum is . . .

A. The septal branch of the superior labial branch of the facial artery.

Q. The septal branch of the superior labial artery anastomoses with a septal branch from the anterior ethmoidal artery and with a branch of . . .

A. The sphenopalatine branch of the maxillary artery.

Q. The anastomosis between the septal branch of the anterior ethmoidal artery, the septal branch of the superior labial artery, and the sphenopalatine artery takes place on . . .

A. The medial wall of the vestibule of the nose.

Q. This area is known as . . .

A. Kiesselbach's area. It is notable because it is a frequent site of epistaxis (nose bleeds).

Q. In Figure 3-40, identify A.

A. The orbital plate of the frontal bone.

Q. In Figure 3-40, identify B.

A. The frontal air sinus. It opens via the frontonasal duct (the ethmoidal infundibulum) into the anterior part of the middle meatus of the nose.

Q. The ethmoidal labyrinth consists of . . .

A. A complex of paranasal sinuses enclosed in the lateral part of the ethmoid bone. They are divided into three groups of sinuses that are defined by where they open into the nasal cavity.

Q. In Figure 3-40, identify C.

A. The anterior ethmoidal sinuses. They open into the ethmoidal infundibulum, and hence into the middle meatus of the nose.

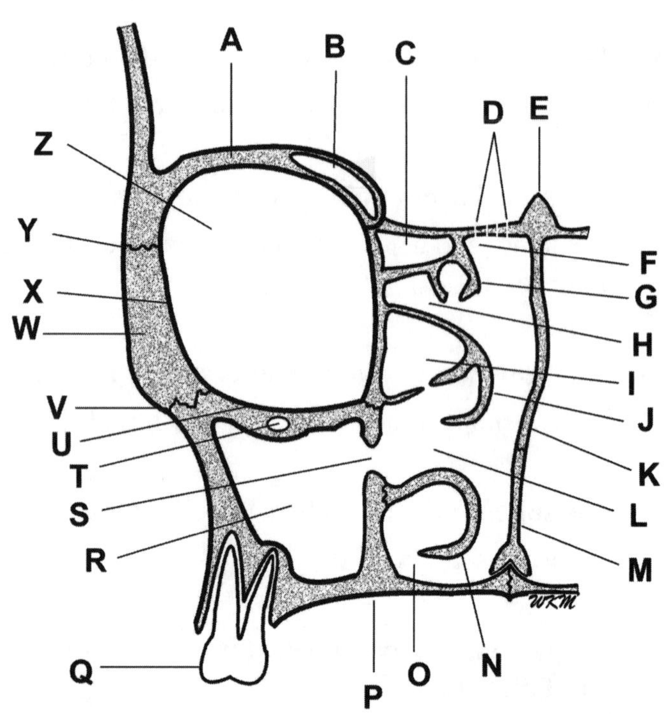

Figure 3-40 Coronal Section Through the Nasal Cavity, the Paranasal Sinuses, and the Orbit

Q. In Figure 3-40, identify D.

A. The cribriform plate of the ethmoid bone.

Q. The apertures in the cribriform plate of the ethmoid are for the passage of . . .

A. Olfactory nerve fibers.

Q. In Figure 3-40, identify E.

A. The crista galli of the ethmoid bone. The anterior end of the falx cerebri is attached to it.

Q. In Figure 3-40, identify F.

A. The sphenoethmoidal recess. The sphenoidal sinus drains into it.

Q. In Figure 3-40, identify G.

A. The superior concha. It is part of the ethmoidal labyrinth.

Q. In Figure 3-40, identify H.

A. The superior meatus of the nose. Only the posterior ethmoidal sinuses drain into it.

Q. In Figure 3-40, identify I.

A. The middle ethmoidal sinuses.

Q. In Figure 3-40, identify J.

A. The middle concha of the nose. It is part of the ethmoidal labyrinth.

Q. In Figure 3-40, identify K.

A. The perpendicular plate of the ethmoid bone. It forms a large part of the nasal septum.

Q. In Figure 3-40, identify L.

A. The middle meatus of the nose. The frontal sinus, the anterior ethmoidal sinuses, the middle ethmoidal sinuses, and the maxillary sinus all open into the middle meatus.

Q. In Figure 3-40, identify M.

A. The vomer. This bone forms the posteroinferior part of the nasal septum.

Q. In Figure 3-40, identify N.

A. The inferior nasal concha. Unlike the middle and superior nasal conchae, it is a separate bone.

Q. In Figure 3-40, identify O.

A. The inferior meatus of the nose. The nasolacrimal duct opens into it anteriorly. The pharyngotympanic tube opens into the lateral wall of the nasopharynx at the posterior end of the inferior meatus. To canulate the pharyngotympanic tube, the canula is passed along the inferior meatus.

Q. In Figure 3-40, identify P.

A. The hard palate. At this point, it consists of the palatal process of the maxilla.

Q. In Figure 3-40, identify Q.

A. The second molar.

Q. In Figure 3-40, identify R.

A. The maxillary sinus. It opens into the hiatus semilunaris in the middle meatus of the nose.

Q. In Figure 3-40, identify S.

A. The opening of the maxillary sinus. Note that it is high on the anterior part of the medial wall of the sinus. This makes drainage difficult in the erect position.

Q. In Figure 3-40, identify T.

A. The infraorbital canal. It carries the infraorbital nerve and its accompanying vessels from the pterygopalatine fossa to the cheek.

Q. In Figure 3-40, identify U.

A. The orbital plate of the maxilla. Posteriorly, it is thin and may be fractured by a blow to the globe of the eye. The inferior rectus muscle is often trapped by this fracture, resulting in immobility of the globe and double vision.

Q. In Figure 3-40, identify V.

A. The zygomaticomaxillary suture. It is readily palpable through the skin.

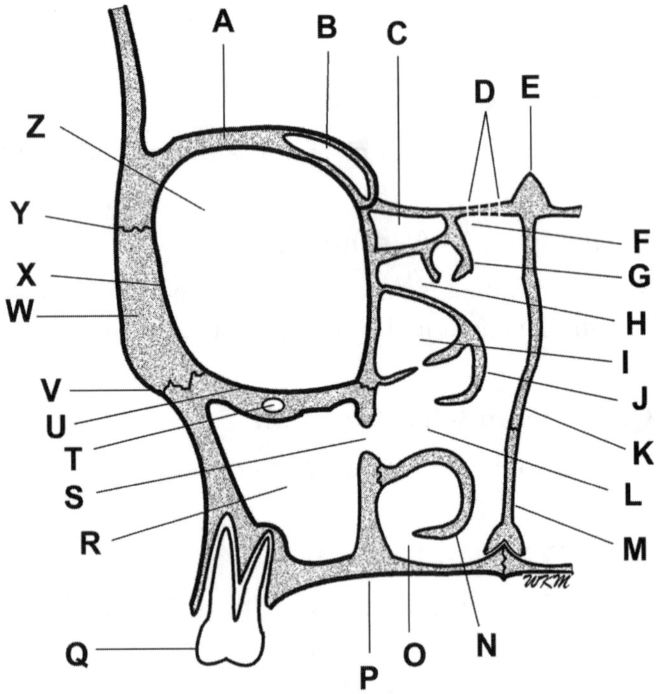

Figure 3-40 Coronal Section Through the Nasal Cavity, the Paranasal Sinuses, and the Orbit

Q. In Figure 3-40, identify W.

A. The zygoma.

Q. In Figure 3-40, identify X.

A. The orbital plate of the zygoma.

Q. In Figure 3-40, identify Y.

A. The zygomaticofrontal suture. It is readily palpable through the skin.

Q. In Figure 3-40, identify Z.

A. The orbit.

THE MOUTH

Q. The vestibule of the mouth is . . .

A. The narrow space between the lips and the cheeks, the gingivae (gums), and the teeth.

Q. When the teeth are clenched, the largest opening between the vestibule and the oral cavity proper is . . .

A. Posterior to the third molar. When treatment of a fractured mandible requires wiring the upper and lower teeth together, this opening is used for liquid feeding.

Q. The vestibule can be subdivided into an anterior region and a posterior region. They are . . .

A. The labial (labiogingival) sulcus, which is between the lips and the gums, and the buccal (buccogingival) sulcus, which is between the cheeks and the gums, respectively.

Q. The muscles of the lips and cheek (the muscles of facial expression) are supplied by branches of the . . .

A. Facial nerve.

Q. The mucous membrane of the vestibule below the level of a line from the angle of the mouth to the external auditory meatus is supplied by . . .

A. The buccal nerve, which is a branch of the mandibular nerve, and the mental nerve. The mental nerve is the continuation of the inferior alveolar nerve, which is itself a branch of the mandibular division of the trigeminal nerve.

Q. The mucous membrane of the vestibule above the level of a line from the angle of the mouth to the external auditory meatus is supplied by . . .

A. The zygomaticofacial nerve, the infraorbital nerve, and the superior alveolar nerves. They are all branches of the maxillary nerve.

Q. The glands that open into the vestibule of the mouth are . . .

A. The labial glands, the buccal glands, and the parotid glands.

Q. The parotid duct, after running horizontally and superficially across the masseter muscle, opens into the vestibule of the mouth opposite . . .

A. The second upper molar. To reach the vestibule of the mouth, the duct penetrates the buccal fat pad and the buccinator muscle. The group of buccal glands that surround this opening are often called the molar glands.

Q. The opening of the parotid duct into the vestibule is marked by . . .

A. The parotid papilla. Redness and swelling of the parotid papilla is often the first sign of mumps (viral infective parotitis).

Q. The oral cavity proper lies within the teeth and the gingivae. It has a roof, a floor, and lateral walls. It is continuous posteriorly, through the oropharyngeal isthmus, with . . .

A. The oropharynx.

Q. The oropharyngeal isthmus is defined laterally by . . .

A. The palatoglossal folds. They overlie the palatoglossal muscles extending from the sides of the soft palate to the sides of the back of the tongue.

Q. The nerve supply of the palatoglossus is . . .

A. The pharyngeal plexus. All of the palatine muscles, with the exception of the tensor palati muscle, are supplied by this plexus. Its fibers probably originate in the cranial part of the accessory nerve, but they travel via the pharyngeal branch of the vagus nerve.

Q. The nerve supply of the tensor palati muscle is . . .

A. The mandibular division of the trigeminal nerve. It also supplies the tensor tympani muscle.

Q. The roof of the oral cavity consists of the hard palate and the soft palate. Their sensory innervation is by . . .

A. The greater and the lesser palatine branches of the maxillary nerve. They also carry secretomotor fibers to the palatine mucous glands.

Q. The floor of the mouth is composed of the dorsum of the tongue in the midline and laterally by . . .

A. The linguogingival sulcus.

Q. The mucosa of the lateral wall of the linguogingival sulcus covers . . .

A. The mylohyoid muscle.

Q. The mucosa of the medial wall of the linguogingival sulcus covers . . .

A. The hyoglossus muscle.

Q. Between the mylohyoid and hyoglossus muscles, deep to the linguogingival fold of mucosa, lie . . .

A. The deep part of the submandibular gland, its duct, and the lingual nerve. This nerve winds around the duct inferiorly, passing from its lateral to its medial side. The deepest structures in this interval are the hypoglossal nerve and its accompanying vein, the vena comitans nervi hypoglossi.

Q. The vena comitans nervi hypoglossi originates from . . .

A. The deep lingual vein. It originates below the tip of the tongue, where it is easily visible.

Q. General sensation from the anterior two-thirds of the dorsum of the tongue is provided by . . .

A. The lingual nerve.

Q. Taste sensation to the anterior two-thirds of the dorsum of the tongue is also carried by the lingual nerve. These fibers leave the lingual nerve via . . .

A. The chorda tympani nerve to reach the facial nerve. Their cell bodies are in the geniculate ganglion of the facial nerve.

Q. The chorda tympani nerve also carries secretomotor fibers to . . .

A. The submandibular salivary gland and to the sublingual salivary gland. It also supplies the mucous glands in the floor of the mouth.

Q. Sensory innervation to the posterior one-third of the dorsum of the tongue is by . . .

A. The glossopharyngeal (ninth cranial) nerve. This nerve carries both general sensation and taste from the posterior one-third of the tongue.

Q. The only muscle supplied by the glossopharyngeal nerve is . . .

A. The stylopharyngeus muscle.

Q. The parasympathetic fibers to the submandibular gland synapse in . . .

A. The submandibular ganglion.

Q. The preganglionic parasympathetic fibers originate from . . .

A. The facial nerve.

Q. The preganglionic fibers to the submandibular glands reach the lingual nerve, and hence the submandibular ganglion, via . . .

A. The chorda tympani nerve.

Q. The hypoglossal nerve supplies all . . .

A. The intrinsic and the extrinsic muscles of the tongue, with the exception of the palatoglossus muscle, which is supplied by the pharyngeal plexus.

Q. Anteriorly, the floor of the linguogingival sulcus is formed by . . .

A. The genioglossus muscle. It lies in contact with, but is superior to, the geniohyoid muscle, which separates it from the anterior part of the mylohyoid muscle.

Q. Also, anteriorly, in the floor of the sulcus lie . . .

A. The submandibular ducts and their papillae and the sublingual salivary glands.

Q. The mucous membrane of the anterior two-thirds of the tongue, that part anterior to the sulcus terminalis, is supplied by . . .

A. The lingual nerve.

Q. The taste fibers from the anterior two-thirds of the tongue travel, at first, with the lingual nerve. They then leave it to join the facial nerve via . . .

A. The chorda tympani nerve.

Q. The muscles of the anterior two-thirds of the tongue are supplied by . . .

A. The hypoglossal nerve. All of the intrinsic and the extrinsic muscles of the tongue, with the exception only of the palatoglossus muscle, are supplied by the hypoglossal nerve.

Q. The mucous membrane of the posterior one-third of the tongue and of the oropharynx is innervated by . . .

A. The glossopharyngeal nerve.

Q. The sensory innervation of the anterior surface of the epiglottis is via . . .

A. The glossopharyngeal nerve.

Q. The sensory innervation of the posterior surface of the epiglottis is via . . .

A. The internal laryngeal branch of the superior laryngeal branch of the vagus nerve.

Q. The muscles of the posterior one-third of the tongue are innervated by . . .

A. The hypoglossal nerve. All the intrinsic and extrinsic muscles of the tongue, with the exception of the palatoglossus muscle, which is supplied by the pharyngeal plexus, are supplied by the hypoglossal nerve.

Q. In Figure 3-41, identify A.

A. The body of the mandible.

Q. In Figure 3-41, identify B.

A. The geniohyoid muscle. It arises from the inferior mandibular spine (the inferior genial tubercle) and inserts onto the body of the hyoid bone.

Q. In Figure 3-41, identify C.

A. The genioglossus muscle. It arises from the superior mandibular spine (the superior genial tubercle). The genioglossus muscle is the muscle responsible for protrusion of the tongue.

Q. In Figure 3-41, identify D.

A. The body and the greater cornu of the hyoid bone.

Q. In Figure 3-41, identify E.

A. The hyoglossus muscle.

Q. In Figure 3-41, identify F.

A. The vallecula. It serves to collect saliva in the intervals between swallowing.

Q. In Figure 3-41, identify G.

A. The epiglottis.

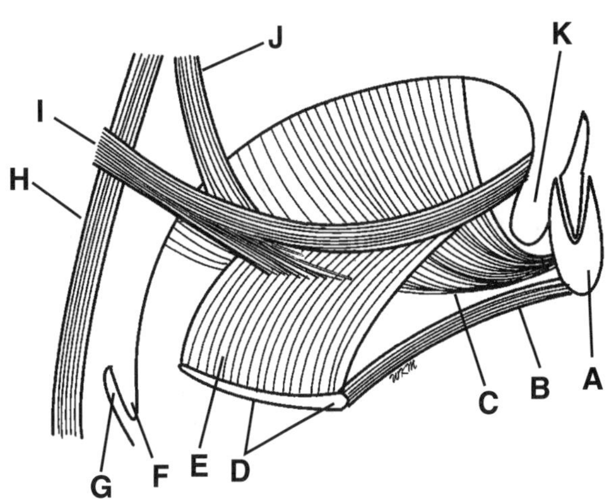

Figure 3-41 The Extrinsic Muscles of the Tongue, Right Lateral Aspect

Q. In Figure 3-41, identify H.

A. The palatopharyngeus muscle. It arises from the side of the soft palate. With the stylopharyngeus muscle and the salpingopharyngeus muscle, it is inserted into the posterior border of the lamina of the thyroid cartilage. The palatopharyngeus muscles are each covered by a mucosal fold. They form the palatopharyngeal arch (posterior pillars of the fauces).

Q. In Figure 3-41, identify I.

A. The styloglossus muscle. It divides anteriorly into a straight part and an oblique portion, which intermingle with the hyoglossus muscle.

Q. In Figure 3-41, identify J.

A. The palatoglossus muscle. The palatoglossal muscles are each covered by a mucosal fold. They form the palatoglossal arch (anterior pillars of the fauces).

Q. The tonsillar fossa lies between . . .

A. The palatoglossal and the palatopharyngeal arches. The palatine tonsil, the "tonsil," lies within it.

Q. In Figure 3-41, identify K.

A. The linguogingival sulcus. Water soluble tablets are rapidly absorbed from this sulcus; thus it is often used when rapid absorption of medication is required. For example, nitroglycerine tablets, which are used to treat coronary artery spasms, are placed here.

Q. In Figure 3-42, identify A.

A. The avascular median fibrous septum of the tongue. It is used as an avascular plane to minimize bleeding from the tongue during surgical hemiglossectomy.

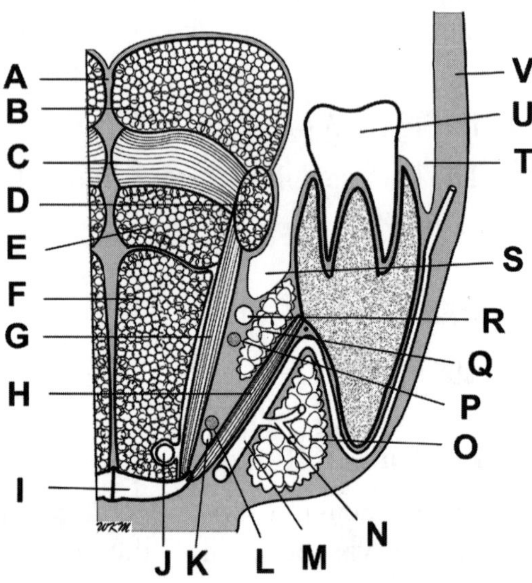

Figure 3-42 The Floor of the Mouth, Coronal Section

Q. In Figure 3-42, identify B.

A. The intrinsic superior longitudinal muscle of the tongue.

Q. In Figure 3-42, identify C.

A. The intrinsic transverse muscle of the tongue.

Q. In Figure 3-42, identify D.

A. The styloglossus muscle. It is a true extrinsic muscle of the tongue.

Q. In Figure 3-42, identify E.

A. The intrinsic inferior longitudinal muscle of the tongue.

Q. The nerve supply of the intrinsic muscles of the tongue is by . . .

A. The hypoglossal nerve. The hypoglossal nerve supplies all of the intrinsic and extrinsic muscles of the tongue except the palatoglossus muscle, which, despite its name, is a muscle of the soft palate.

Q. In Figure 3-42, identify F.

A. The genioglossus muscle.

Q. In Figure 3-42, identify G.

A. The hyoglossus muscle.

Q. In Figure 3-42, identify H.

A. The mylohyoid muscle. It extends from the front of the body of the hyoid bone to the mylohyoid line on the mandible. Its medial fibers interlace with those of the opposite side to form a median raphe and complete the floor of the mouth.

Q. The innervation of the mylohyoid muscle is by . . .

A. The nerve to the mylohyoid. It originates from the inferior alveolar branch of the mandibular division of the trigeminal nerve. It can be seen, unlabelled, in Figure 3-42, in the angle between the mylohyoid muscle and the mandible.

Q. The other muscle supplied by the nerve to the mylohyoid muscle is . . .

A. The anterior belly of the digastric muscle, in which the nerve terminates.

Q. The posterior belly of the digastric muscle is supplied by . . .

A. The facial nerve.

Q. In Figure 3-42, identify I.

A. The body of the hyoid bone.

Q. In Figure 3-42, identify J.

A. The lingual artery. It is a branch of the external carotid artery.

Q. In Figure 3-42, identify K.

A. The venae comitans nervi hypoglossi. The lingual artery runs deep to the hyoglossus muscle; the venae comitans run with the hypoglossal nerve in the interval between the hyoglossus muscle and the mylohyoid muscle.

Q. In Figure 3-42, identify L.

A. The hypoglossal nerve.

Q. In Figure 3-42, identify M.

A. The facial artery. It ascends on the medial side of the submandibular salivary gland, loops over its superior border, and then descends between it and the mandible. It causes a groove in the inferior border of the mandible. At this point, the artery can be readily palpated.

Q. In Figure 3-42, identify N.

A. The branch of the facial artery to the submandibular salivary gland.

Q. In Figure 3-42, identify O.

A. The larger, superficial part of the submandibular salivary gland. Its smaller, deeper part lies deep to the mylohyoid muscle on the surface of the hyoglossus muscle (see Figure 3-43).

Q. In Figure 3-42, identify P.

A. The lingual nerve.

Q. In Figure 3-42, identify Q.

A. The sublingual salivary gland. It lies anterior to the deep part of the submandibular gland and has numerous ducts that open into the linguogingival sulcus.

Q. In Figure 3-42, identify R.

A. The submandibular duct.

Q. In Figure 3-42, identify S.

A. The linguogingival sulcus.

Q. In Figure 3-42, identify T.

A. The labiogingival sulcus.

Q. In Figure 3-42, identify U.

A. The crown of the second lower molar.

Q. In Figure 3-42, identify V.

A. The cheek.

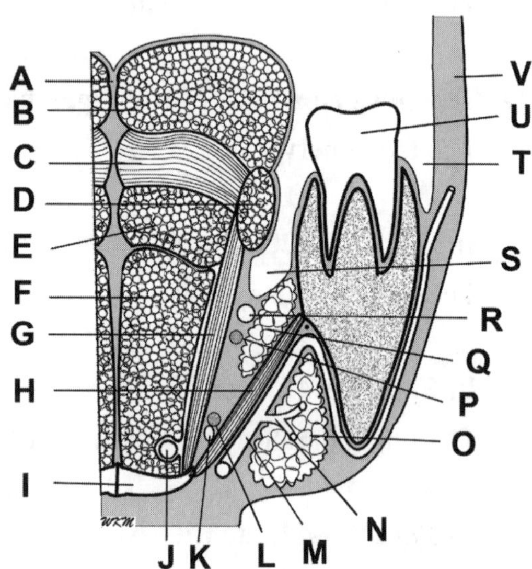

Figure 3-42 The Floor of the Mouth, Coronal Section

Q. In Figure 3-43, identify A.

A. The sublingual papilla. The submandibular duct opens at its apex.

Q. In Figure 3-43, identify B.

A. The lingual nerve. At this point, it is carrying both taste and general sensation from the anterior two-thirds of the tongue. It is also carrying postganglionic secretomotor fibers to the sublingual salivary gland and to mucous glands on the tongue and in the linguogingival sulcus. Notice that it crosses the submandibular duct twice.

Q. In Figure 3-43, identify C.

A. The duct of the submandibular salivary gland.

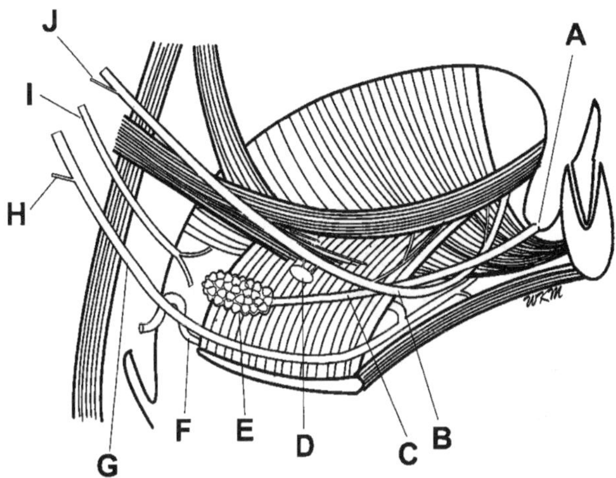

Figure 3-43 The Nerves of the Tongue, Right Lateral Aspect

Q. In Figure 3-43, identify D.

A. The submandibular parasympathetic ganglion. Preganglionic parasympathetic fibers synapse here. The resulting postganglionic fibers are secretomotor to the submandibular and sublingual salivary glands and to mucous glands in the floor of the mouth.

Q. In Figure 3-43, identify E.

A. The deep part of the submandibular salivary gland. It is continuous with the larger superficial part of the submandibular gland, which extends around the posterior border of the mylohyoid muscle onto its superficial surface.

Q. In Figure 3-43, identify F.

A. The characteristic upward loop of the lingual artery at the point where it is crossed by the hypoglossal nerve. It then leaves the nerve to run deep to the hyoglossus muscle.

Q. In Figure 3-43, identify G.

A. The hypoglossal nerve. It supplies all of the intrinsic and all of the true extrinsic muscles of the tongue. Although it can be seen giving a branch to the geniohyoid muscle, these latter nerve fibers have originated from the anterior primary ramus of the first cervical nerve.

Q. In Figure 3-43, identify H.

A. The branch from the first cervical nerve to the hypoglossal nerve.

Q. In Figure 3-43, identify I.

A. The glossopharyngeal nerve. It crosses the floor of the tonsillar fossa to reach the side of the posterior one-third of the tongue, to which it supplies taste fibers. It also supplies the fibers that carry general sensation from the posterior one-third of the tongue and the oropharynx.

Q. In Figure 3-43, identify J.

A. The chorda tympani nerve. It arises from the facial nerve in the middle ear and supplies parasympathetic and taste fibers to the lingual nerve.

THE PHARYNX

Q. In Figure 3-44, identify A.

A. The mastoid process.

Q. In Figure 3-44, identify B.

A. The styloid process of the petrous temporal bone. The stylohyoid ligament passes from its tip to the lesser cornu of the hyoid bone.

Q. The three muscles arising from the styloid process are . . .

A. The styloglossus muscle, the stylohyoid muscle, and the stylopharyngeus muscle.

Q. The nerves that supply these muscles are . . .

A. The hypoglossal nerve, supplying the styloglossus muscle; the facial nerve, supplying the stylohyoid muscle; and the glossopharyngeal nerve, supplying the stylopharyngeus muscle.

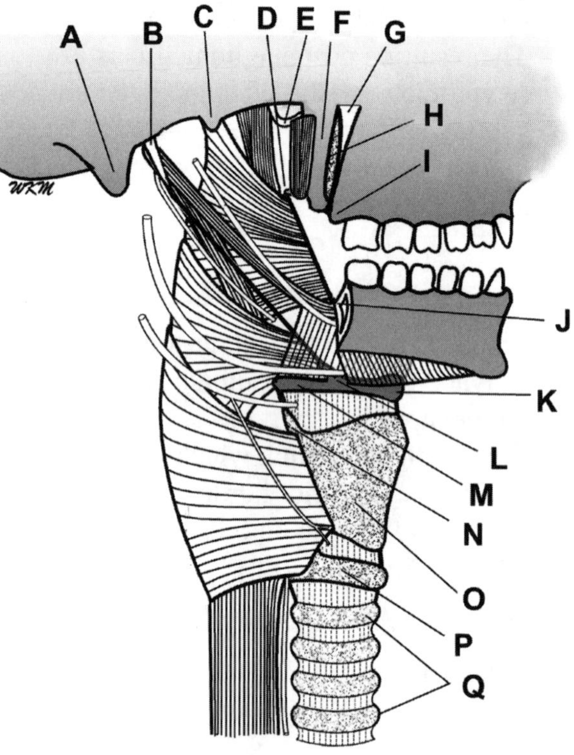

Figure 3-44 Lateral View of the Pharynx and Larynx, Skeletal Elements

Q. In Figure 3-44, identify C.

A. The pharyngeal tubercle of the occipital bone. The tubercle is a midline structure, and the posterior raphe of the pharyngeal constrictor muscles attaches to it.

Q. In Figure 3-44, identify D.

A. The pterygoid hamulus. The tendon of the tensor palati muscle loops around this "pulley" to join its aponeurosis. The pterygomandibular raphe, which provides the origin for the superior constrictor muscle of the pharynx and the buccinator muscle, is attached to its tip.

Q. In Figure 3-44, identify E.

A. The cartilage of the pharyngotympanic tube.

Q. In Figure 3-44, identify F.

A. The lateral surface of the medial pterygoid plate. It is the origin of the tensor palati muscle.

Q. In Figure 3-44, identify G.

A. The pterygomaxillary fissure. It leads into the pterygopalatine fossa. The maxillary artery enters the pterygopalatine fossa through this fissure. The maxillary nerve enters the pterygopalatine fossa via the foramen rotundum.

Q. In Figure 3-44, identify H.

A. The cut surface of the lateral pterygoid plate.

Q. In Figure 3-44, identify I.

A. The tuberosity of the maxilla. It provides attachment for part of the buccinator muscle.

Q. In Figure 3-44, identify J.

A. The posterior end of the mylohyoid line on the medial (lingual) surface of the mandible. It provides the inferior attachment of the pterygomandibular raphe.

Q. In Figure 3-44, identify K.

A. The body of the hyoid bone. Its upper border is covered by the fibers of the mylohyoid muscle, which arise from its anterior surface.

Q. In Figure 3-44, identify L.

A. The base of the lesser cornu of the hyoid bone. It is obscured by the origin of the hyoglossus muscle, which arises from its lateral surface.

Q. In Figure 3-44, identify M.

A. The greater cornu of the hyoid bone.

Q. In Figure 3-44, identify N.

A. The superior horn of the thyroid cartilage. It is attached to the tip of the greater cornu of the hyoid bone by the lateral thyrohyoid ligament.

Q. In Figure 3-44, identify O.

A. The right lamina of the thyroid cartilage. Its oblique line provides attachment for the inferior pharyngeal constrictor muscle posteriorly, the thyrohyoid muscle superiorly, and the sternothyroid muscle inferiorly. The laryngeal prominence can be seen on its anterior border. It is much more obvious in adult males than in females and children. The change in the thyroid cartilages, which causes this increased prominence in the pubescent male, results in lengthening the vocal cords and hence the deepening and “breaking” of the juvenile male voice.

Q. In Figure 3-44, identify P.

A. The anterior arch of the cricoid cartilage.

Q. In Figure 3-44, identify Q.

A. The first four cartilaginous rings of the trachea.

Q. In Figure 3-45, identify A.

A. The styloglossus muscle. It arises from the anterolateral surface of the styloid process of the temporal bone.

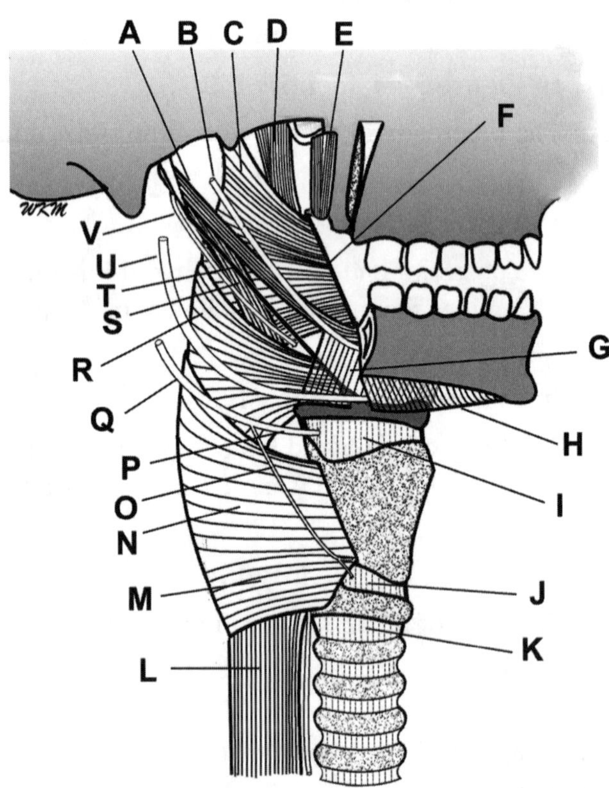

Figure 3-45 Lateral View of the Pharynx and the Larynx: Membranes, Muscles, and Nerves

Q. In Figure 3-45, identify B.

A. The lingual nerve. It is sensory to the anterior two-thirds of the tongue.

Q. In Figure 3-45, identify C.

A. The superior constrictor muscle of the pharynx.

Q. In Figure 3-45, identify D.

A. The levator palatae muscle. It is seen through the triangular interval in the lateral pharyngeal wall, which is closed by the pharyngobasilar fascia. The pharyngobasilar fascia is penetrated by the nasopharyngeal opening of the pharyngotympanic tube. The levator palatae muscle is supplied by the pharyngeal plexus.

Q. In Figure 3-45, identify E.

A. The tensor palati muscle. Its tendon winds around the pterygoid hamulus to be inserted into the side of the soft palate.

Q. The nerve supply of the tensor palati is . . .

A. The mandibular division of the trigeminal nerve. The tensor tympani muscle is supplied by the same nerve.

Q. In Figure 3-45, identify F.

A. The pterygomandibular raphe. Posteriorly, it gives origin to the superior constrictor muscle of the pharynx. The buccinator muscle, which forms the lateral wall of the oral cavity, arises from the anterior margin of the raphe.

Q. In Figure 3-45, identify G.

A. The hyoglossus muscle. The lingual nerve crosses it superiorly, and the hypoglossal nerve crosses it inferiorly. Both these nerves and the submandibular duct lie between the hyoglossus muscle and the mylohyoid muscle.

Q. In Figure 3-45, identify H.

A. The mylohyoid muscle. The two mylohyoid muscles meet in the midline and form a raphe under the chin. Together they form the floor of the oral cavity.

Q. The nerve supply of the mylohyoid muscle is . . .

A. The mylohyoid branch of the inferior alveolar nerve, which is itself a branch of the mandibular division of the trigeminal nerve.

Q. In Figure 3-45, identify I.

A. The thyrohyoid membrane. It is thickened posteriorly to form the lateral thyrohyoid ligament and in the midline to form the median thyrohyoid ligament.

Q. In Figure 3-45, identify J.

A. The lateral cricothyroid ligament. The right and left cricothyroid ligaments meet anteriorly, in the midline, to form the median cricothyroid ligament. It is the elective site for establishing an emergency surgical airway. This procedure is sometimes called a tracheotomy, but it is really a cricothyrotomy.

Q. In Figure 3-45, identify K.

A. The cricotracheal ligament.

Q. In Figure 3-45, identify L.

A. The esophagus.

Q. In Figure 3-45, identify M.

A. The cricopharyngeal part of the inferior constrictor muscle. It may act as a mild sphincter of the pharynx. Its hypertrophy is believed to be the cause of an acquired pharyngeal diverticulum (pouch), which is referred to as "Zenker's diverticulum."

Q. In Figure 3-45, identify N.

A. The thyropharyngeal part of the inferior constrictor muscle.

Q. In Figure 3-45, identify O.

A. The external laryngeal branch of the superior laryngeal nerve.

Q. In Figure 3-45, identify P.

A. The internal laryngeal branch of the superior laryngeal nerve.

Q. The internal laryngeal nerve enters the larynx through . . .

A. The posterior part of the thyrohyoid membrane to enter the larynx between the middle and inferior constrictor muscles of the pharynx.

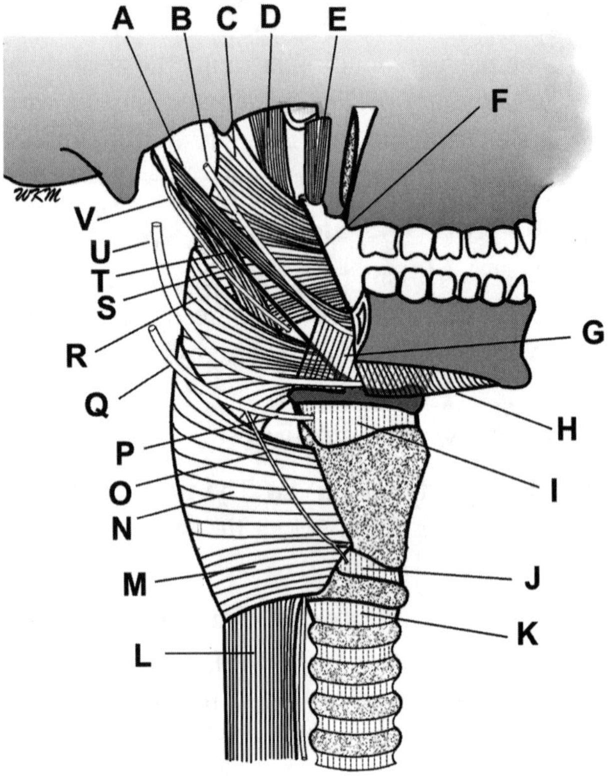

Figure 3-45 Lateral View of the Pharynx and the Larynx: Membranes, Muscles, and Nerves

Q. The internal laryngeal branch of the superior laryngeal nerve supplies . . .

A. The mucous membrane of the larynx and the pharynx from the epiglottis to the glottis.

Q. In Figure 3-45, identify Q.

A. The superior laryngeal branch of the vagus nerve. It is accompanied by the superior thyroid branch of the external carotid artery.

Q. In Figure 3-45, identify R.

A. The middle constrictor muscle of the pharynx.

Q. In Figure 3-45, identify S.

A. The stylopharyngeus muscle. It is inserted into the posterior border of the lamina of the thyroid cartilage.

Q. Besides the stylopharyngeus muscle, two other muscles are inserted into the posterior border of the lamina of the thyroid cartilage. They are . . .

A. The salpingopharyngeus muscle and the palatopharyngeus muscle.

Q. In Figure 3-45, identify T.

A. The stylohyoid ligament. Its inferior attachment to the lesser cornu of the hyoid bone is obscured by the origin of the hyoglossus muscle.

Q. In Figure 3-45, identify U.

A. The hypoglossal nerve. It supplies all of the intrinsic and extrinsic muscle of the tongue.

Q. The hypoglossal nerve reaches the tongue by running in the angle between the origins of . . .

A. The mylohyoid muscle and the hyoglossus muscles.

Q. The palatoglossus muscle is neither an intrinsic or extrinsic muscle of the tongue. It is a muscle of the pharynx, as is the levator palatae muscle, so they are both supplied via . . .

A. The pharyngeal plexus. It has been suggested that the fibers from the pharyngeal plexus to the palatoglossus muscle and levator palatae muscle may originate only from the cranial part of the accessory nerve rather than from the vagus nerve.

Q. In Figure 3-45, identify V.

A. The glossopharyngeal nerve. It winds around the lower border of the stylopharyngeus muscle to enter the oropharynx between the middle and superior constrictor muscles of the pharynx.

Q. The nerve supply of the stylopharyngeus muscle is . . .

A. The glossopharyngeal nerve. It is thought to be the only muscle supplied by the glossopharyngeal nerve, although this nerve also contributes branches to the pharyngeal plexus.

Q. Besides the stylopharyngeus muscle, the glossopharyngeal nerve supplies . . .

A. General sensation and taste fibers to the posterior one-third of the tongue and the oropharynx.

Q. The nerve supply of the constrictor muscles of the pharynx is from . . .

A. The pharyngeal plexus. Although the pharyngeal nerves appear to originate from the vagus nerve, they probably obtain most of their fibers from the cranial part of the accessory (11th cranial) nerve.

THE LARYNX

Q. All of the laryngeal muscles, with the exception of the cricothyroid muscle, which is supplied by the external laryngeal nerve, are supplied by . . .

A. The recurrent laryngeal nerve. The nerve also supplies the mucous membrane of the larynx below the glottis.

Q. The recurrent laryngeal nerve is closely associated with . . .

A. The inferior thyroid artery.

Q. Damage to both recurrent laryngeal nerves during a thyroidectomy leads to . . .

A. Difficulty with speaking, as well as difficulty with breathing, due to the unopposed action of the cricothyroid muscles. The dyspnoea may be severe enough to require intubation.

Q. Unopposed action of the cricothyroid muscles results in . . .

A. Tightening and adduction of the vocal ligaments.

Q. The cricothyroid muscles are supplied by . . .

A. The external laryngeal branches of the superior laryngeal nerves.

Q. Paralysis of both cricothyroid muscles results in . . .

A. Inability to sing a high note.

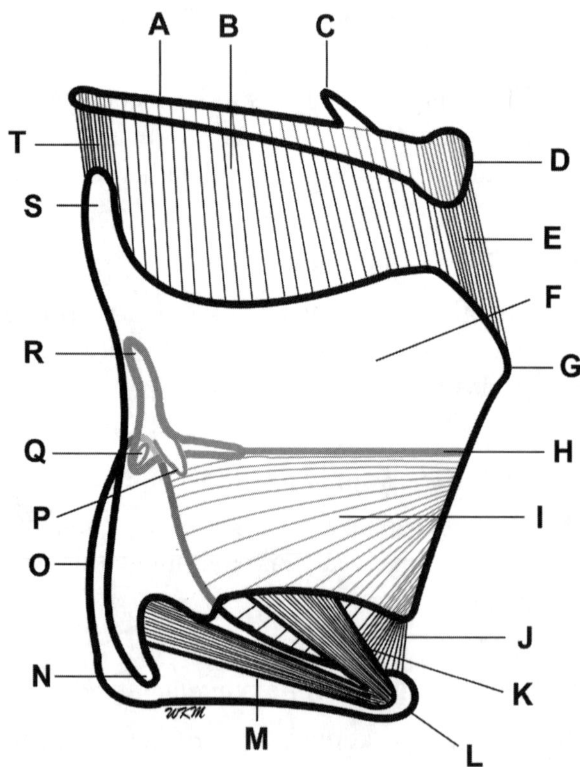

Figure 3-46 The Laryngeal Skeleton, Right Lateral Aspect

Q. In Figure 3-46, identify A.

A. The greater cornu of the hyoid bone. It is readily palpable and is frequently broken during manual strangulation.

Q. In Figure 3-46, identify B.

A. The thyrohyoid membrane. It is perforated posteriorly by the internal laryngeal nerve and by the superior laryngeal vessels.

Q. In Figure 3-46, identify C.

A. The lesser cornu of the hyoid bone. The stylohyoid ligament is attached to its apex.

Q. In Figure 3-46, identify D.

A. The body of the hyoid bone. It lies at the level of the fourth cervical vertebra.

Q. In Figure 3-46, identify E.

A. The median thyrohyoid ligament. It is much thicker than the thyrohyoid membrane. Both are attached to the upper margin of the posterior (deep) surface of the hyoid bone, from which they are separated by a bursa.

Q. In Figure 3-46, identify F.

A. The right lamina of the thyroid cartilage.

Q. In Figure 3-46, identify G.

A. The laryngeal prominence. It is readily palpable, particularly in men. In the male it becomes increasingly prominent as puberty continues into manhood, and the voice "breaks."

Q. In Figure 3-46, identify H.

A. The anterior attachment of the right vocal ligament. Posteriorly, it is attached to the tip of the vocal process of the right arytenoid cartilage.

Q. In Figure 3-46, identify I.

A. The right lateral cricothyroid ligament. Its upper part is seen through the right lamina of the thyroid cartilage. It is also known as the cricovocal membrane, because its upper margin is thickened to form the vocal ligament.

Q. In Figure 3-46, identify J.

A. The thick median (anterior) cricothyroid ligament.

Q. In Figure 3-46, identify K.

A. The "straight" part of the cricothyroid muscle.

Q. In Figure 3-46, identify L.

A. The anterior arch of the cricoid cartilage.

Q. In Figure 3-46, identify M.

A. The "oblique" part of the cricothyroid muscle.

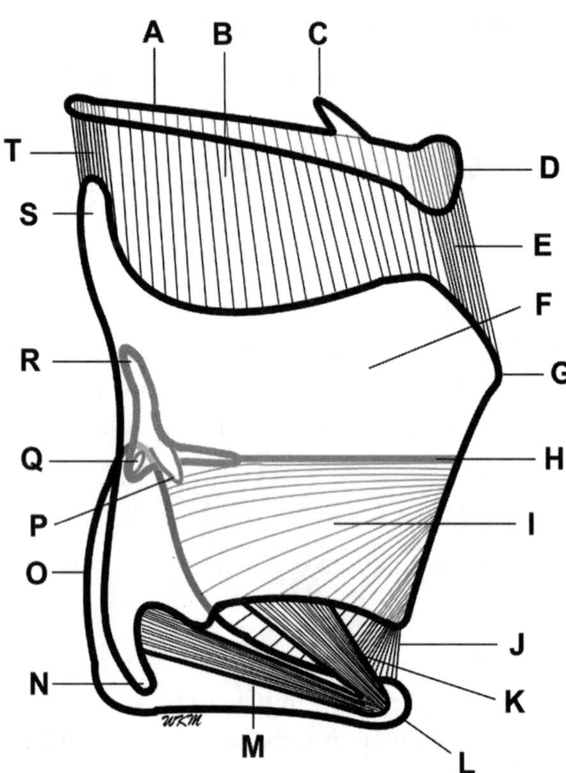

Figure 3-46 The Laryngeal Skeleton, Right Lateral Aspect

Q. The action of the cricothyroid muscle is to tighten . . .

A. The vocal ligaments by rotating the cricoid cartilage with respect to the thyroid cartilage. The movement takes place at the synovial cricothyroid articulation.

Q. The nerve supply of the cricothyroid muscle is . . .

A. The external laryngeal branch of the superior laryngeal nerve. It runs with the superior thyroid artery. It is at risk during ligature of that artery, as performed during a thyroidectomy.

Q. In Figure 3-46, identify N.

A. The inferior horn of the thyroid cartilage. It articulates with the lateral edge of the lamina of the cricoid cartilage and allows pivoting of the thyroid cartilage on the cricoid cartilage.

Q. In Figure 3-46, identify O.

A. The lamina of the cricoid cartilage. It articulates superiorly with the arytenoid cartilage.

Q. In Figure 3-46, identify P.

A. The muscular process of the arytenoid cartilage. Both the posterior and the lateral cricoarytenoid muscles gain attachment to it.

Q. In Figure 3-46, identify Q.

A. The articulation between the arytenoid cartilage and the cricoid cartilage. The shapes of the articular facets are such that lateral rotation of the arytenoid cartilage on the cricoid cartilage is accompanied by a lateral sliding movement of the arytenoid cartilage. This movement further opens the glottis.

Q. In Figure 3-46, identify R.

A. The superior process of the right arytenoid cartilage, as seen through the right lamina of the thyroid cartilage

Q. In Figure 3-46, identify S.

A. The right superior horn of the thyroid cartilage.

Q. In Figure 3-46, identify T.

A. The right lateral thyrohyoid ligament.

Q. In Figure 3-47, identify A.

A. The epiglottis, sectioned in the midline.

Q. In Figure 3-47, identify B.

A. The elastic hyoepiglottic ligament.

Q. In Figure 3-47, identify C.

A. The body of the hyoid bone, sectioned in the midline.

Q. In Figure 3-47, identify D.

A. The median thyrohyoid ligament.

Q. In Figure 3-47, identify E.

A. The thyroid cartilage sectioned in the midline.

Q. In Figure 3-47, identify F.

A. The right vestibular ligament.

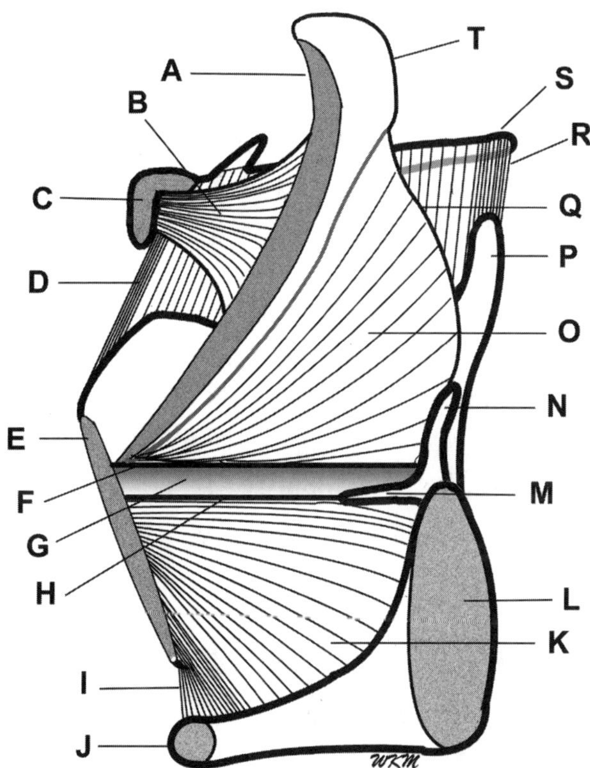

Figure 3-47 The Laryngeal Skeleton, Sagittal Section

Q. In Figure 3-47, identify G.

A. The ventricle of the larynx. Each saccule of the larynx extends upward from it between the vestibular folds and the thyroid cartilage. They contain numerous mucous glands, whose secretions serve to lubricate the vocal folds.

Q. In Figure 3-47, identify H.

A. The right vocal ligament.

Q. In Figure 3-47, identify I.

A. The median cricothyroid ligament. This site is often used for creating an emergency surgical airway. The procedure is often called an emergency tracheotomy, but it is really a cricothyrotomy.

Q. In Figure 3-47, identify J.

A. The sagittally cut anterior arch of the cricoid cartilage.

Q. In Figure 3-47, identify K.

A. The lateral cricothyroid ligament. It is also known as the cricovocal membrane. The thickened, free, upper margin of the lateral cricothyroid ligament is the vocal ligament.

Q. In Figure 3-47, identify L.

A. The sagittally cut lamina of the thyroid cartilage.

Q. In Figure 3-47, identify M.

A. The vocal process of the arytenoid cartilage.

Q. In Figure 3-47, identify N.

A. The superior process of the arytenoid cartilage. The margin of the aryepiglottic fold is attached to its apex.

Q. In Figure 3-47, identify O.

A. The quadrangular membrane.

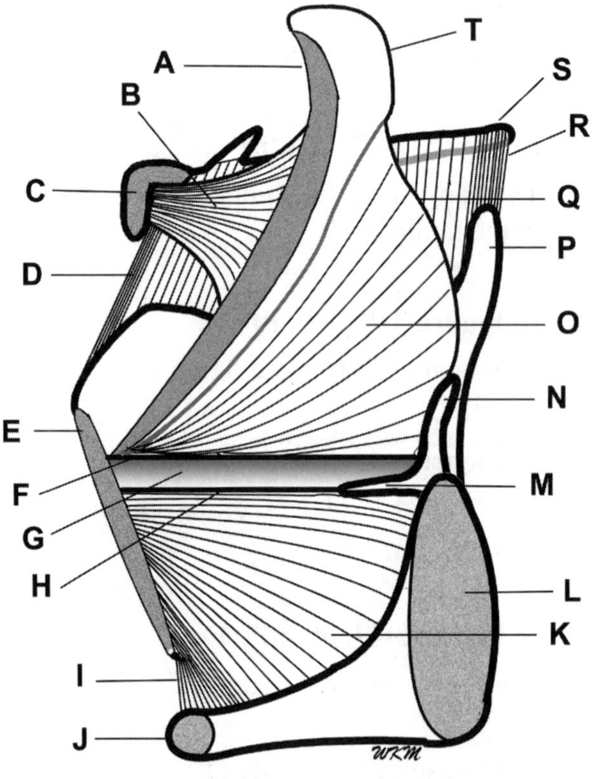

Figure 3-47 The Laryngeal Skeleton, Sagittal Section

Q. In Figure 3-47, identify P.

A. The superior cornu of the thyroid cartilage.

Q. In Figure 3-47, identify Q.

A. The margin of the aryepiglottic fold. It contains two small cartilages: the corniculate and the cuneiform cartilages.

Q. In Figure 3-47, identify R.

A. The thickened lateral thyrohyoid ligament.

Q. In Figure 3-47, identify S.

A. The greater cornu of the hyoid bone.

Q. In Figure 3-47, identify T.

A. The free margin of the epiglottis.

Q. In Figure 3-48, identify A.

A. The posterior (pharyngeal) surface of the epiglottis. The anterior surface of the upper part of the epiglottis forms the posterior wall of the vallecula.

Q. In Figure 3-48, identify B.

A. The left greater cornu of the hyoid bone. It is attached to the superior horn of the left thyroid lamina by the left lateral thyrohyoid ligament.

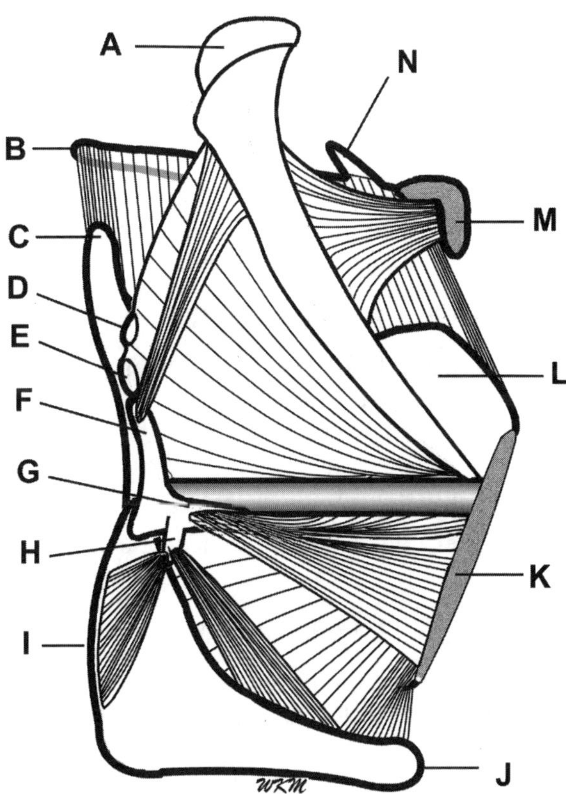

Figure 3-48 Larynx Dissection, Right Aspect: Bones and Cartilages

Q. In Figure 3-48, identify C.

A. The superior horn of the left thyroid lamina.

Q. In Figure 3-48, identify D.

A. The right cuneiform cartilage. It is a small wedge-shaped cartilage in the margin of the aryepiglottic fold. During laryngoscopy, it is often visible as a small white nodule.

Q. In Figure 3-48, identify E.

A. The corniculate cartilage. It articulates with the superior horn of the arytenoid cartilage. It is easily seen during laryngoscopy.

Q. In Figure 3-48, identify F.

A. The superior process of the right arytenoid cartilage. The right aryepiglottic fold is attached to its tip.

Q. In Figure 3-48, identify G.

A. The vocal process of the right arytenoid cartilage. The vocal ligament is the thickened superior margin of the lateral cricothyroid ligament, which is also named the conus elasticus. The vocal ligament is attached to the tip of the vocal process of the arytenoid cartilage. The vocalis muscle lies parallel to it, on its lateral side.

Q. In Figure 3-48, identify H.

A. The lateral, muscular process of the right arytenoid cartilage. The right posterior cricoarytenoideus muscle and the right lateral cricoarytenoideus muscle are attached to its tip.

Q. In Figure 3-48, identify I.

A. The posterior surface of the lamina of the cricoid cartilage. It gives origin to the right posterior cricoarytenoideus muscle.

Q. In Figure 3-48, identify J.

A. The anterior arch of the cricoid cartilage.

Q. In Figure 3-48, identify K.

A. The thyroid cartilage. It has been sectioned in the midline.

Q. In Figure 3-48, identify L.

A. The left lamina of the thyroid cartilage.

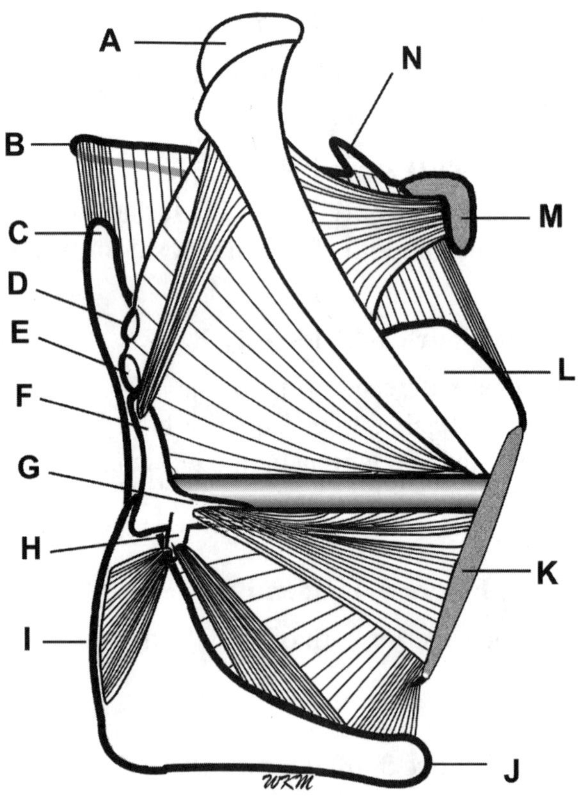

Figure 3-48 Larynx Dissection, Right Aspect: Bones and Cartilages

Q. In Figure 3-48, identify M.

A. The body of the hyoid bone. It has been sectioned in the midline. The hyoid bone can be considered to be the skeleton of the tongue.

Q. In Figure 3-48, identify N.

A. The lesser cornu of the hyoid bone. It is suspended from the skull by the right stylohyoid ligament.

Q. In Figure 3-49, identify A.

A. The thyrohyoid membrane.

Q. In Figure 3-49, identify B.

A. The left lateral cricothyroid ligament. It is the thickened posterior margin of the cricothyroid membrane.

Q. In Figure 3-49, identify C.

A. The aryepiglotticus muscle. It is largely responsible for closing the laryngeal inlet during swallowing.

Q. In Figure 3-49, identify D.

A. The right quadrangular ligament. It has the aryepiglotticus muscle on its lateral surface and is covered with mucous membrane. Together, these structures constitute the aryepiglottic fold. The right and left aryepiglottic folds are largely responsible for closing the larynx during swallowing.

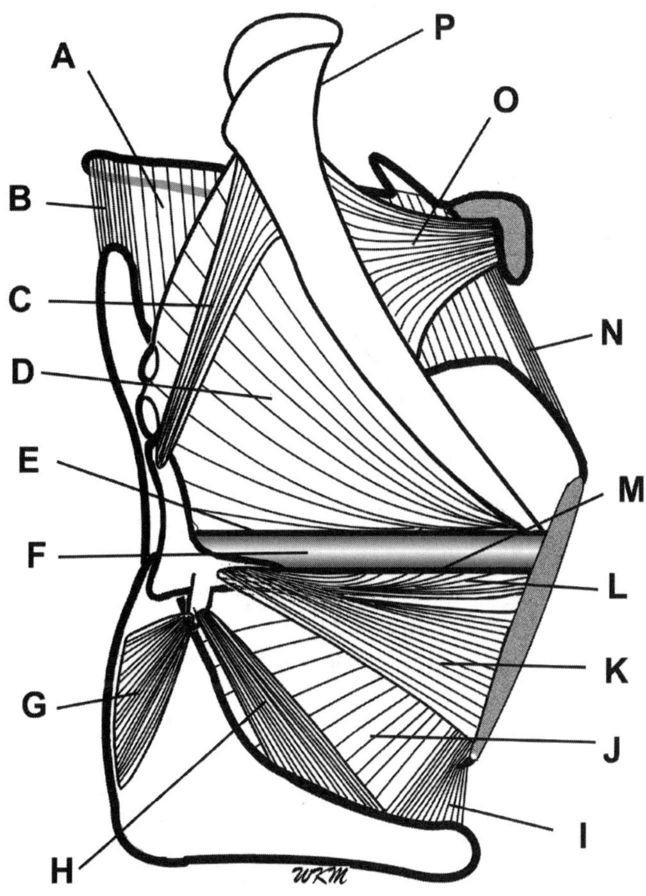

Figure 3-49 Larynx Dissection, Right Aspect: Ligaments and Muscles

Q. In Figure 3-49, identify E.

A. The vestibular fold.

Q. In Figure 3-49, identify F.

A. The opening of the sinus, leading into the saccule of the larynx. It opens into the median ventricle of the larynx between the vocal and vestibular folds.

Q. In Figure 3-49, identify G.

A. The posterior cricoarytenoideus muscle. Its posterior pull on the muscular process of the arytenoid cartilage *abducts* the ipsilateral vocal ligament by rotating the arytenoid cartilage.

Q. In Figure 3-49, identify H.

A. The lateral cricoarytenoideus muscle. Its anterior pull on the muscular process of the arytenoid cartilage *adducts* the ipsilateral vocal ligament.

Q. The nerve supply of the lateral cricoarytenoideus muscles is . . .

A. The recurrent laryngeal branch of the vagus nerve.

Q. The only muscle of the larynx that is not supplied by the recurrent laryngeal nerve is . . .

A. The cricothyroid muscle. It is supplied by the external laryngeal branch of the superior laryngeal branch of the vagus nerve.

Q. In Figure 3-49, identify I.

A. The median cricothyroid ligament.

Q. In Figure 3-49, identify J.

A. The right lateral cricothyroid ligament (the conus elasticus, the cricovocal membrane). Its free edge, superiorly, is the vocal ligament.

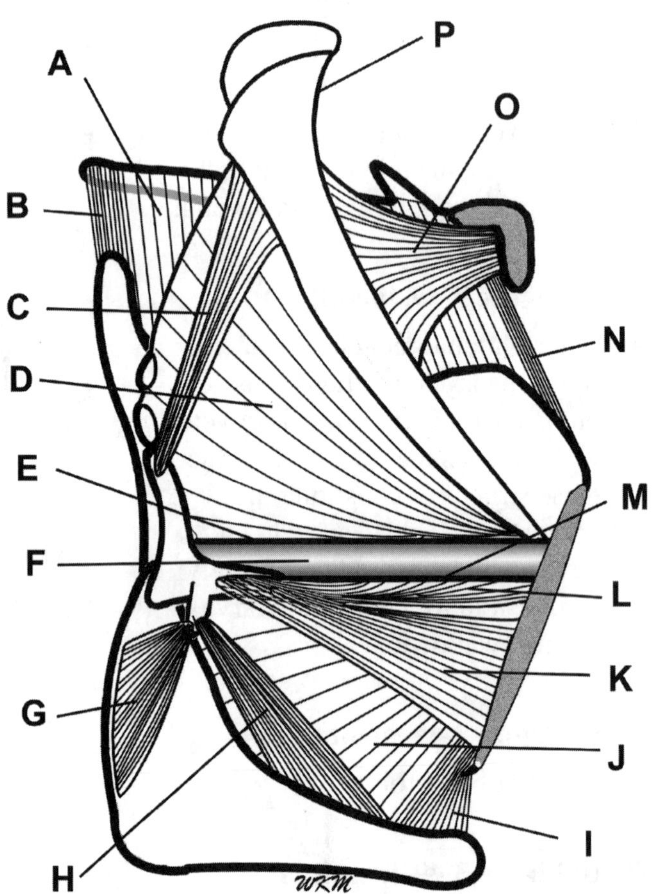

Figure 3-49 Larynx Dissection, Right Aspect: Ligaments and Muscles

Q. In Figure 3-49, identify K.

A. The right thyroarytenoideus muscle. Its medial border is the vocalis muscle. The main bulk of the muscle slackens the vocal ligament.

Q. In Figure 3-49, identify L.

A. The right vocalis muscle. It is considered to be part of the thyroarytenoideus muscle. However, its posterior fibers, arising from the arytenoid cartilage, are inserted into the vocal ligament. They serve to shorten the effective length of the vocal ligament and to tighten its anterior part, hence raising the pitch of the voice.

Q. In Figure 3-49, identify M.

A. The right vocal ligament.

Q. In Figure 3-49, identify N.

A. The median thyrohyoid ligament.

Q. In Figure 3-49, identify O.

A. The elastic hyoepiglottic ligament.

Q. In Figure 3-49, identify P.

A. The lingular surface of the epiglottis. It forms the posterior wall of the vallecula.

Q. In Figure 3-50, identify A.

A. The greater cornu of the hyoid bone.

Q. In Figure 3-50, identify B.

A. The epiglottic tubercle. The aryepiglottic folds come together at this point to close off the larynx during swallowing. The mucosa changes from the oral, stratified epithelium to the respiratory, ciliated columnar epithelium.

Q. In Figure 3-50, identify C.

A. The free margin of the epiglottis.

Q. In Figure 3-50, identify D.

A. The thyrohyoid membrane.

Q. In Figure 3-50, identify E.

A. The margin of the aryepiglottic fold.

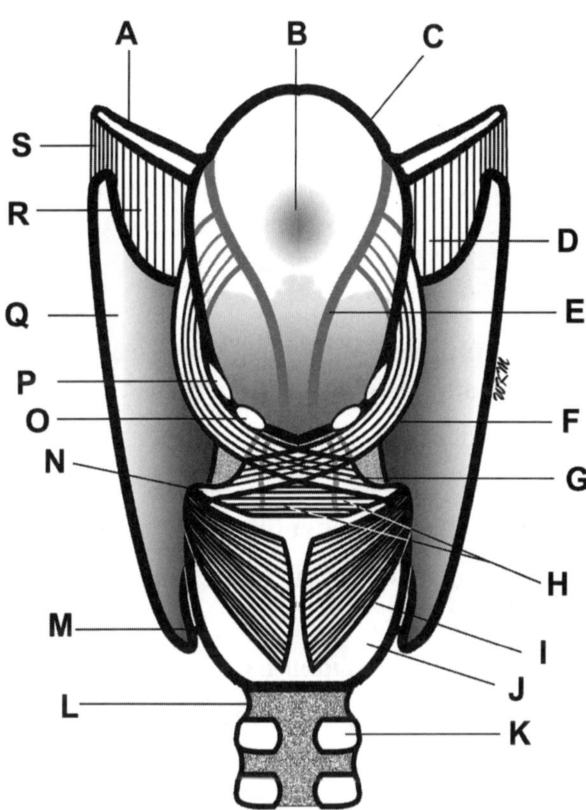

Figure 3-50 The Larynx and Epiglottis, Posterior Aspect

Q. In Figure 3-50, identify F.

A. The aryepiglotticus muscle. It passes in the aryepiglottic fold to be inserted into the lateral margin of the epiglottis.

Q. In Figure 3-50, identify G.

A. The right arytenoideus obliquus muscle. It runs from the posterior surface of the muscular process of the right arytenoid cartilage to the tip of the superior process of the left arytenoid cartilage. Many of its fibers are continued into the aryepiglottic fold and constitute the aryepiglotticus muscle.

Q. In Figure 3-50, identify H.

A. The single transverse arytenoid muscle.

Q. The function of the transverse arytenoid muscle and the aryepiglotticus muscles is to close . . .

A. The aditus to the larynx during swallowing by approximating the aryepiglottic folds to the epiglottic tubercle.

Q. In Figure 3-50, identify I.

A. The posterior cricoarytenoideus muscle. It arises from the posterior surface of the lamina of the cricoid cartilage. It attaches to the tip of the muscular process of the arytenoid cartilage.

Q. The function of the posterior cricoarytenoideus muscle is to . . .

A. Abduct the vocal folds.

Q. In Figure 3-50, identify J.

A. The lamina of the cricoid cartilage.

Q. In Figure 3-50, identify K.

A. The first ring of the trachea.

Q. In Figure 3-50, identify L.

A. The cricotracheal membrane.

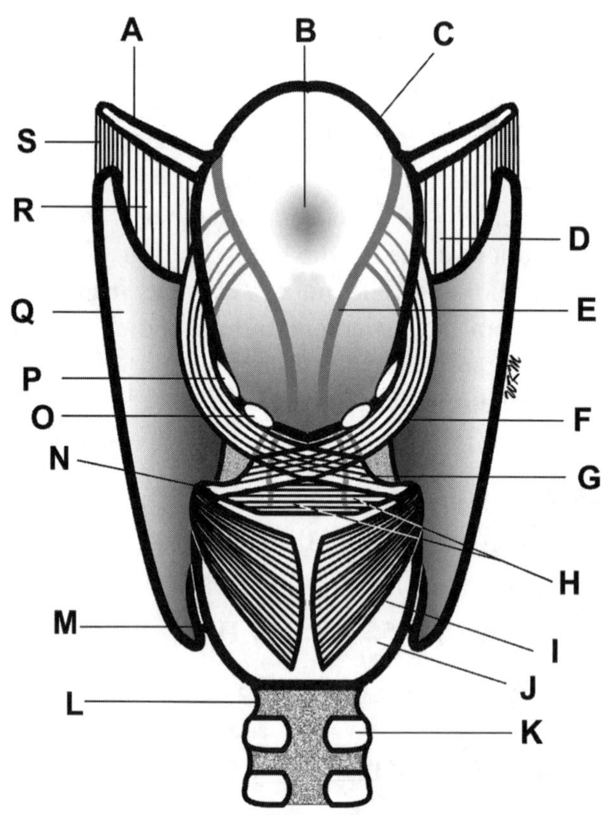

Figure 3-50 The Larynx and Epiglottis, Posterior Aspect

Q. In Figure 3-50, identify M.

A. The articulation between the inferior cornu of the thyroid cartilage and the side of the cricoid cartilage.

Q. In Figure 3-50, identify N.

A. The attachment of the posterior cricoarytenoideus muscle to the muscular process of the arytenoid cartilage.

Q. In Figure 3-50, identify O.

A. The corniculate cartilage. It articulates with the tip of the superior process of the arytenoid cartilage and is embedded in the margin of the aryepiglottic fold.

Q. In Figure 3-50, identify P.

A. The cuneiform cartilage. Both the cuneiform cartilage and the corniculate cartilage are visible during laryngoscopy.

Q. In Figure 3-50, identify Q.

A. The left lamina of the thyroid cartilage.

Q. In Figure 3-50, identify R.

A. The thyrohyoid membrane.

Q. In Figure 3-50, identify S.

A. The lateral cricothyroid ligament.

Q. In Figure 3-51, identify A.

A. The vestibule or aditus to the larynx.

Q. In Figure 3-51, identify B.

A. The quadrangular membrane. Its free edge forms the vestibular folds.

Q. In Figure 3-51, identify C.

A. The sinus (saccule) of the larynx.

Q. In Figure 3-51, identify D.

A. The ventricle of the larynx.

Q. In Figure 3-51, identify E.

A. The vocal ligament.

Q. In Figure 3-51, identify F.

A. The lateral cricothyroid ligament. It is also known as the conus elasticus or the cricovocal membrane.

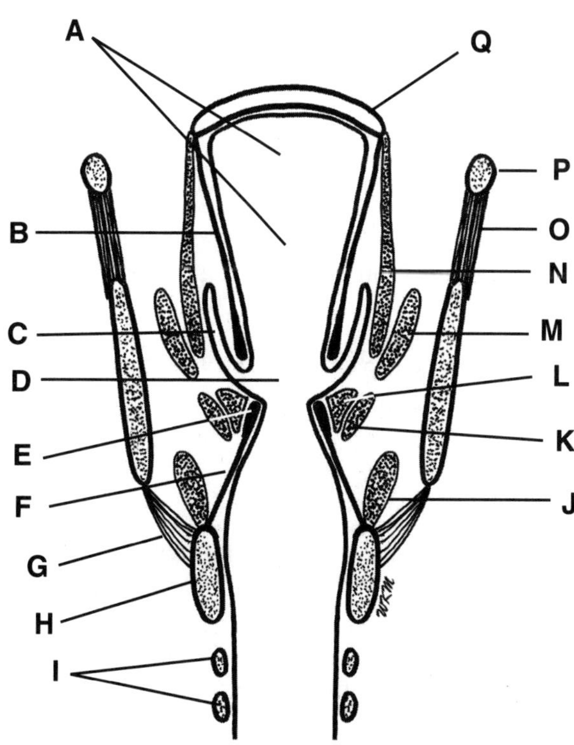

Figure 3-51 A Coronal Section Through the Larynx

Q. In Figure 3-51, identify G.

A. The cricothyroid muscle. It tightens the vocal ligaments.

Q. In Figure 3-51, identify H.

A. The cricoid cartilage in section.

Q. In Figure 3-51, identify I.

A. The upper two rings of the trachea.

Q. In Figure 3-51, identify J.

A. The lateral cricoarytenoideus muscle. It adducts the vocal ligaments.

Q. In Figure 3-51, identify K.

A. The inferior thyroarytenoideus muscle. It slackens the vocal ligaments.

Q. In Figure 3-51, identify L.

A. The vocalis muscle. It reduces the length of the vocal ligaments available for vibration.

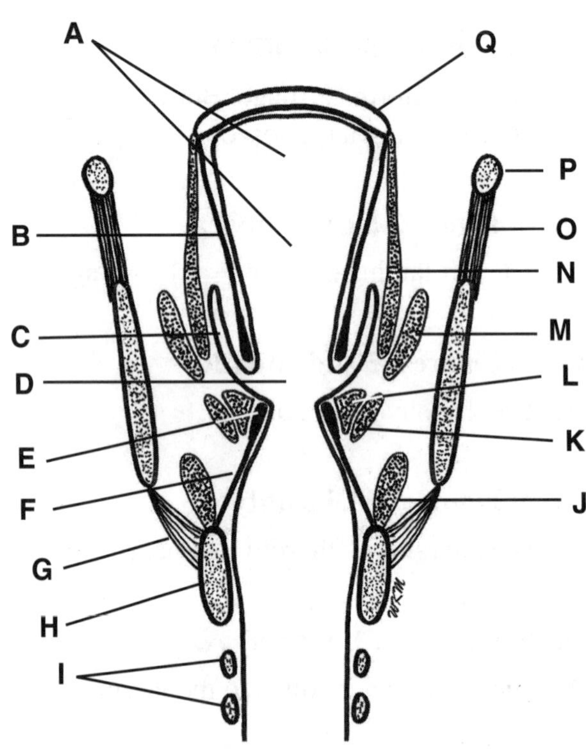

Figure 3-51 A Coronal Section Through the Larynx

Q. In Figure 3-51, identify M.

A. The superior, upper part of the thyroarytenoideus muscle. Many of its fibers continue into the aryepiglottic fold to reach the epiglottis. They help to open the aditus to the larynx.

Q. In Figure 3-51, identify N.

A. The aryepiglotticus muscle. It is largely responsible for closing the aditus to the larynx.

Q. In Figure 3-51, identify O.

A. The lateral thyrohyoid ligament.

Q. In Figure 3-51, identify P.

A. The tip of the greater cornu of the hyoid bone.

Q. In Figure 3-51, identify Q.

A. The epiglottis. It diverts the flow of saliva from the vallecula to the piriform fossa.

Chapter 4

The Thorax

THE THORACIC WALLS

Q. The inlet of the thorax is a plane that extends anteriorly from the neck of the 1st rib to the suprasternal notch. The vertebral level of the suprasternal notch is . . .

A. The lower border of the body of the 2nd thoracic vertebra.

Q. The vertebral level of the manubriosternal junction is . . .

A. The lower border of the body of the 4th thoracic vertebra.

Q. In the lateral part of the intercostal spaces, the fibers of the external intercostal muscles run downward and forward from . . .

A. The rib above to the rib below.

Q. Anteriorly, the external intercostal muscles are replaced by . . .

A. The anterior intercostal membranes.

Q. The external intercostal muscles contract during . . .

A. Inspiration. However, the most significant muscle of inspiration is the diaphragm.

Q. In the lateral part of the intercostal spaces, the fibers of the internal intercostal muscles run downward and backward from . . .

A. The rib above to the rib below.

Q. Posteriorly, the internal intercostal muscles are replaced by . . .

A. The posterior intercostal membranes.

Q. The internal intercostal muscles contract during . . .

A. Expiration. There is considerable disagreement in the literature concerning the actions of all of the intercostal muscles. However, they certainly provide an efficient method of closing the intervals between the ribs without impeding rib movement.

Q. The deepest layer of intercostal muscles is . . .

A. The innermost intercostal muscles. By analogy with the abdominal muscles, as evidenced by their embryologic development, the innermost intercostal muscles are sometimes called the transversus thoracis muscles.

Q. The innermost intercostals are incomplete. They are most prominent laterally in . . .

A. The midthoracic region.

Q. The significance of the innermost intercostal muscles lies in their relationship to . . .

A. The intercostal nerves and the intercostal vessels. As in the abdomen, the intercostal nerves and vessels lie between the second and third layers of the muscles of the wall of the thoracic cavity.

Q. The innermost intercostal muscles, the intercostals intima, are separated from the parietal pleura, the layer of pleura that lines the wall of the thoracic cavity, by . . .

A. The endothoracic fascia.

Q. The intercostal muscles receive their nerve supply from . . .

A. The intercostal nerves.

Q. The intercostal nerves are . . .

A. The anterior (ventral) primary rami of the 1st through 11th thoracic spinal nerves.

Q. The three categories of nerve fibers carried by the intercostal nerves are . . .

A. Those sensory to the skin and the pleura; those motor to the voluntary somatic muscles; and the autonomic postganglionic sympathetic nerve fibers to the sweat glands.

Q. The intercostal nerves run around the thoracic wall in the intercostal spaces between the internal intercostal muscles and the intercostales intima muscles. Each nerve travels in . . .

A. The subcostal groove on the inferior surface of the rib above. They are separated from the parietal pleura by the innermost intercostal muscles.

Q. The intercostal nerves are separated from the ribs by . . .

A. The intercostal arteries and veins. The veins lie next to the ribs. The arteries separate the veins from the nerves. This is the common relationship of *Nerves, Arteries, and Veins.*

Q. The structures supplied by the sensory branches of the 1st through the 6th thoracic intercostal nerves are . . .

A. The skin and the parietal pleura.

Q. In addition to the skin and the parietal pleura, the thoracoabdominal intercostal nerves (the 7th through the 11th thoracic anterior primary rami) supply . . .

A. The parietal peritoneum of the abdominal cavity. They also supply the abdominal muscles.

Q. The branches of the intercostal nerves are . . .

A. The collateral branches, the lateral cutaneous branches, the anterior cutaneous branches, and, of course, the muscular branches to both the thoracic wall and the abdominal wall.

Q. The collateral branches of the intercostal nerves are small. Each arises posteriorly and runs along . . .

A. The superior border of the appropriate rib inferior to the intercostal space.

Q. The lateral cutaneous branches penetrate the outer intercostal muscles in the midaxillary line to reach the skin. Each branch then divides into . . .

A. Anterior and posterior branches.

Q. The lateral cutaneous branch of the 2nd intercostal nerve becomes . . .

A. The intercostobrachial nerve of the appropriate side. Its main distribution is to the medial side of the upper arm.

Q. The anterior cutaneous branch reaches the skin not far from the midline. It then divides into . . .

A. Medial and lateral branches.

Q. The intercostal nerves are commonly divided into three groups: the thoracic nerves, the thoracoabdominal nerves, and the subcostal nerve. The thoracic group is . . .

A. The 1st through the 6th intercostal nerves. They do not reach the abdominal wall. The lateral branches of the first two intercostal nerves supply the axilla and the medial side of the upper arm. They are the intercostobrachial nerves.

Q. The thoracoabdominal nerves are . . .

A. The 7th through the 11th thoracic anterior (ventral) primary rami. They supply both the thorax and the abdomen.

Q. The subcostal nerves are . . .

A. The anterior primary rami of the 12th thoracic nerves. Because they do not lie between ribs, they are not true intercostal nerves. They only supply abdominal structures.

Q. Anterior to the sternocostalis muscle (the anterior part of the transversus thoracis muscles) and situated between it and the internal intercostal muscles lies a large artery running superoinferiorly. It is . . .

A. The internal thoracic artery. Its original name was the internal mammary artery because it gives three branches that run through the 2nd, 3rd, and 4th intercostal spaces to the female breast. These branches enlarge markedly throughout pregnancy. During lactation, they become very large. When lactation is completed, they return almost to the prepregnant state. In the male, they are much smaller. They are, however, enlarged in gynecomastia, a condition of female-type breasts in the male.

Q. In addition to the mammary branches, the internal thoracic artery gives rise to . . .

A. The anterior intercostal arteries. These are the branches to the anterior part of the intercostal spaces.

Q. The internal thoracic artery originates in the neck from . . .

A. The first part of the subclavian artery.

Q. The internal thoracic artery terminates by dividing into two branches. They are . . .

A. The musculophrenic artery and the superior epigastric artery. The musculophrenic artery follows the attachment of the diaphragm to the costal margin. The superior epigastric artery descends down the abdominal wall, lying in the posterior part of the rectus sheath.

Q. The superior epigastric artery anastomoses with . . .

A. The inferior epigastric artery. The inferior epigastric artery originates from the external iliac artery.

THE PLEURA AND THE LUNGS

Q. The thoracic cavity is divided into right and left halves by . . .

A. The mediastinum, the median partition.

Q. Each pleural cavity is lined by a serous membrane, the parietal pleura. The parietal pleura is divided into . . .

A. The costal pleura, the mediastinal pleura, and the diaphragmatic pleura. The costal pleura lines the thoracic wall. The mediastinal pleura covers the mediastinum. The diaphragmatic pleura covers the superior surface of the diaphragm.

Q. A similar serous membrane covers the lungs. It is known as . . .

A. The visceral pleura. It is firmly attached to the lungs.

Q. The visceral pleura is continuous with the mediastinal pleura around . . .

A. The lung root, the hilum of the lung.

Q. The nerves supplying the parietal pleura are . . .

A. The intercostal nerves and the phrenic nerves. The parietal pleura is sensitive to normal somatic sensory stimuli, such as cutting, pricking, and similar stimuli.

Q. The nerves supplying the visceral pleura are . . .

A. The autonomic nerves. The visceral pleura is sensitive only to stretching.

Q. Between the parietal and visceral layers of pleura is . . .

A. A small quantity of serous fluid. It serves as a lubricant to allow the smooth contraction and expansion of the lungs during respiration.

Q. The visceral and the parietal layers of pleura are kept in contact by . . .

A. The pressure of the atmosphere.

Q. The right lung is slightly larger and heavier than the left lung because the heart occupies a significant part of the left side of the thoracic cavity. The right lung weighs . . .

A. A little over 600 grams. The left lung weighs a little less than that amount.

Q. The relative density of the lungs is . . .

A. Less than 1.0. The lungs float readily in water. However, the lungs of a stillborn baby sink in water. The lungs of a stillborn baby do not contain air and therefore appear to be solid. On section, they appear to be glandular, resembling fetal lungs.

Q. The lungs are normally attached to the mediastinum only at . . .

A. The lung root. Here, the bronchi, the vessels, and the nerves enter or leave the lung from the mediastinum. However, pathological adhesions between the visceral pleura and the parietal pleura are often present elsewhere, for example, at the lung apex in the elderly. They are often due to old, healed, tubercular disease.

Q. Each lung is described as having an apex, a base, a mediastinal surface, and a costal surface. Two of these are convex. They are . . .

A. The apex and the costal surfaces.

Q. In Figure 4-1, identify A.

A. The lung apex. It is part of the upper lobe and projects above the first rib into the root of the neck. Here it can be percussed and auscultated.

Q. In Figure 4-1, identify B.

A. The shallow impression on the lung made by the esophagus. Note that it is interrupted by the deep groove on the lung made by the arch of the unpaired azygos vein.

Q. In Figure 4-1, identify C.

A. The area of the lung related to the trachea.

Q. In Figure 4-1, identify D.

A. The oblique fissure. Note that both the posterior end and the anterior end of the fissure are marked. The oblique fissure separates the upper lobe and the middle lobe of the lung from the lower lobe of the lung.

Q. In Figure 4-1, identify E.

A. The apex of the inferior lobe of the right lung.

Q. In Figure 4-1, identify F.

A. The impression on the lung made by the azygos vein. It arches posteriorly immediately above the hilum of the lung.

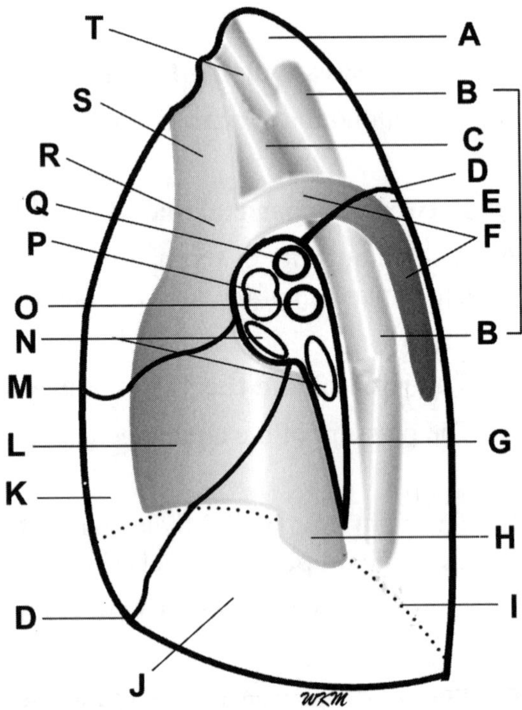

Figure 4-1 The Right Lung, Medial Aspect

Q. In Figure 4-1, identify G.

A. The pulmonary ligament. It is a fold of pleura that connects the visceral and parietal layers of the pleura. The line of pleural reflection continues upward to enclose the lung vessels and the bronchi.

Q. In Figure 4-1, identify H.

A. The short but marked impression on the lung made by the inferior vena cava.

Q. In Figure 4-1, identify I.

A. The rounded inferior medial margin of the lung. It lies between the medial and the diaphragmatic surfaces.

Q. In Figure 4-1, identify J.

A. The large diaphragmatic impression on the base of the right lung. At this point, the diaphragm separates the right lung base from the underlying right lobe of the liver.

Q. In Figure 4-1, identify K.

A. The middle lobe of the right lung.

Q. In Figure 4-1, identify L.

A. The cardiac impression. It is caused mainly by the right atrium.

Q. In Figure 4-1, identify M.

A. The horizontal fissure. It separates the middle lobe from the superior lobe of the right lung.

Q. In Figure 4-1, identify N.

A. The superior and the inferior pulmonary veins. They are the most anterior vessel and the most inferior vessel, respectively, in the root of the right lung.

Q. In Figure 4-1, identify O.

A. The hyparterial bronchus. It serves both the inferior and middle lobes of the right lung.

Q. In Figure 4-1, identify P.

A. The right pulmonary artery. It is divided into superior and inferior branches.

Q. In Figure 4-1, identify Q.

A. The eparterial bronchus. It serves only the superior lobe of the right lung.

Q. In Figure 4-1, identify R.

A. The impression on the right lung made by the superior vena cava.

Q. In Figure 4-1, identify S.

A. The impression caused by the superior vena cava as it divides into the right and the left brachiocephalic veins. The right brachiocephalic vein continues superiorly, grooving the lung. The left brachiocephalic vein crosses to the left, posterior to the manubrium sterni.

Q. In Figure 4-1, identify T.

A. The marked groove made by the right subclavian artery across the apex of the right lung.

Q. The important nerve that lies on the lateral surface of the superior vena cava, between it and the lung, is . . .

A. The right phrenic nerve. It continues inferiorly, lying on the surface of the right atrium, to penetrate the diaphragm immediately to the right of the inferior vena cava.

Q. In Figure 4-2, identify A.

A. The apex of the left lung.

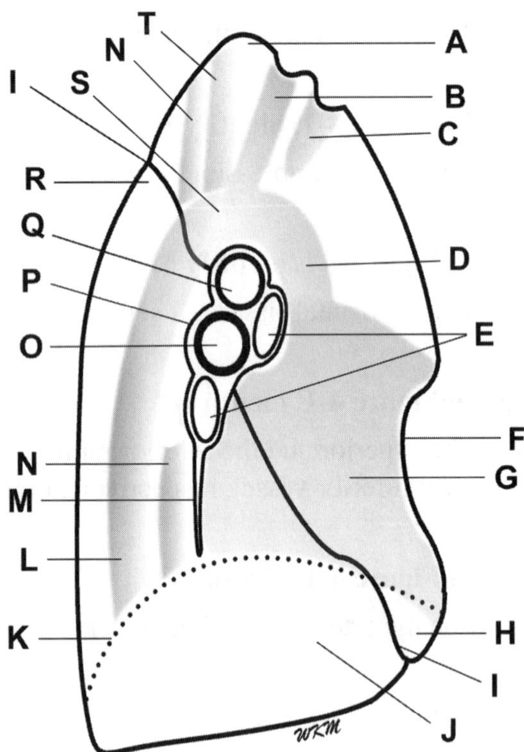

Figure 4-2 The Left Lung, Medial Aspect

Q. In Figure 4-2, identify B.

A. The groove and the impression made by the left subclavian artery .

Q. In Figure 4-2, identify C.

A. The groove and the impression caused by the left brachiocephalic vein.

Q. In Figure 4-2, identify D.

A. The impression due to the ascending aorta.

Q. In Figure 4-2, identify E.

A. The left superior pulmonary vein and the left inferior pulmonary vein.

Q. In Figure 4-2, identify F.

A. The cardiac notch. This is the area where the apex of the heart, contained in the pericardial sac, comes directly in contact with the thoracic wall without intervening lung tissue. This is why the cardiac impulse can be so readily palpated at this location.

Q. In Figure 4-2, identify G.

A. The "cardiac impression." It is caused mainly by the left ventricle.

Q. In Figure 4-2, identify H.

A. The lingula. This structure is only present on the left lung. It is part of the upper lobe. It is considered to be shaped like a tongue.

Q. In Figure 4-2, identify I.

A. The oblique fissure of the left lung. Note that both the inferior end of the oblique fissure and the superior end of the oblique fissure are identified.

Q. In Figure 4-2, identify J.

A. The diaphragmatic surface (the base) of the left lung.

Q. In Figure 4-2, identify K.

A. The rounded junction between the mediastinal and the diaphragmatic surfaces of the lung.

Q. In Figure 4-2, identify L.

A. The groove for the descending aorta.

Q. In Figure 4-2, identify M.

A. The left pulmonary ligament. It is the fold of pleura below the hilus of the left lung. It connects the visceral and the parietal pleura.

Q. In Figure 4-2, identify N.

A. The impression on the left lung caused by the left margin of the esophagus. The esophagus also is in contact with the left lung above and behind the arch of the aorta, posterior to the trachea. This latter area is also marked **N.**

Q. In Figure 4-2, identify O.

A. The left main bronchus.

Q. In Figure 4-2, identify P.

A. The reflection of the visceral pleura onto the left lung root. It becomes parietal pleura over the mediastinum.

Q. In Figure 4-2, identify Q.

A. The left pulmonary artery.

Q. In Figure 4-2, identify R.

A. The apex of the lower lobe of the left lung.

Q. In Figure 4-2, identify S.

A. The impression of the arch of the aorta.

Q. In Figure 4-2, identify T.

A. A faint impression caused by the trachea.

THE HEART

Q. The heart and the great vessels are enclosed in a protective fibrous sac. This sac is called . . .

A. The fibrous pericardium.

Q. Inside the fibrous pericardium, the heart is enclosed in a serous sac. The serous membrane lining the fibrous pericardium is . . .

A. The parietal layer of the serous pericardium.

Q. The thin serous layer covering the myocardium of the heart is . . .

A. The visceral layer of the serous pericardium.

Q. The sensory innervation of both the parietal layer of the serous pericardium and of the fibrous pericardium is derived from . . .

A. Both phrenic nerves.

Q. The phrenic nerves originate from . . .

A. The anterior primary rami of the 3rd, 4th, and 5th cervical nerves.

Q. When myocardial infarction affects the whole thickness of the myocardium, and therefore also involves the visceral layer of serous pericardium, the overlying parietal pericardium becomes secondarily involved by contact with the underlying visceral pericardium. This will result in referred pain in . . .

A. The neck and shoulder. They are supplied by the same cervical anterior primary rami.

Q. The visceral layer of pericardium and the myocardium are innervated by . . .

A. The autonomic nervous system.

Q. These sensory autonomic nerve fibers are segmentally derived. The spinal nerves involved are . . .

A. The 2nd, 3rd, and 4th thoracic spinal nerves.

Q. Therefore, the pain from myocardial damage often will be felt . . .

A. As a band around the upper chest. It may also be perceived as “heaviness” in the same area.

Q. In Figure 4-3, identify A.

A. The aorta.

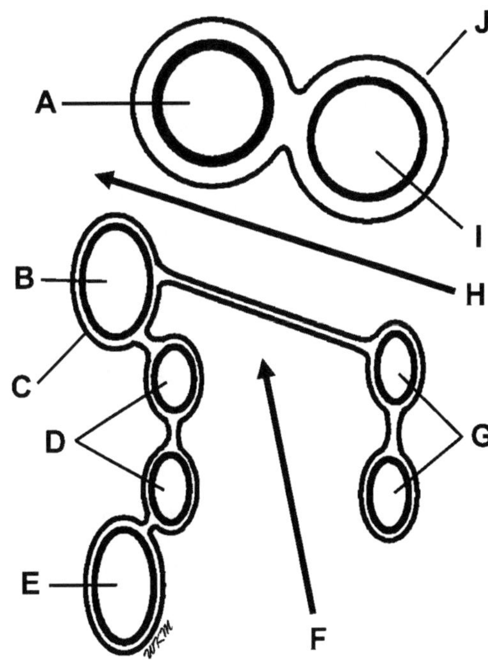

Figure 4-3 The Transverse and Oblique Pericardial Sinuses

Q. In Figure 4-3, identify B.

A. The superior vena cava.

Q. In Figure 4-3, identify C.

A. The reflection of the pericardium onto the superior vena cava.

Q. In Figure 4-3, identify D.

A. The right pulmonary veins.

Q. In Figure 4-3, identify E.

A. The inferior vena cava.

Q. In Figure 4-3, identify F.

A. The oblique pericardial sinus. It is posterior to the left atrium and anterior to the esophagus.

Q. In Figure 4-3, identify G.

A. The left pulmonary veins.

Q. In Figure 4-3, identify H.

A. The transverse pericardial sinus.

Q. In Figure 4-3, identify I.

A. The pulmonary trunk.

Q. In Figure 4-3, identify J.

A. The reflection of the pericardium onto the pulmonary trunk.

Q. The visceral and parietal pericardium are continuous at only two places. These areas of continuity occur where the major vessels enter or leave the heart. The arterial connection between the parietal and visceral pericardium surrounds . . .

A. The aorta and the pulmonary trunk.

Q. The connection between the visceral and the parietal pericardium at the venous end of the heart surrounds . . .

A. The superior and inferior vena cava and the right and the left groups of pulmonary veins.

Q. This grouping of the veins creates a blind-ended sinus in the serous pericardial sac behind the heart. This sinus is . . .

A. The oblique sinus of the pericardium.

Q. The anterior wall of the oblique sinus of the pericardium is . . .

A. The visceral layer of pericardium. It covers the posterior wall of the left atrium.

Q. Posterior to the oblique sinus, behind the parietal and fibrous pericardium, lies . . .

A. The esophagus. A barium swallow shown on a lateral chest X-ray will outline the left atrium. This is still the most economical way to evaluate the size of the left atrium.

Q. When the pericardial sac is opened, a finger can be inserted posterior to the aorta and the pulmonary trunk and anterior to the superior vena cava. This sinus, which is open at both ends, is . . .

A. The transverse sinus of the pericardium. The aorta and the pulmonary trunk can be compressed between a finger in this sinus, and the thumb placed on the anterior surface of the aorta and the pulmonary trunk. This maneuver is used by cardiac surgeons to occlude temporarily both the aorta and the pulmonary trunk.

Q. The posterior surface, or base, of the heart is separated from the vertebral column by . . .

A. The esophagus.

Q. The chamber that forms the base of the heart is . . .

A. The left atrium.

Q. The anterior (sternocostal) surface of the heart is separated from the sternum in the midline by . . .

A. The thymus prior to puberty in the young and the thymic remnants in adults. Laterally, the thin anterior margin of each lung intervenes to a varying extent between the costal cartilages and the fibrous pericardium.

Q. The anterior surface of the heart consists mainly of . . .

A. The right ventricle.

Q. The chamber of the heart that largely constitutes the right surface and the right margin of the heart is . . .

A. The right atrium.

Q. The two chambers that make up the left surface of the heart are . . .

A. The left auricle and the left ventricle. The latter makes up the greater part of this surface.

Q. The apex of the heart is formed by . . .

A. The tip of the left ventricle.

Q. The inferior surface of the fibrous pericardium is fused with the central tendon of the diaphragm. The chamber of the heart that forms its diaphragmatic surface is . . .

A. The left ventricle.

Q. The right coronary artery arises from the right (anterior) aortic sinus. It runs forward between . . .

A. The pulmonary trunk and the right auricle to reach the atrioventricular groove.

Q. The right coronary artery runs in the atrioventricular groove around . . .

A. The right margin of the heart to the junction of the atrioventricular groove with the posterior interventricular groove.

Q. The vein that accompanies the right coronary artery around the right margin of the heart is . . .

A. The small cardiac vein.

Q. The main tributary of the small cardiac vein is . . .

A. The right marginal vein.

Q. The right coronary artery follows the atrioventricular groove to its intersection with the posterior interventricular groove. Here, it anastomoses with . . .

A. The terminal branch of the circumflex branch of the left coronary artery.

Q. In about 65 percent of cases, the blood supply to the sinuatrial node is . . .

A. The main atrial (nodal) branch of the right coronary artery.

Q. In Figure 4-4, identify A.

A. The superior vena cava. It opens into the right atrium.

Q. In Figure 4-4, identify B.

A. The ascending aorta.

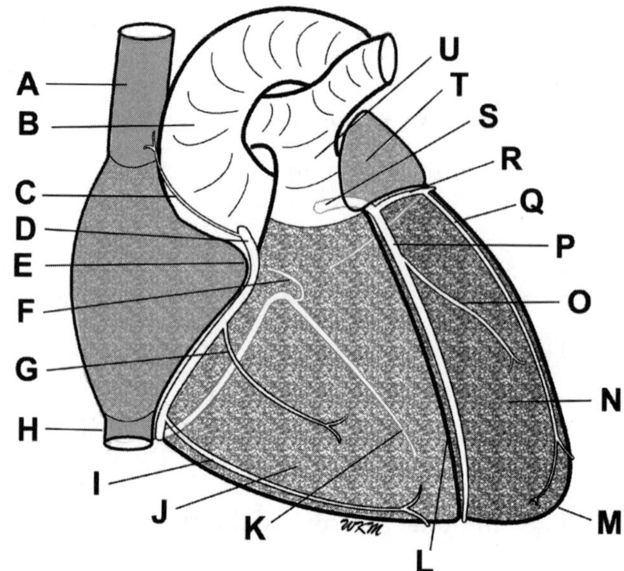

Figure 4-4 The Coronary Arteries, Anterior Aspect

Q. In Figure 4-4, identify C.

A. The sinuatrial artery, the first branch of the right coronary artery.

Q. In Figure 4-4, identify D.

A. The right coronary artery. It arises from the right (anterior) aortic sinus. The least confusing terminology for the remaining two aortic sinuses is the left (left-posterior) aortic sinus from which the left coronary artery originates and the noncoronary (right-posterior) sinus.

Q. In Figure 4-4, identify E.

A. The auricle of the right atrium. It often overlaps the emerging right coronary artery.

Q. In Figure 4-4, identify F.

A. The atrioventricular nodal branch of the right coronary artery. It is on the posterior surface of the heart.

Q. In Figure 4-4, identify G.

A. An anterior ventricular branch of the right coronary artery.

Q. In Figure 4-4, identify H.

A. The inferior vena cava. It empties into the right atrium

Q. In Figure 4-4, identify I.

A. The right marginal artery.

Q. In Figure 4-4, identify J.

A. The right ventricle.

Q. In Figure 4-4, identify K.

A. The posterior interventricular branch of the right coronary artery. It runs in the posterior interventricular groove, but does not supply much of the interventricular septum. After the atrioventricular node is supplied, usually by the right coronary artery, the conducting system of the heart is supplied by the anterior descending branch of the left coronary artery.

Q. In Figure 4-4, identify L.

A. The anterior interventricular sulcus.

Q. In Figure 4-4, identify M.

A. The apex of the heart. It is formed by the left ventricle.

Q. In Figure 4-4, identify N.

A. The left ventricle.

Q. In Figure 4-4, identify O.

A. The diagonal branch of the anterior interventricular branch of the left coronary artery.

Q. In Figure 4-4, identify P.

A. The anterior descending interventricular branch of the left coronary artery. It supplies most of the interventricular septum, including the atrioventricular bundle. It does not usually supply the atrioventricular node.

Q. In Figure 4-4, identify Q.

A. The left marginal artery.

Q. In Figure 4-4, identify R.

A. The circumflex branch of the left coronary artery.

Q. In Figure 4-4, identify S.

A. The origin of the left coronary artery from the left coronary (left posterior) aortic sinus.

Q. In Figure 4-4, identify T.

A. The left auricle.

Q. In Figure 4-4, identify U.

A. The pulmonary trunk.

Q. In Figure 4-5, identify A.

A. The coronary sinus. It drains into the right atrium, immediately to the left of the inferior vena cava. Its orifice is guarded by a semilunar valve. The coronary sinus is derived embryologically from the left horn of the sinus venosus. Its wall contains cardiac muscle.

Q. In Figure 4-5, identify B.

A. The small cardiac vein. Running with the right coronary artery around the right border of the heart, it follows the right atrioventricular groove to end in the coronary sinus.

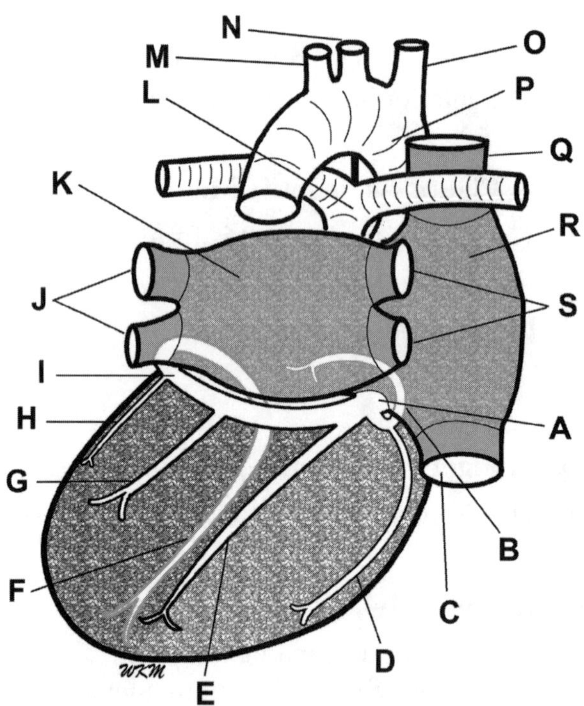

Figure 4-5 The Cardiac Veins, Posteroinferior Aspect

Q. In Figure 4-5, identify C.

A. The inferior vena cava.

Q. In Figure 4-5, identify D.

A. The right marginal vein. It may open independently into the coronary sinus.

Q. In Figure 4-5, identify E.

A. The middle cardiac vein. It lies in the posterior interventricular groove, accompanying the posterior interventricular branch of the right coronary artery.

Q. In Figure 4-5, identify F.

A. The great cardiac vein. It commences at the apex of the heart and ascends in the anterior interventricular groove. It accompanies the descending interventricular branch of the left coronary artery. It winds around the left border of the heart together with the circumflex branch of the left coronary artery to terminate as the left end of the coronary sinus.

Q. In Figure 4-5, identify G.

A. The posterior vein of the left ventricle.

Q. In Figure 4-5, identify H.

A. The left marginal vein.

Q. In Figure 4-5, identify I.

A. The commencement of the coronary sinus. It lies in the posterior atrioventricular groove.

Q. In Figure 4-5, identify J.

A. The superior left pulmonary vein and the inferior left pulmonary vein.

Q. In Figure 4-5, identify K.

A. The posterior surface of the left atrium. It is separated from the esophagus by the oblique pericardial sinus. A barium swallow with a lateral thoracic X-ray often is used to visualize it.

Q. In Figure 4-5, identify L.

A. The pulmonary trunk. It is connected to the undersurface of the arch of the aorta by the ligamentum arteriosum, the ductus arteriosus of the fetus. It divides into the right and left pulmonary arteries.

Q. In Figure 4-5, identify M.

A. The left subclavian artery.

Q. In Figure 4-5, identify N.

A. The left common carotid artery.

Q. In Figure 4-5, identify O.

A. The brachiocephalic artery. It subsequently divides into the right subclavian artery and the right common carotid artery.

Q. In Figure 4-5, identify P.

A. The beginning of the arch of the aorta.

Q. In Figure 4-5, identify Q.

A. The superior vena cava.

Q. In Figure 4-5, identify R.

A. The right atrium.

Q. In Figure 4-5, identify S.

A. The right superior pulmonary vein and the right inferior pulmonary vein.

Q. In addition to the nodal artery, the branches of the right coronary artery are . . .

A. The anterior atrial arteries, the posterior atrial arteries, the anterior ventricular arteries, the large right marginal artery, and the posterior ventricular arteries.

Q. The largest posterior ventricular branch of the right coronary artery is . . .

A. The posterior interventricular branch.

Q. The posterior interventricular branch of the right coronary artery supplies . . .

A. The posterior part of the interventricular septum and the atrioventricular node. However, the atrioventricular bundle is supplied by a branch from the left coronary artery.

Q. The vein that accompanies the posterior interventricular branch of the right coronary artery is . . .

A. The middle cardiac vein. It enters the coronary sinus just before the sinus opens into the posterior aspect of the right atrium, immediately to the left of the opening of the inferior vena cava.

Q. The left coronary artery, which is the larger of the two coronary arteries, arises from the left posterior aortic sinus. It passes forward between . . .

A. The pulmonary trunk and the left auricle.

Q. The anterior descending interventricular branch of the left coronary artery supplies most of the interventricular septum, including the atrioventricular bundle. It gives off one large named branch to the anterior wall of the left ventricle. This branch is . . .

A. The diagonal artery.

Q. The vein that accompanies the anterior descending interventricular branch of the left coronary artery is . . .

A. The great cardiac vein.

Q. The left coronary artery continues in the atrioventricular groove around the left margin of the heart. It is now called . . .

A. The circumflex branch of the left coronary artery.

Q. The vein that accompanies the circumflex branch of the left coronary artery around the left margin of the heart is . . .

A. The continuation of the great cardiac vein.

Q. At the left margin of the heart, the circumflex artery gives off a branch. This branch is . . .

A. The left marginal artery.

Q. The vein that accompanies the left marginal artery is . . .

A. The left marginal vein.

Q. The left marginal vein joins . . .

A. The great cardiac vein, which now becomes the coronary sinus.

Q. The coronary sinus is formed by the union of the great cardiac vein and the left marginal vein. Its four other important tributaries are . . .

A. The oblique vein of the left atrium, which is the remnant of the embryonic left superior vena cava; the posterior vein of the left ventricle; the middle cardiac vein; and the small cardiac veins.

Q. The circumflex branch of the left coronary artery continues around the atrioventricular groove to its junction with the posterior interventricular groove. Here it anastomoses with . . .

A. The right coronary artery. It turns inferiorly into the posterior interventricular groove.

Q. The right coronary artery usually supplies the sinuatrial node and the atrioventricular node. These nodes are the "pacemakers" of the heart. This arrangement of the blood supply to the "pacemakers" of the heart is known as . . .

A. Right coronary dominance.

Q. In about 40% of hearts, the circumflex branch of the left coronary artery is enlarged and continues down the posterior interventricular groove to replace the corresponding branch of the right coronary artery. It will then supply the atrioventricular node as well as the conducting system. This arrangement is known as . . .

A. Left coronary dominance.

Q. Interruption of the conducting system of the heart, or a "heart block," which is a situation that allows the ventricles to adopt their own intrinsic rhythm of approximately 30 beats a minute, is most likely to be the result of thrombosis of . . .

A. The right coronary artery. This vessel most commonly supplies the cardiac pacemaking system.

Q. A partial heart block, which results in the two ventricles beating asynchronously, is most likely caused by thrombosis of . . .

A. The left coronary artery. It supplies the conducting bundle. However, the damage to the left ventricular myocardium usually overshadows the damage to the conducting system.

Q. The terminal branches of the coronary arteries supply . . .

A. The endocardial surface of the myocardium.

Q. Following a coronary thrombosis, the myocardium most severely affected is . . .

A. The endocardial region of the myocardium. The small, peripheral, terminal branches of the coronary arteries, which supply the subendocardial myocardium, are the most likely to be occluded during a coronary thrombosis.

Q. In Figure 4-6, identify A.

A. The left atrium.

Q. In Figure 4-6, identify B.

A. The right atrium.

Q. In Figure 4-6, identify C.

A. The fossa ovalis. It is the site of the closure of the fetal foramen ovale from fusion of the septum primum and the septum secundum after birth.

Q. In Figure 4-6, identify D.

A. The superior vena cava.

Q. In Figure 4-6, identify E.

A. The right superior and inferior pulmonary veins.

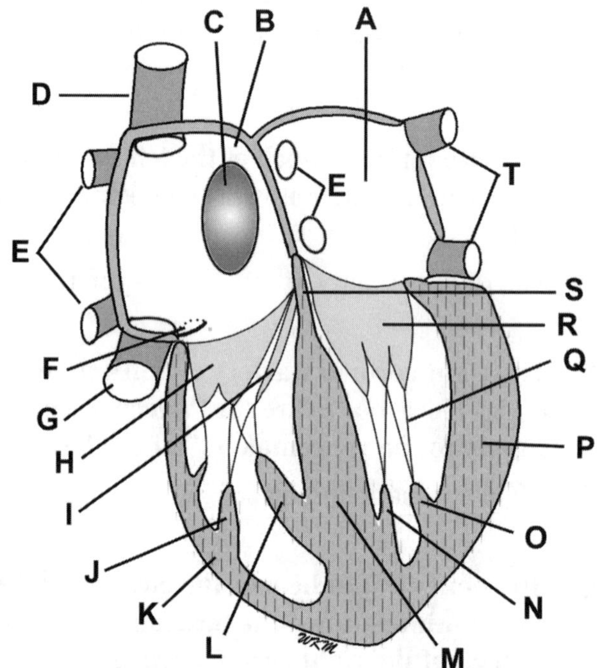

Figure 4-6 Diagrammatic Coronal Section of the Heart, Posterior Segment

Q. In Figure 4-6, identify F.

A. The opening of the coronary sinus.

Q. In Figure 4-6, identify G.

A. The inferior vena cava.

Q. In Figure 4-6, identify H.

A. The posterior leaflet (posterior cusp) of the tricuspid valve.

Q. In Figure 4-6, identify I.

A. The septal leaflet (septal cusp) of the tricuspid valve.

Q. In Figure 4-6, identify J.

A. The posterior papillary muscle of the right ventricle.

Q. In Figure 4-6, identify K.

A. The wall of the right ventricle.

Q. In Figure 4-6, identify L.

A. The septal papillary muscle of the right ventricle. It arises in association with the septomarginal trabeculae, the so-called moderator band.

Q. In Figure 4-6, identify M.

A. The interventricular septum.

Q. In Figure 4-6, identify N.

A. The posteromedial (posterior) papillary muscle of the left ventricle.

Q. In Figure 4-6, identify O.

A. The anterolateral (anterior) papillary muscle of the left ventricle.

Q. In Figure 4-6, identify P.

A. The wall of the left ventricle. In the normal adult heart, it is approximately three times as thick as the wall of the right ventricle.

Q. In Figure 4-6, identify Q.

A. A chorda tendineae. The chordae tendineae connect the papillary muscles to the leaflets (cusps) of the mitral valve and the tricuspid valves.

Q. In Figure 4-6, identify R.

A. The posterior leaflet (posterior cusp) of the mitral valve.

Q. In Figure 4-6, identify S.

A. The tendinous part of the interventricular septum. This is the site of closure of the embryonic interventricular foramen.

Q. In Figure 4-6, identify T.

A. The superior and the inferior left pulmonary veins.

EXAMINATION OF THE HEART

Q. In Figure 4-7, identify A.

A. The left and the right common carotid arteries.

Q. In Figure 4-7, identify B.

A. The left internal jugular vein.

Q. In Figure 4-7, identify C.

A. The left clavicle.

Q. In Figure 4-7, identify D.

A. The left subclavian artery.

Q. In Figure 4-7, identify E.

A. The aortic "knuckle," which is a consistent shadow on X-rays. It is the junction of the arch and the descending aorta.

Q. In Figure 4-7, identify F.

A. The left pulmonary artery.

Q. In Figure 4-7, identify G.

A. The left auricle.

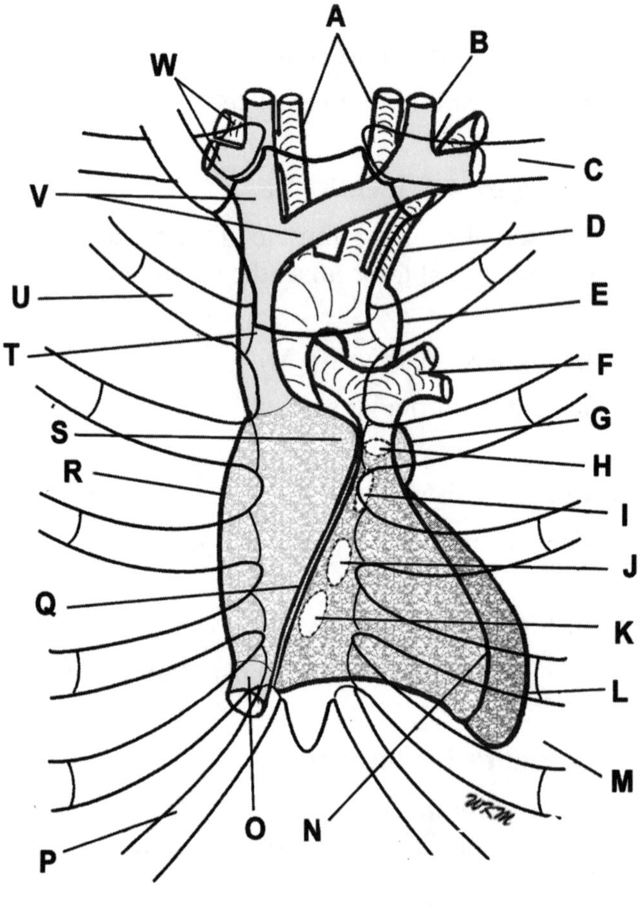

Figure 4-7 Surface Projection of the Heart

Q. In Figure 4-7, identify H.

A. The surface marking of the pulmonary valve.

Q. In Figure 4-7, identify I.

A. The surface marking of the aortic valve.

Q. In Figure 4-7, identify J.

A. The surface marking of the left atrioventricular (mitral, bicuspid) valve.

Q. In Figure 4-7, identify K.

A. The surface marking of the right atrioventricular (tricuspid) valve.

Q. In Figure 4-7, identify L.

A. The left ventricle. It forms the apex and the left margin of the heart.

Q. In Figure 4-7, identify M.

A. The 5th intercostal space.

Q. In Figure 4-7, identify N.

A. The anterior interventricular groove, or sulcus.

Q. In Figure 4-7, identify O.

A. The inferior vena cava.

Q. In Figure 4-7, identify P.

A. The right 7th costal cartilage.

Q. In Figure 4-7, identify Q.

A. The atrioventricular groove.

Q. In Figure 4-7, identify R.

A. The right atrium. It forms the right border of the heart.

Q. In Figure 4-7, identify S.

A. The right auricle.

Q. In Figure 4-7, identify T.

A. The superior vena cava.

Q. In Figure 4-7, identify U.

A. The right 2nd costal cartilage. The 2nd costal cartilages articulate with the sternum at the manubriosternal junction (the angle of Louis).

Q. In Figure 4-7, identify V.

A. The right and the left brachiocephalic veins.

Q. In Figure 4-7, identify W.

A. The right subclavian vein and the right subclavian artery.

Q. The area where stenotic murmurs generated by a constricted pulmonary valve can be heard best is . . .

A. The left 2nd interspace, close to the sternum. These systolic murmurs are very rare. They essentially occur only in congenital pulmonary stenosis, congenital narrowing of the pulmonary artery, and in those congenital conditions in which an abnormal volume of blood passes through a normal size pulmonary artery, such as occurs in patients with a significant congenital ventricular septal defect.

Q. The area where stenotic murmurs generated by a constricted aortic valve can be heard best is . . .

A. The 2nd interspace to the right of the sternum. These systolic murmurs are quite common. They usually result from calcification of the aortic valve leaflets in arteriosclerotic heart disease.

Q. The area where stenotic murmurs generated by a constricted mitral valve can be heard best is . . .

A. Just medial to the apex of the heart. These diastolic murmurs are quite common. They usually result from previous rheumatic heart disease.

Q. The area where stenotic murmurs generated by a constricted tricuspid valve can be heard best is . . .

A. The lower end of the sternum. These diastolic murmurs are extremely rare.

Q. Stenotic murmurs are generated by . . .

A. Turbulent blood flow through the narrowed opening.

Q. Regurgitant murmurs result from . . .

A. Incompetent "leaky" valves.

Q. These murmurs will be heard best . . .

A. Upstream from the site of the damaged valve.

Q. Venae cordis minimae are small veins that open directly into all of . . .

A. The chambers of the heart. It is possible that they may contribute to the nutrition of the myocardium following coronary thrombosis. This suggestion has resulted in recent attempts to increase the nutrition of the myocardium through the use of lasers to drill small channels through the endocardium into the myocardium.

THE MEDIASTINUM

Q. The mediastinum is the flexible partition between the two sides of the thorax. Its superior boundary is . . .

A. The thoracic inlet.

Q. The inferior boundary of the mediastinum is . . .

A. The diaphragm.

Q. The lateral limits of the mediastinum are . . .

A. The right and the left mediastinal pleura.

Q. The mediastinum contains . . .

A. The heart, the great vessels, the trachea, the esophagus, the vagus nerve, the phrenic nerve, and a number of smaller structures, including the lymph nodes. All are of major clinical importance.

Q. The mediastinum is arbitrarily divided into the superior and the inferior mediastina by a plane that extends from . . .

A. The manubriosternal junction, anteriorly, to the lower border of the 4th thoracic vertebra, posteriorly.

Q. The major structures in the superior mediastinum are . . .

A. The great vessels, the trachea, and the esophagus.

Q. The superior mediastinum is often described as having an arterial side and a venous side. The venous side is . . .

A. The right side. It contains the superior vena cava, the right brachiocephalic vein, the arch of the azygos vein, the right superior intercostal vein, and the right phrenic nerve.

Q. The arterial (left) side of the superior mediastinum contains . . .

A. The aortic arch, the left subclavian artery, the common carotid arteries, the left vagus nerve and its branch, the recurrent laryngeal nerve, the left phrenic nerve, and the left superior intercostal vein.

Q. The central part of the superior mediastinum contains . . .

A. The left brachiocephalic vein, the trachea, the esophagus, the thoracic duct, the right vagus nerve, and the left recurrent laryngeal nerve.

Q. The inferior mediastinum extends from the manubriosternal junction, anteriorly, and to the lower border of the body of the 4th thoracic vertebra, posteriorly. Inferiorly, it extends to . . .

A. The central tendon of the diaphragm.

Q. The inferior mediastinum is divided into three regions. They are . . .

A. The anterior, the middle, and the posterior mediastina.

Q. The anterior mediastinum, lying between the sternum and the pericardium, contains . . .

A. The sternopericardial ligaments, an occasional lymph node, and, in the young, the thymus. In the adult, only degenerate remnants of the thymus can be found.

Q. The middle mediastinum extends from the anterior mediastinum to the anterior surface of the esophagus. It contains . . .

A. The pericardium and its contents, the tracheal bifurcation, both the main bronchi and their associated lymph nodes, and the right and left phrenic nerves.

Q. The contents of the pericardium can be divided into an inferior and a posterior group. From right to left, the superior group is made up of . . .

A. The superior vena cava, the aorta, and the pulmonary trunk.

Q. Posterior to the superior part of the pericardial cavity, but still within the middle mediastinum, are . . .

A. The bifurcation of the trachea, both the main bronchi, and the superior and the inferior groups of tracheobronchial lymph nodes.

Q. The inferior region of the pericardial cavity is occupied by . . .

A. The heart. The base of the heart, comprising the left atrium, lies posteriorly.

Q. From their respective lung roots, the left and right, superior and inferior pulmonary veins open into . . .

A. The left and right margins of the left atrium.

Q. The posterior mediastinum lies between the vertebral column and the middle mediastinum. Apart from lymph nodes, all of its contents are oriented . . .

A. Longitudinally.

Q. The most anterior structure in the posterior mediastinum is . . .

A. The esophagus.

Q. The vessels in the posterior mediastinum are . . .

A. The descending aorta, the azygos vein, the hemiazygos vein, the accessory hemiazygos vein, and the thoracic duct.

Q. The branches of the descending aorta are . . .

A. The intercostal arteries, the bronchial arteries, and the esophageal arteries.

Q. The paired branches of the descending thoracic aorta are . . .

A. The intercostal arteries. The esophageal and the bronchial arteries are midline visceral branches to the respiratory and the alimentary systems.

Q. The nerves in the posterior mediastinum are . . .

A. The vagus nerves and the greater and the lesser splanchnic nerves.

Q. The splanchnic nerves contain . . .

A. Myelinated preganglionic sympathetic and visceral afferent fibers.

Q. The greater splanchnic nerves originate from . . .

A. The 5th through the 9th sympathetic chain ganglia.

Q. The lesser splanchnic nerves originate in . . .

A. The 10th and 11th thoracic sympathetic ganglia.

Q. The least splanchnic nerves originate in . . .

A. The 12th thoracic sympathetic ganglion.

Q. The splanchnic nerves leave the thorax through . . .

A. The crura of the diaphragm.

Q. The preganglionic fibers in the splanchnic nerves synapse in . . .

A. The celiac ganglion and the aorticorenal ganglia.

Q. In Figure 4-8, identify A.

A. The brachiocephalic artery.

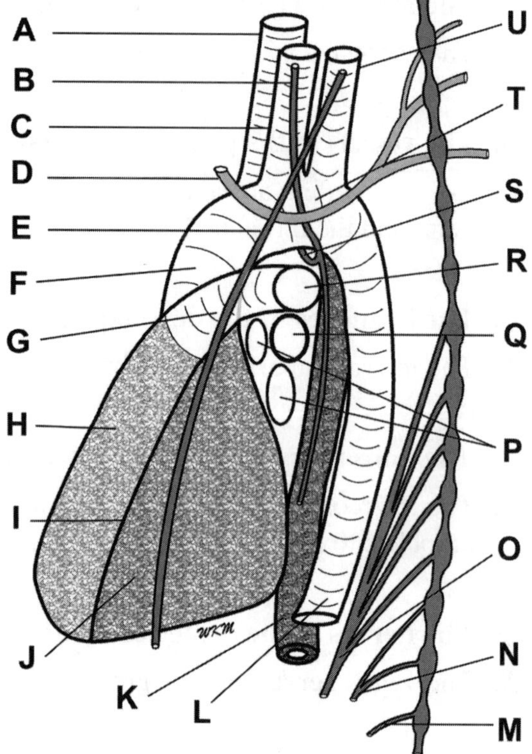

Figure 4-8 The Mediastinum, Left Aspect

Q. In Figure 4-8, identify B.

A. The left vagus nerve. It crosses the arch of the aorta deep to the superior intercostal vein.

Q. In Figure 4-8, identify C.

A. The left common carotid artery.

Q. In Figure 4-8, identify D.

A. The left superior intercostal vein. It drains the 2nd, 3rd, and 4th intercostal spaces and terminates by entering the left brachiocephalic vein.

Q. In Figure 4-8, identify E.

A. The left phrenic nerve. It has crossed the left vagus nerve and the left superior intercostal vein superficially, lying between them and the mediastinal pleura.

Q. In Figure 4-8, identify F.

A. The ascending aorta.

Q. In Figure 4-8, identify G.

A. The pulmonary trunk.

Q. In Figure 4-8, identify H.

A. The right ventricle.

Q. In Figure 4-8, identify I.

A. The anterior interventricular groove.

Q. In Figure 4-8, identify J.

A. The left ventricle.

Q. In Figure 4-8, identify K.

A. The esophagus. Before the esophagus pierces the diaphragm, both the left and right vagus nerves divide to form a plexus around it. The left vagus nerve forms most of the anterior esophageal plexus, and the right vagus nerve forms most of the posterior esophageal plexus.

Q. In Figure 4-8, identify L.

A. The descending aorta.

Q. In Figure 4-8, identify M.

A. The least splanchnic nerve. It arises from the 12th thoracic sympathetic ganglion.

Q. In Figure 4-8, identify N.

A. The lesser splanchnic nerve. It arises from the 10th and the 11th thoracic sympathetic chain ganglia.

Q. In Figure 4-8, identify O.

A. The greater splanchnic nerve. It arises from the 5th through the 9th thoracic sympathetic ganglia.

Q. In Figure 4-8, identify P.

A. The left superior pulmonary vein and the left inferior pulmonary vein. They are the most anterior and the most inferior structures, respectively, in the left lung root.

Q. In Figure 4-8, identify Q.

A. The left main bronchus. It is the most prominent structure in the root of the lung.

Q. In Figure 4-8, identify R.

A. The left pulmonary artery.

Q. In Figure 4-8, identify S.

A. The recurrent laryngeal branch of the left vagus nerve.

Q. In Figure 4-8, identify T.

A. The arch of the aorta.

Q. In Figure 4-8, identify U.

A. The left subclavian artery.

Q. In Figure 4-9, identify A.

A. The esophagus.

Q. In Figure 4-9, identify B.

A. The trachea. It divides between the arch of the azygos vein and the arch of the aorta into the right and left principal bronchi.

Q. In Figure 4-9, identify C.

A. The right vagus nerve. Note that it lies medial to the arch of the azygos vein and that it forms a plexus on the posterior surface of the esophagus. It is identified twice.

Q. In Figure 4-9, identify D.

A. The right phrenic nerve. Note that it is superficial, lying on the right side of the superior vena cava, and then continues down the right side of the right atrium and onto the surface of the inferior vena cava. It is identified twice.

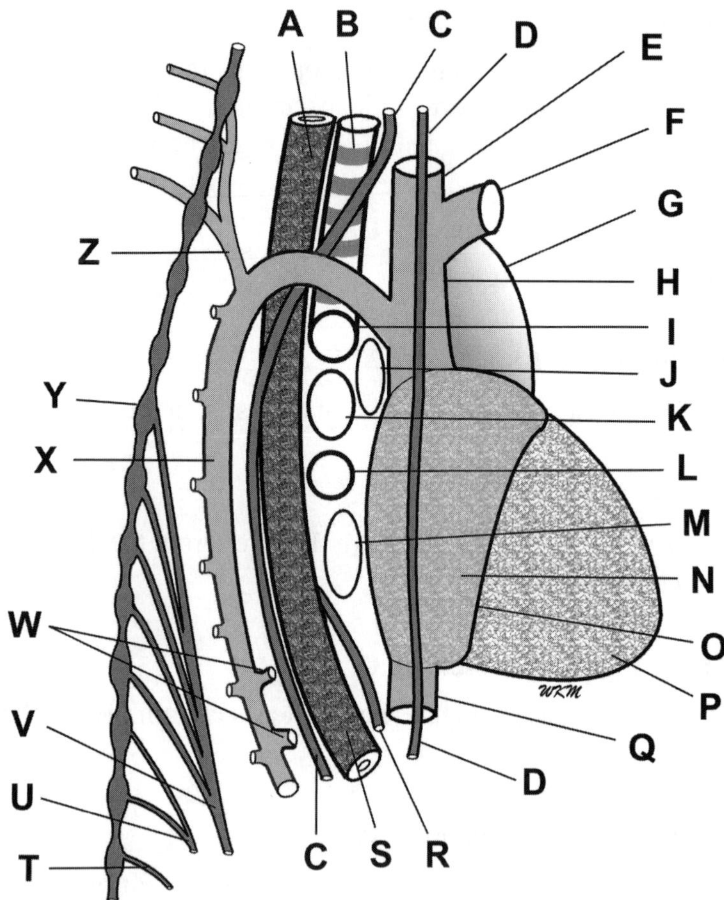

Figure 4-9 The Mediastinum, Right Aspect

Q. In Figure 4-9, identify E.

A. The right brachiocephalic vein.

Q. In Figure 4-9, identify F.

A. The left brachiocephalic vein. It crosses to the left, posterior to the manubrium sternum. In women and children, it may reach as high as the suprasternal notch, where it may be vulnerable to injury during a low tracheotomy.

Q. In Figure 4-9, identify G.

A. The right side of the ascending aorta.

Q. In Figure 4-9, identify H.

A. The superior vena cava.

Q. In Figure 4-9, identify I.

A. The eparterial bronchus.

Q. In Figure 4-9, identify J.

A. The right superior pulmonary vein.

Q. In Figure 4-9, identify K.

A. The right pulmonary artery.

Q. In Figure 4-9, identify L.

A. The hyparterial bronchus. It is only present in the hilus of the right lung. There is no eparterial bronchus to the left lung. The left pulmonary artery is the most superior structure in the root of the left lung.

Q. In Figure 4-9, identify M.

A. The right inferior pulmonary vein. The inferior pulmonary veins are always the inferior structures in the lung roots.

Q. In Figure 4-9, identify N.

A. The right atrium. It forms the greater part of the right border of the heart. The right ventricle forms mainly the sternocostal surface of the heart.

Q. In Figure 4-9, identify O.

A. The right atrioventricular groove. The right coronary artery lies within it.

Q. In Figure 4-9, identify P.

A. The right ventricle.

Q. In Figure 4-9, identify Q.

A. The inferior vena cava. The right phrenic nerve (**D**) passes through the diaphragm in company with the inferior vena cava.

Q. In Figure 4-9, identify R.

A. The left vagus nerve. It forms a plexus on the anterior wall of the esophagus.

Q. In Figure 4-9, identify S.

A. The esophagus. It veers to the left to pierce the diaphragm to the left of the midline.

Q. In Figure 4-9, identify T.

A. The least splanchnic nerve. It ends in the renal autonomic plexus.

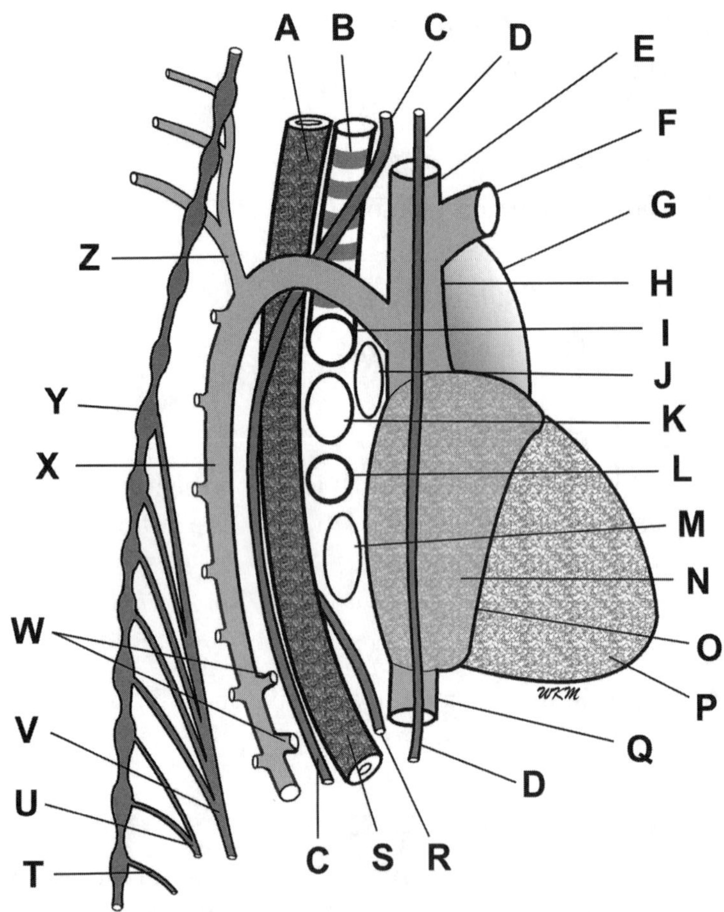

Figure 4-9 The Mediastinum, Right Aspect

Q. In Figure 4-9, identify U.

A. The lesser splanchnic nerve. It terminates in the celiac and aorticorenal plexuses.

Q. In Figure 4-9, identify V.

A. The greater splanchnic nerve. It terminates mainly in the celiac plexus.

Q. In Figure 4-9, identify W.

A. The accessory hemiazygos vein and the hemiazygos vein. The accessory hemiazygos vein drains the 5th to the 8th left intercostal spaces. The hemiazygos vein drains the lower-left intercostal spaces.

Q. In Figure 4-9, identify X.

A. The azygos vein.

Q. In Figure 4-9, identify Y.

A. The 5th right sympathetic chain ganglion. It is the highest root of the greater splanchnic nerve. The highest chain ganglion depicted is the inferior cervical ganglion.

Q. In Figure 4-9, identify Z.

A. The right superior intercostal vein.

Q. In Figure 4-10, identify A.

A. The visceral and parietal layers of pleura.

Q. In Figure 4-10, identify B.

A. The sympathetic chain. It is lying on the neck of the 4th rib.

Q. In Figure 4-10, identify C.

A. The right vagus nerve.

Q. In Figure 4-10, identify D.

A. The arch of the azygos vein. At this level, it arches anteriorly to join the superior vena cava (**E**).

Q. In Figure 4-10, identify F.

A. The right phrenic nerve. Notice that it lies lateral to the superior vena cava (**E**).

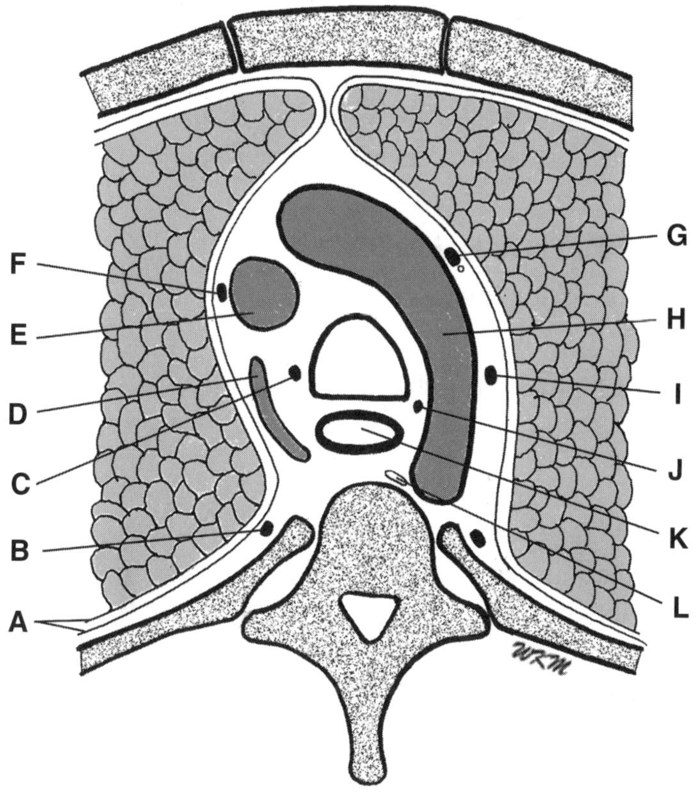

Figure 4-10 Transverse Section of the Thorax (T4), Inferior Aspect

Q. In Figure 4-10, identify G.

A. The left phrenic nerve. It is lying lateral to the aortic arch (**H**) and is accompanied by the small pericardiacophrenic artery.

Q. In Figure 4-10, identify I.

A. The left vagus nerve. It is crossing the lateral side of the arch of the aorta posterior to the phrenic nerve.

Q. In Figure 4-10, identify J.

A. The left recurrent laryngeal nerve in the groove between the trachea and esophagus.

Q. In Figure 4-10, identify K.

A. The esophagus.

Q. In Figure 4-10, identify L.

A. The thoracic duct. It has just crossed over from the right of the mid-line to the left of the mid-line.

RADIOLOGY OF THE THORAX

Q. In Figure 4-11, identify A.

A. The trachea. It is deviated to the right due to the presence of the aorta.

Q. In Figure 4-11, identify B.

A. The right pulmonary artery.

Q. In Figure 4-11, identify C.

A. The right atrium.

Q. In Figure 4-11, identify D.

A. The right inferior pulmonary veins.

Q. In Figure 4-11, identify E.

A. The margin of the right breast.

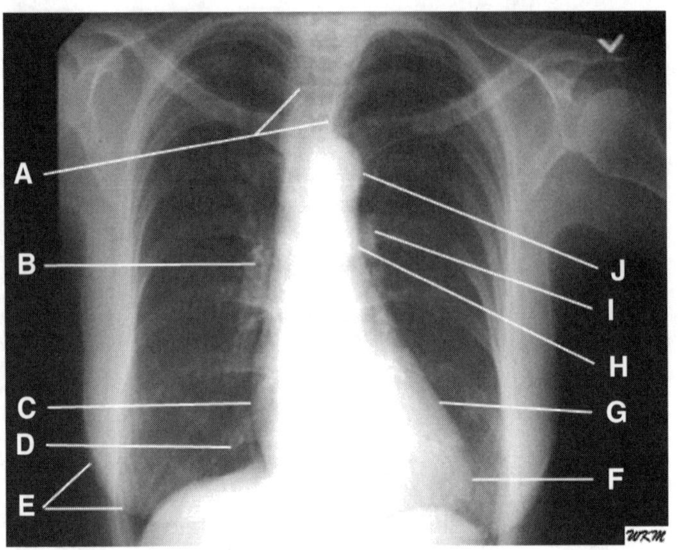

Figure 4-11 PA X-ray of the Thorax in Inspiration

Q. In Figure 4-11, identify F.

A. The apex of the heart, the tip of the left ventricle.

Q. In Figure 4-11, identify G.

A. The left ventricle.

Q. In Figure 4-11, identify H.

A. The pulmonary trunk.

Q. In Figure 4-11, identify I.

A. The left pulmonary artery.

Q. In Figure 4-11, identify J.

A. The aortic "knuckle." It is the outline of the beginning of the descending aorta.

Q. In Figure 4-12, identify A.

A. Air in the trachea. The radiological density varies as the trachea crosses the vertebrae and the intervertebral disks. The vertebral bodies are denser than the intervertebral disks.

Q. In Figure 4-12, identify B.

A. The right principal bronchus. Intrapulmonary bronchi cannot normally be seen in normal X-rays.

Q. In Figure 4-12, identify C.

A. The right pulmonary artery.

Q. In Figure 4-12, identify D.

A. The right inferior pulmonary veins.

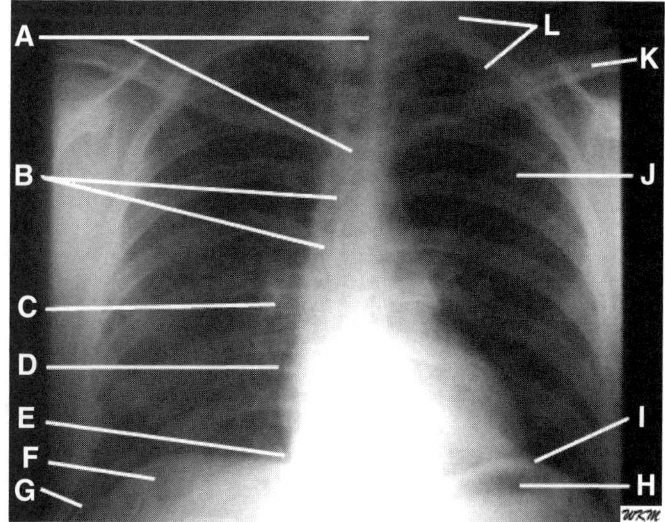

Figure 4-12 PA X-ray of the Thorax, Lung Fields

Q. In Figure 4-12, identify E.

A. The mediastinodiaphragmatic angle. At this point, the inferior vena cava penetrates the diaphragm.

Q. In Figure 4-12, identify F.

A. The liver. It lies beneath the right cupola of the diaphragm.

Q. In Figure 4-12, identify G.

A. The right costodiaphragmatic recess.

Q. In Figure 4-12, identify H.

A. Gas in the fundus of the stomach.

Q. In Figure 4-12, identify I.

A. The left cupola of the diaphragm.

Q. In Figure 4-12, identify J.

A. The anterior end of the left 2nd rib.

Q. In Figure 4-12, identify K.

A. The left clavicle.

Q. In Figure 4-12, identify L.

A. The left 1st rib.

Q. In Figure 4-13, identify A.

A. The trachea.

Q. In Figure 4-13, identify B.

A. The carina of the trachea.

Q. In Figure 4-13, identify C.

A. The left principal bronchus.

Q. In Figure 4-13, identify D.

A. The left lower lobe bronchus.

Q. In Figure 4-13, identify E.

A. The right principal bronchus. Note that it is more in line with the trachea than is the left principal bronchus. For this reason, inhaled foreign bodies, such as primary teeth, peanuts, and so on, lodge more frequently in the right lower lobe bronchus.

Q. In Figure 4-13, identify F.

A. The right upper lobe bronchus.

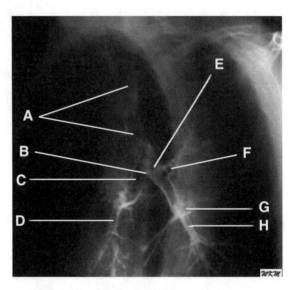

Figure 4-13 Bronchogram

Q. In Figure 4-13, identify G.

A. The middle lobe bronchus.

Q. In Figure 4-13, identify H.

A. The right lower lobe bronchus.

Q. In city dwellers, the network of thin black or dark grey lines often found on the surface of adult lungs under the pleura is due to . . .

A. The presence of carbon particles in the lung lymphatic vessels. The pulmonary lymph nodes also show the presence of carbon. In coal miners, the lungs may be completely black, the so-called "Black Lung" pneumoconiosis.

Q. In Figure 4-14, identify A.

A. Air in the trachea.

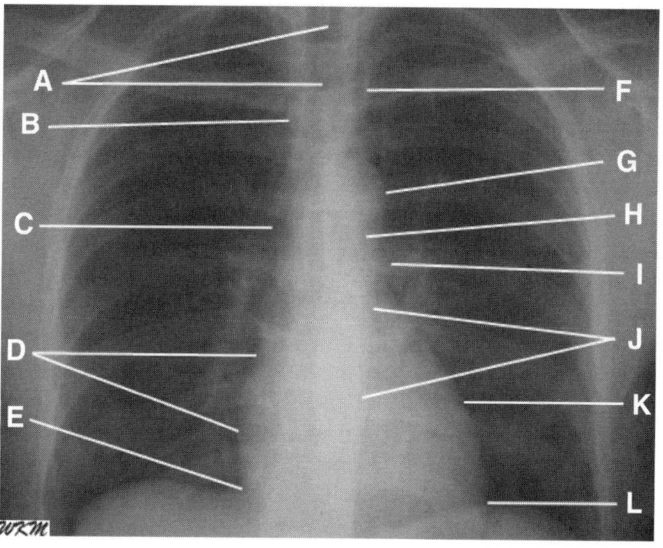

Figure 4-14 PA X-ray of the Outline of the Heart

Q. In Figure 4-14, identify B.

A. The superior vena cava at the union of the left and the right brachiocephalic veins.

Q. In Figure 4-14, identify C.

A. The right primary bronchus.

Q. In Figure 4-14, identify D.

A. The right atrium.

Q. In Figure 4-14, identify E.

A. The inferior vena cava.

Q. In Figure 4-14, identify F.

A. The left sternoclavicular joint.

Q. In Figure 4-14, identify G.

A. The termination of the arch of the aorta. It is called the aortic "knuckle."

Q. In Figure 4-14, identify H.

A. The pulmonary trunk and the left pulmonary artery.

Q. In Figure 4-14, identify I.

A. The left auricle.

Q. In Figure 4-14, identify J.

A. The descending aorta. It is seen as it descends posterior to the heart.

Q. In Figure 4-14, identify K.

A. The left ventricle.

Q. In Figure 4-14, identify L.

A. The apex of the heart. At this point, the cardiac impulse, which is caused by the left ventricle, can be palpated. It is sometimes referred to as the "apex beat" of the heart.

Q. In Figure 4-15, the catheter at point A is in . . .

A. The left brachiocephalic vein.

Q. Therefore, the catheter must have been inserted into . . .

A. The left subclavian vein.

Q. In Figure 4-15, the catheter at point B is in . . .

A. The superior vena cava.

Q. In Figure 4-15, the end of the catheter at point C is coiled in . . .

A. The right ventricle.

Q. In Figure 4-15, identify vessel D.

A. The right superior pulmonary vein.

Q. In Figure 4-15, the catheter at point E is in . . .

A. The right atrium.

Q. In Figure 4-15, identify vessel F.

A. The right inferior pulmonary vein.

Q. In Figure 4-15, identify vessel G.

A. The ascending aorta.

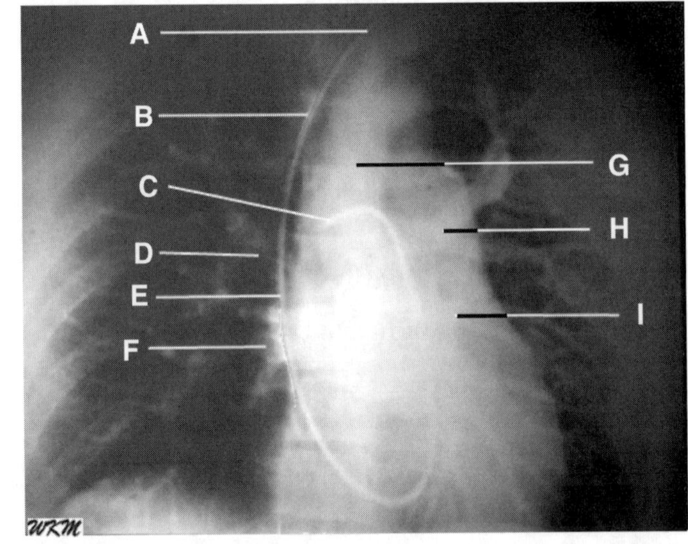

Figure 4-15 Pulmonary Venogram

Q. In Figure 4-15, identify vessel H.

A. The left superior pulmonary vein.

Q. The shadow of the left superior pulmonary veins is obscured by residual contrast media in . . .

A. The pulmonary trunk.

Q. In Figure 4-15, identify vessel I.

A. The left inferior pulmonary vein.

Q. In Figure 4-16, identify A.

A. The right dome of the diaphragm.

Q. In Figure 4-16, identify B.

A. A cardiac catheter. At this point, it is in the inferior vena cava. Its tip has reached the right atrium.

Q. The catheter has probably been inserted through . . .

A. The right femoral vein. The right common iliac vein joins the inferior vena cava at a less acute angle than the left common iliac vein.

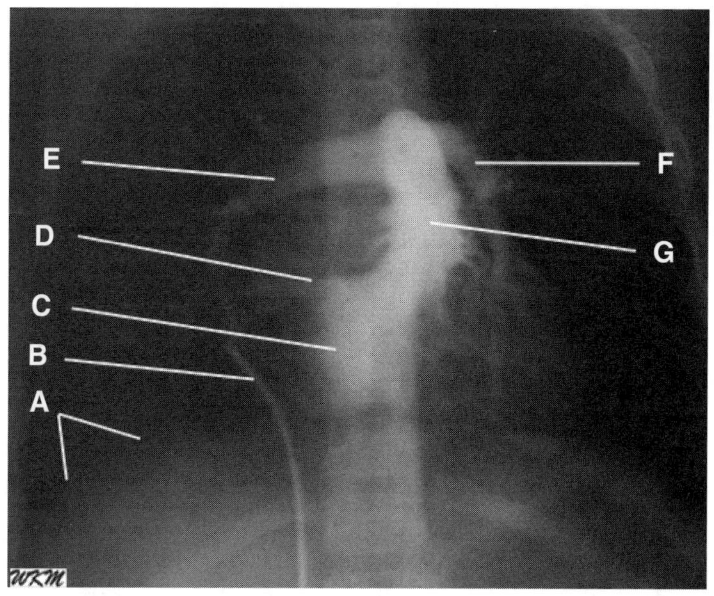

Figure 4-16 Pulmonary Arteriogram

Q. In Figure 4-16, identify C.

A. The contracting right ventricle.

Q. In Figure 4-16, identify D.

A. The closed right atrioventricular (tricuspid) valve.

Q. In Figure 4-16, identify E.

A. The right pulmonary artery. Note that it is much longer than the left pulmonary artery.

Q. The pulmonary trunk is displaced, as usual, to the left of the midline by . . .

A. The arch of the aorta.

Q. In Figure 4-16, identify F.

A. The left pulmonary artery.

Q. In Figure 4-16, identify G.

A. The pulmonary trunk.

Q. In Figure 4-17, identify A.

A. The trachea. In infants and children, it is smaller than it is in adults. Inhalation of a small object, such as a fragment of a peanut, is a common cause of accidental death in infants.

Q. In Figure 4-17, identify B.

A. The right principal bronchus. Its close alignment with the trachea makes it a common site for lodgment of foreign bodies in both children and adults. A common example in children is an inhaled primary tooth at or after the age of five. At about this age, the "milk" central incisors are shed. They will be replaced by the permanent incisors.

Q. In Figure 4-17, identify C.

A. The left principal bronchus. It is longer and clearly more oblique than the right bronchus. During early embryonic development of the normal fetal heart and lungs, the left bronchus is required to pass under the arch of the aorta to allow proper development of the left bronchial system and lung. By week 12, respiratory movements with movement of the contained fluid commence. This allows development of the normal respiratory mechanisms.

Q. In Figure 4-17, identify D.

A. The right atrium. It is very prominent in infants.

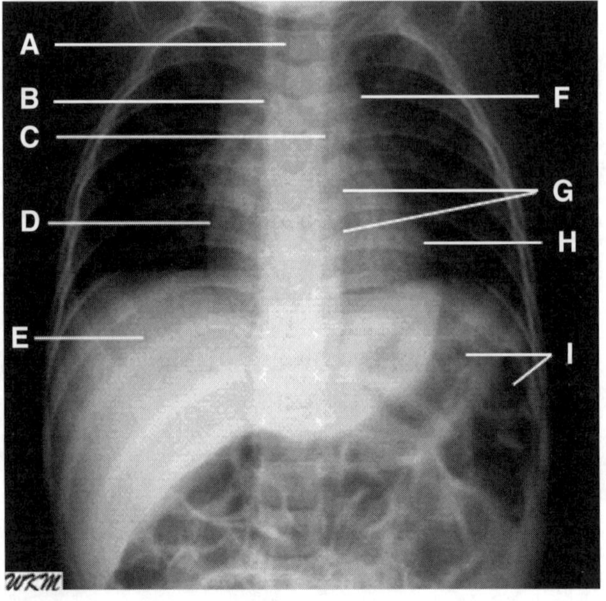

Figure 4-17 AP X-ray of Nine Month-Old Infant

Q. In Figure 4-17, identify E.

A. The liver.

Q. In Figure 4-17, identify F.

A. The arch of the aorta.

Q. In Figure 4-17, identify G.

A. The descending aorta.

Q. In Figure 4-17, identify H.

A. The left ventricle.

Q. In Figure 4-17, identify I.

A. Gas in the splenic flexure of the colon.

Q. In Figure 4-18, identify A.

A. The right subclavian vein.

Q. In Figure 4-18, identify B.
A. The right brachiocephalic vein.

Q. In Figure 4-18, identify C.
A. The superior vena cava.

Q. In Figure 4-18, identify D.
A. The right atrioventricular orifice.

Q. In Figure 4-18, identify E.
A. The right atrium.

Q. In Figure 4-18, identify F.
A. The inferior vena cava.

Q. In Figure 4-18, identify G.
A. The right and the left lobes of the liver.

Q. In Figure 4-18, identify H.
A. The left brachiocephalic vein.

Q. In Figure 4-18, identify I.
A. The ascending aorta.

Q. In Figure 4-18, identify J.
A. The pulmonary trunk.

Q. In Figure 4-18, identify K.
A. The left ventricle.

Q. In Figure 4-19, identify A.
A. The superior vena cava.

Q. In Figure 4-19, identify B.
A. The ascending aorta.

Q. In Figure 4-19, identify C.
A. The pulmonary trunk.

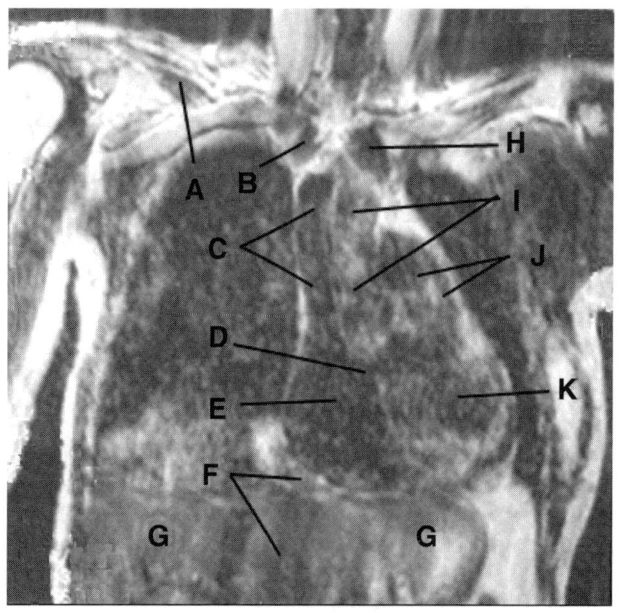

Figure 4-18 Coronal MRI of the Thorax

Q. In Figure 4-19, identify D.

A. The left main bronchus.

Q. In Figure 4-19, identify E.

A. The descending aorta.

Q. In Figure 4-19, identify F.

A. The esophagus.

Q. In Figure 4-19, identify G.

A. The right pulmonary artery.

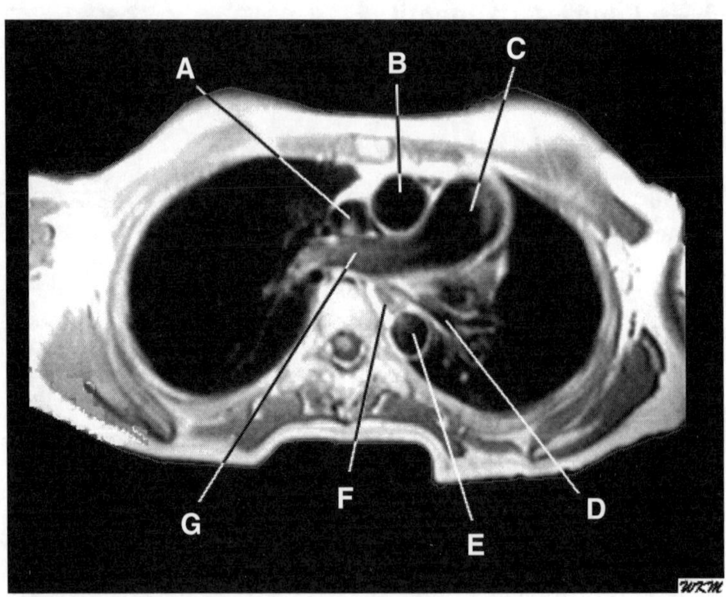

Figure 4-19 Transverse MRI of the Thorax

Q. In Figure 4-20, identify A.

A. A mammary implant. They make the diagnosis of mammary carcinoma very difficult.

Q. In Figure 4-20, identify B.

A. The superior vena cava opening into the right atrium.

Q. In Figure 4-20, identify C.

A. The aortic sinuses.

Q. In Figure 4-20, identify D.

A. The pulmonary trunk.

Q. In Figure 4-20, identify E.

A. The left ventricle.

Q. In Figure 4-20, identify F.

A. The descending aorta.

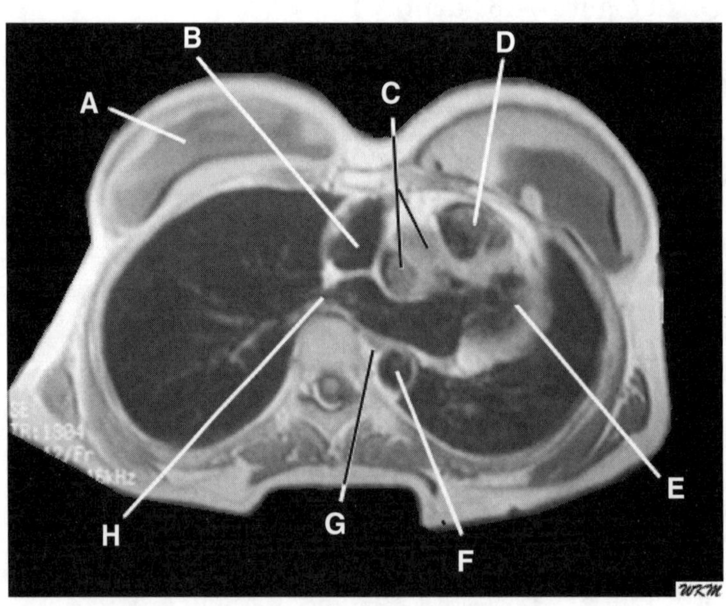

Figure 4-20 Transverse MRI of the Thorax

Q. In Figure 4-20, identify G.

A. The esophagus.

Q. In Figure 4-20, identify H.

A. The superior right pulmonary vein opening into the left atrium.

Chapter 5

The Abdomen

THE ABDOMINAL WALL, THE INGUINAL CANAL, AND THE TESTIS

Q. The anterior abdominal wall extends from the xiphisternal articulation to the symphysis pubis. Its cutaneous innervation is provided by the lateral and the anterior branches of . . .

A. The 7th through 11th thoracic (thoracoabdominal) nerves; the 12th thoracic (subcostal) nerves; and the iliohypogastric and ilioinguinal nerves, which are branches of the 1st lumbar nerves.

Q. The epigastric (supraumbilical) region is supplied by . . .

A. The 7th, 8th, and 9th thoracic anterior primary rami. This is the same segmental innervation as that of the stomach and of most of the small intestine.

Q. The cutaneous supply of the umbilical region comes from . . .

A. The anterior primary rami of the 10th thoracic nerves. This is the same segmental innervation as that of the distal small intestine, the appendix, the testis, and the ovary. This innervation is of significance because pain sensations from each of these organs, which are carried by visceral afferent fibers, are referred to the area of skin supplied by the same segmental nerves.

Q. The hypogastric region is supplied by . . .

A. The 11th thoracic nerves, the 12th thoracic (subcostal) nerves, and the 1st lumbar (iliohypogastric) nerves. This is the same segmental innervation as that of the large intestine.

Q. The blood supply of the abdominal wall originates from four major sources. They are . . .

A. The internal thoracic arteries, via their superior epigastric branches; the aorta, via its lower intercostal and lumbar branches; the external iliac arteries, via their deep circumflex iliac and deep inferior epigastric branches; and the femoral arteries, via their superficial circumflex iliac and superficial inferior epigastric branches.

Q. Four major muscles are on each side of the abdominal wall. They are . . .

A. The obliquus externus abdominis muscle, the obliquus internus abdominis muscle, the transversus abdominis muscle, and the rectus abdominis muscle.

Q. In Figure 5-1, identify A.

A. The obliquus externus abdominis muscle. Its fibers run medially, downward and forward.

Q. In Figure 5-1, identify B.

A. The aponeurosis of the obliquus externus abdominis muscle.

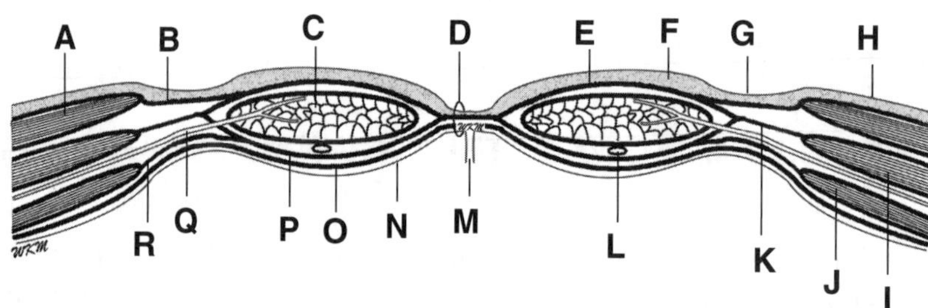

Figure 5-1 The Abdominal Wall above the Umbilicus, Horizontal Section

Q. In Figure 5-1, identify C.

A. The rectus abdominis muscle.

Q. In Figure 5-1, identify D.

A. The linea alba, the white line. It is the thinnest part of the abdominal wall. Because it is avascular, it is the easiest and quickest way to open the abdomen during surgery.

Q. In Figure 5-1, identify E.

A. The anterior layer of the sheath of the rectus abdominis muscle. It is firmly attached to the rectus abdominis muscle and to the tendinous intersections of that muscle. The clear visibility of these intersections is a matter of pride in the male body-building community.

Q. In Figure 5-1, identify F.

A. The fatty layer of subcutaneous tissue. It can reach thicknesses of 4 inches (10 cm) or more in the obese.

Q. In Figure 5-1, identify G.

A. The linea semilunaris. The linea semilunaris is a vertical linear depression in the abdominal wall at the lateral margin of each of the rectus abdominis muscles. It is the line where the obliquus externus abdominis muscle, the obliquus internus abdominis muscle, and the transversus abdominis muscle all become aponeurotic.

Q. In Figure 5-1, identify H.

A. The skin.

Q. In Figure 5-1, identify I.

A. The obliquus internus abdominis muscle. Its fibers run at right angles to the obliquus externus abdominis muscle.

Q. In Figure 5-1, identify J.

A. The transversus abdominis muscle.

Q. In Figure 5-1, identify K.

A. The aponeurosis of the obliquus internus abdominis muscle.

Q. In Figure 5-1, identify L.

A. The superior epigastric artery. It is one of the two terminal branches of the internal thoracic artery. The other terminal branch is the musculophrenic artery.

Q. In Figure 5-1, identify M.

A. The falciform ligament. It is a fold of peritoneum that runs to the liver from the anterior abdominal wall above the umbilicus. In the fetus, its free edge contains the umbilical vein. After birth, this vessel becomes fibrous and persists as the ligamentum teres hepatis.

Q. In Figure 5-1, identify N.

A. The parietal layer of the peritoneum.

Q. In Figure 5-1, identify O.

A. The transversalis fascia.

Q. In Figure 5-1, identify P.

A. The posterior layer of the rectus sheath. It is not attached to the intersections of the rectus abdominis muscle.

Q. In Figure 5-1, identify Q.

A. The 9th thoracic nerve. The 7th through the 11th thoracic nerves, the thoracoabdominal nerves, supply both intercostal and abdominal muscles. In the abdomen, they run around the body wall between the transversus abdominis muscles and the obliquus internus abdominis muscles. They supply the skin and all the muscles of the abdominal wall.

Q. In Figure 5-1, identify R.

A. The aponeurosis of the transversus abdominis muscle.

Q. Two abdominal muscles gain attachment to the external surfaces of the ribs and/or the costal cartilages. They are . . .

A. The obliquus externus abdominis muscle, which is attached to the costal cartilages/ribs 5–12, and the rectus abdominis muscle, which is attached to the 5th, 6th, and 7th costal cartilages.

Q. The muscle attached to the costal margin is . . .

A. The obliquus internus abdominis muscle. It is attached to the margins of the costal cartilages and ribs 7 through 12. The transversus abdominis muscle is attached to the inner surfaces of the costal cartilages and ribs 7 through 12, interdigitating with the diaphragm.

Q. The superior attachment of the obliquus externus abdominis muscle is . . .

A. The outer surfaces and lower borders of the lower eight ribs and costal cartilages. It interdigitates with the serratus anterior muscle.

Q. The posterior margin of the obliquus externus abdominis muscle is . . .

A. Not attached. The posterior border is free.

Q. Inferiorly, the obliquus externus abdominis muscle is attached to . . .

A. The anterior half of the outer lip of the iliac crest, to the anterior superior iliac spine, and to the pubic tubercle.

Q. Between the anterior superior iliac spine and the pubic tubercle, the unattached aponeurotic fibers of the obliquus externus abdominis muscle curl inward to form . . .

A. The inguinal ligament. Just lateral to the pubic tubercle, these fibers curve posteriorly to form the lacuna ligament. They continue along the superior ramus of the pubis as the pectinate ligament.

Q. Medially, the fibers of the obliquus externus abdominis muscle become aponeurotic along a line descending from the tip of the 9th costal cartilage. They then pass anterior to the edge of . . .

A. The vertical rectus abdominis muscle. They then join with the superficial part of the internal oblique aponeurosis and end in the midline by interlacing with the fibers of the obliquus externus abdominis muscle of the opposite side.

Q. The interlacing fibers of the two obliquus externus abdominis muscles form . . .

A. The linea alba. It is called this because it is avascular and white.

Q. The muscle fibers of the obliquus externus abdominis muscles extend anteriorly, that is medially, for a variable distance, but never extend medially beyond . . .

A. The vertical line, which extends downward from the tip of the 9th costal cartilage. They do not extend inferiorly below the level of the anterior superior iliac spine.

Q. The rectus abdominis muscles arise superiorly from the outer surface of . . .

A. The 5th, 6th, and 7th costal cartilages. The attachment of the lateral muscle fibers is to the 5th costal cartilage, the attachment of the intermediate fibers is to the 6th costal cartilage, and the attachment of the medial fibers is to the 7th costal cartilage at its articulation with the sternum.

Q. The rectus abdominis muscles are attached inferiorly to . . .

A. The pubic tubercles and to the pubic symphysis.

Q. Three horizontal fibrous intersections extend completely through the rectus abdominis muscles. They are the remnants of the fusions of individual embryonic myotomes. The superior intersections are at the level of . . .

A. The xiphisternum.

Q. The inferior fibrous rectus intersections are at the level of . . .

A. The umbilicus. The middle fibrous intersections lie midway between the other two.

Q. The fibrous rectus intersections are firmly attached to . . .

A. The anterior layer of the rectus sheath. The posterior layer of the rectus sheath is only complete superiorly; inferiorly, it is deficient.

Q. The superficial fascia is notorious for its tendency to accumulate fat. The fat cells accumulate in its superficial layer. Hence, the superficial fascia of the abdomen is divided into . . .

A. The superficial fatty layer (fascia of Camper) and the deeper membranous layer (fascia of Scarpa).

Q. The membranous layer of the superficial fascia is attached inferiorly to . . .

A. The iliac crests; to the deep fascia inferior to the inguinal ligaments, sometimes called Holden's lines; and to the pubic tubercles.

Q. In the male, in the midline between the pubic tubercles, the superficial fascia descends to cover . . .

A. The penis and the scrotum. Surrounding the penis, the superficial fascia loses its fatty layer so that only the membranous layer persists. On each side of the penis, the fatty and the membranous layers of the fascia blend. Smooth muscle, the dartos, replaces the superficial fascia over the testis, hence the wrinkled appearance of the scrotum. In the female, the fatty layer persists over the pubis as the mons veneris. Both layers can be followed further into the labia majora.

Q. In Figure 5-2, identify A.

A. The obliquus externus abdominis muscle.

Q. In Figure 5-2, identify B.

A. The aponeurosis of the obliquus externus abdominis muscle.

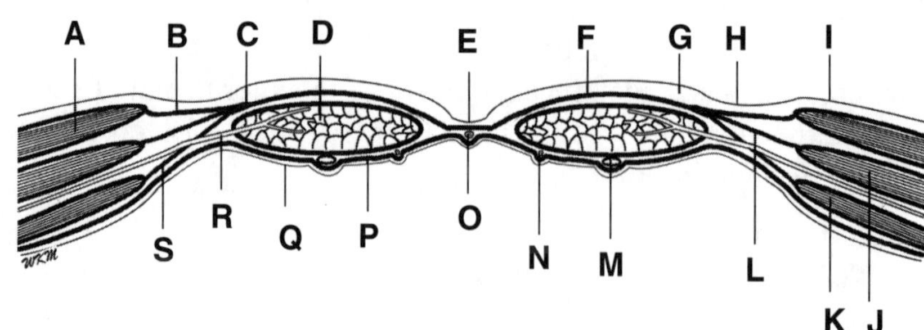

Figure 5-2 The Abdominal Wall below the Arcuate Line, Horizontal Section

Q. In Figure 5-2, identify C.

A. The point of fusion of the aponeuroses of all three lateral muscles of the abdominal wall. The fusion of the three aponeuroses forms the anterior layer of the rectus sheath. Below the arcuate line, the posterior layer of the rectus sheath is absent, and the rectus abdominis muscle is separated from the peritoneum only by the transversalis fascia.

Q. In Figure 5-2, identify D.

A. The rectus abdominis muscle.

Q. In Figure 5-2, identify E.

A. The linea alba.

Q. In Figure 5-2, identify F.

A. The anterior layer of the rectus sheath of the rectus abdominis femoris muscle. At this level, below the arcuate line, it is formed by the fusion of the aponeuroses of all the three lateral abdominal wall muscles.

Q. In Figure 5-2, identify G.

A. Subcutaneous fat in the superficial fascia. Below the umbilicus, fat tends to accumulate even more rapidly in the superficial part of the superficial fascia than it does above the level of the umbilicus. So much so, that, as previously noted, the superficial fascia is often divided anatomically into a superficial fatty layer (fascia of Camper) and a deeper membranous layer (fascia of Scarpa).

Q. In Figure 5-2, identify H.

A. The lower part of the linea semilunaris. It is situated at the lateral margin of each rectus abdominis muscle.

Q. In Figure 5-2, identify I.

A. The skin.

Q. In Figure 5-2, identify J.

A. The obliquus internus abdominis muscle.

Q. In Figure 5-2, identify K.

A. The transversus abdominis muscle.

Q. In Figure 5-2, identify L.

A. The aponeurosis of the obliquus internus abdominis muscle.

Q. In Figure 5-2, identify M.

A. The inferior epigastric artery. It raises the lateral umbilical fold of the parietal peritoneum of the anterior abdominal wall.

Q. In Figure 5-2, identify N.

A. The medial umbilical ligament, the obliterated umbilical artery of the fetus. It raises the medial umbilical fold of the peritoneum of the anterior abdominal wall.

Q. In Figure 5-2, identify O.

A. The median umbilical ligament and its peritoneal fold. The median umbilical ligament is the remnant of the urachus of the fetus. It raises the median umbilical fold of the peritoneum of the anterior abdominal wall.

Q. In Figure 5-2, identify P.

A. The transversalis fascia.

Q. In Figure 5-2, identify Q.

A. The parietal layer of the peritoneum.

Q. In Figure 5-2, identify R.

A. The subcostal nerve.

Q. In Figure 5-2, identify S.

A. The aponeurosis of the transversus abdominis muscle.

Q. The fibers of the obliquus internus abdominis muscles run at right angles to those of the obliquus externus abdominis muscles. The direction of their fibers corresponds with the corresponding muscles of the thorax: the intercostales interna muscles and the intercostales externa muscles. The inferior attachment of each obliquus internus abdominis muscle is often called its origin. The obliquus internus abdominis muscle is attached inferiorly to . . .

A. The lateral two-thirds of the inguinal ligament, to the anterior two-thirds of the iliac crest, and, posteriorly, to the thoracolumbar fascia.

Q. The superior attachment of the obliquus internus abdominis muscle is to . . .

A. The costal margin.

Q. Between the xiphisternum and a point midway between the umbilicus and the pubis, the aponeurosis of the obliquus internus abdominis muscle divides into anterior and posterior layers to enclose . . .

A. The rectus abdominis muscle. The two layers form its sheath.

Q. Below this point, midway between the pubis and the umbilicus, all of the fibers of the obliquus internus abdominis muscle pass anterior to the rectus abdominis muscle. Together with the lower fibers of the transversus abdominis muscle, with which they fuse, they form . . .

A. The conjoint tendon. It is attached to the pubic crest.

Q. The posterior sheath of the rectus abdominis muscle is deficient inferiorly. The inferior margin of the posterior wall of the rectus sheath is called . . .

A. The arcuate line.

Q. The lateral margin of the rectus sheath forms . . .

A. The vertical (curved) linea semilunaris.

Q. The transversus abdominis muscle runs horizontally from its origin but fans out as it passes anteriorly. Its origin is, posterolaterally, from . . .

A. The inner surface of the lower six ribs, the thoracolumbar fascia, the anterior two-thirds of the iliac crest, and the outer one-third of the inguinal ligament.

Q. The fibers of the transversus abdominis muscle, which arise from the inguinal ligament, arch superior to the deep inguinal ring. They fuse with the lower fibers of the obliquus internus abdominis muscle to form . . .

A. The conjoint tendon.

Q. The aponeurotic fibers of the upper part of the transversus abdominis muscle fuse with . . .

A. The aponeurotic superior, posterior fibers of the obliquus internus abdominis muscle.

Q. Together they form . . .

A. The posterior wall of the rectus sheath. They then continue to fuse with the linea alba.

Q. The thoracoabdominal nerves run around the abdominal wall between . . .

A. The obliquus internus abdominis muscles and the transversus abdominis muscles.

Q. To reach and supply the rectus abdominis muscle, they must perforate . . .

A. The posterior layer of the rectus sheath.

Q. The transversus abdominis muscle is separated from the peritoneum by . . .

A. The transversalis fascia.

Q. The testis descends, with the spermatic cord trailing behind it, through the abdominal wall late during fetal life. It first passes through . . .

A. The transversalis fascia, inferomedial to the arched margin of the transversus abdominis muscle.

Q. The "opening" through which the testis passes is . . .

A. The deep inguinal ring.

Q. Medial to the deep inguinal ring lies . . .

A. The deep inferior epigastric artery. From its origin from the external iliac artery, it runs upward and medially to the rectus sheath.

Q. The transversalis fascia continues over the testis and spermatic cord as . . .

A. The internal spermatic fascia.

Q. The internal spermatic fascia, which surrounds the spermatic cord, continues downward and medially, forming the inguinal canal. The deep inguinal ring is guarded anteriorly by . . .

A. Those muscle fibers of the obliquus internus abdominis muscle that arise from the lateral one-half to two-thirds of the inguinal ligament.

Q. In Figure 5-3, identify A.

A. The linea alba. It divides inferiorly into a deep insertion and a superficial insertion. The deep attachment, lying posterior to the rectus abdominis muscle, is inserted into the posterior part of the pubic crest. It is named the adminiculum lineae albae. The superficial attachment is anterior to the rectus abdominis muscle. It is not shown in this diagram.

Q. In Figure 5-3, identify B.

A. The rectus abdominis muscle.

Q. In Figure 5-3, identify C.

A. The transversus abdominis muscle.

Q. In Figure 5-3, identify D.

A. The arcuate line. Inferior to the arcuate line, the aponeurosis of the transversus abdominis muscle and the aponeurosis of the obliquus abdominis internus muscle fuse and pass in front of the rectus abdominis muscle to form the conjoint tendon, the falx inguinale.

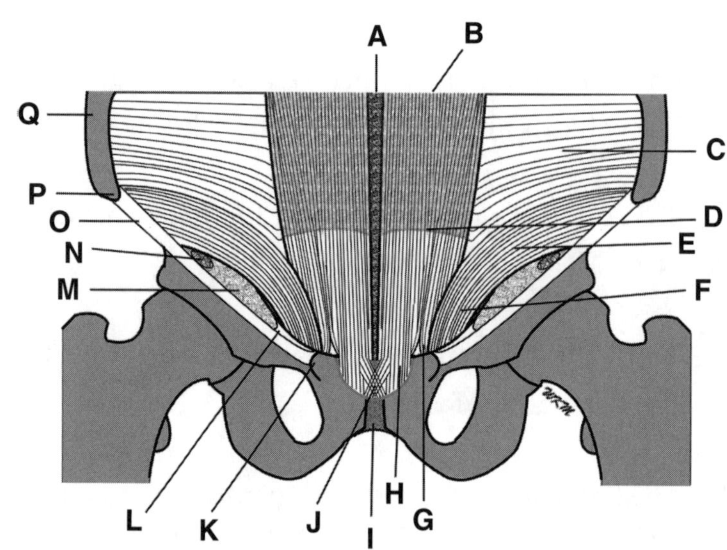

Figure 5-3 The Inguinal Canal, Deep Dissection

Q. In Figure 5-3, identify E.

A. The inferior fibers of the transversus abdominis muscle. These fibers arise from the lateral one-third of the inguinal ligament and join with fibers of the obliquus internus abdominis to form the conjoint tendon, the falx inguinale.

Q. In Figure 5-3, identify F.

A. The conjoint tendon. It is inserted into the crest and medial part of the pecten pubis.

Q. In Figure 5-3, identify G.

A. The lateral tendon of the rectus abdominis muscle. It is attached to the crest of the pubis, deep to the smaller medial tendon of the same muscle and deep to the conjoint tendon.

Q. In Figure 5-3, identify H.

A. The smaller, medial tendon of the rectus abdominis muscle. It is attached to the anterior surface of the symphysis pubis.

Q. In Figure 5-3, identify I.

A. The symphysis pubis.

Q. In Figure 5-3, identify J.

A. The interlacing fibers of the medial tendons of both rectus abdominis muscles.

Q. In Figure 5-3, identify K.

A. The pubic tubercle. It provides attachment for the medial end of the inguinal ligament.

Q. In Figure 5-3, identify L.

A. The lacunar part of the inguinal ligament. It is a posterolateral extension of the medial end of the inguinal ligament, which extends laterally to be attached to the pectineal line of the pubis. Its superior surface forms the floor of the medial end of the inguinal canal.

Q. In Figure 5-3, identify M.

A. The transversalis fascia. It forms the posterior wall of the inguinal canal.

Q. In Figure 5-3, identify N.

A. The deep inguinal ring. The spermatic cord passes through it in the male. In the female, the round ligament of the uterus, a much smaller structure, exits it to reach the labia majora.

Q. In Figure 5-3, identify O.

A. The inguinal ligament. It is the thickened, posteriorly upturned inferior margin of the aponeurosis of the obliquus externus abdominis muscle.

Q. In Figure 5-3, identify P.

A. The anterior superior iliac spine. It is the lateral attachment for the inguinal ligament.

Q. In Figure 5-3, identify Q.

A. The iliac crest.

Q. The spermatic cord passes under the arched lower fibers of the obliquus internus abdominis muscle. As it does so, it obtains a muscular coating. This forms . . .

A. The cremaster muscle.

Q. Other than cardiac muscle, muscles are either smooth or striated. The cremaster muscle is . . .

A. Striated, fast-twitch, muscle. Witness the speed with which the cremasteric reflex elevates the testis when that organ is threatened!

Q. The segment of the spinal cord tested by the cremasteric reflex is . . .

A. The 1st lumbar segment.

Q. The spermatic cord finally "penetrates" the obliquus externus abdominis at the external ring, which is reinforced by medial, lateral, and intercrural fibers. The layer of spermatic fascia acquired at this aperture is . . .

A. The external spermatic fascia.

Q. The nerve that enters the inguinal canal through the deep inguinal ring to supply the cremaster muscle is . . .

A. The genital branch of the genitofemoral nerve.

Q. The nerve that passes through the superficial ring lateral to the spermatic cord is . . .

A. The ilioinguinal nerve.

Q. The superficial inguinal ring is supported posteriorly by . . .

A. The conjoint tendon, the falx inguinale.

Q. The contents of the spermatic cord are . . .

A. The ductus (vas) deferens and its vessels, the testicular artery, the pampiniform plexus of veins, and a plexus of postganglionic sympathetic and visceral afferent nerves.

Q. In the scrotum, in addition to the various layers of spermatic fascia and the dartos muscle, the testis is covered by . . .

A. The tunica vaginalis testis.

Q. There are two layers of the tunica vaginalis testis. They are . . .

A. The visceral (internal) layer and the parietal (external) layer. These layers become continuous posteriorly. The visceral layer covers the thick white protective tunica albuginea testis.

Q. Posterior to the testis lies . . .

A. The epididymis. It is described as having a head (caput), a body (corpus), and a tail (cauda).

Q. On the lateral side, the epididymis is partially separated from the testis by a cleft. This cleft is . . .

A. The sinus of the epididymis.

Q. In Figure 5-4, identify A.

A. The anterior layer of the rectus sheath.

Q. In Figure 5-4, identify B.

A. The aponeurosis of the obliquus internus abdominis muscle. It divides into anterior and posterior laminae, which contribute to the anterior and posterior layers of the sheath of the rectus abdominis muscle.

Q. In Figure 5-4, identify C.

A. The muscle fibers of the upper two-thirds of the obliquus internus abdominis muscle.

Q. In Figure 5-4, identify D.

A. The lower segment of the obliquus internus abdominis muscle. It fuses with the transversus abdominis muscle to form the conjoint tendon, the falx inguinale.

Q. In Figure 5-4, identify E.

A. The deep inguinal ring. It lies under the lower fibers of the obliquus internus abdominis muscle.

Q. In Figure 5-4, identify F.

A. The arched lower fibers of the obliquus internus abdominis muscle. Their contraction is the major factor that prevents herniation of the abdominal contents down the inguinal canal.

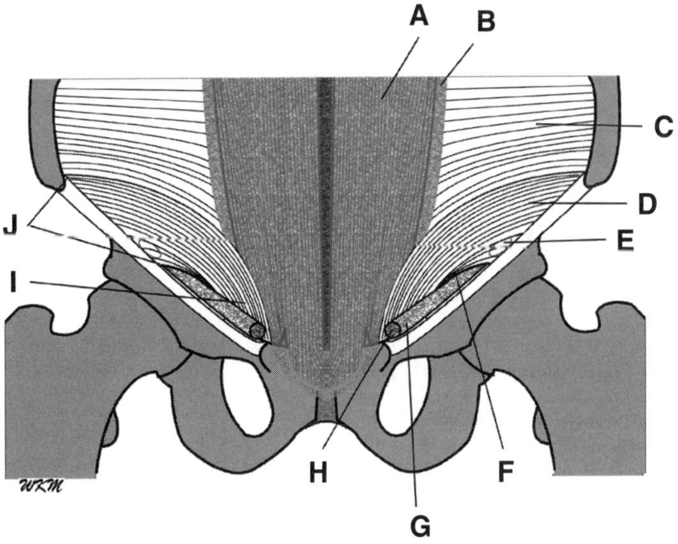

Q. In Figure 5-4, identify G.

A. The spermatic cord in the inguinal canal.

Q. In Figure 5-4, identify H.

A. The sectioned spermatic cord.

Figure 5-4 The Inguinal Canal; Intermediate Dissection

Q. In Figure 5-4, identify I.

A. The conjoint tendon, the falx inguinale.

Q. In Figure 5-4, identify J.

A. The segment of the obliquus internus abdominis muscle that arises from the lateral one-half to two-thirds of the inguinal ligament.

Q. In Figure 5-5, identify A.

A. The linea alba.

Q. In Figure 5-5, identify B.

A. The shadow of the underlying rectus abdominis muscle. It is covered by the anterior layer of the rectus sheath.

Q. In Figure 5-5, identify C.

A. The muscle fibers of the obliquus internus abdominis muscle. They are seen through the aponeurosis of the obliquus externus abdominis muscle.

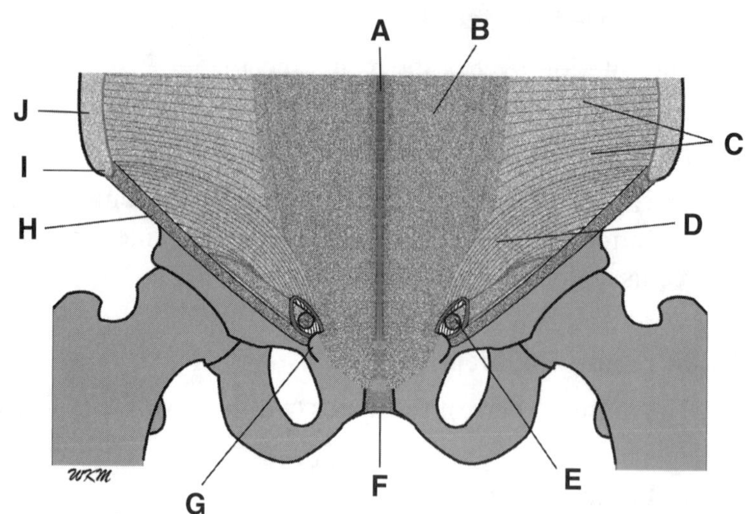

Figure 5-5 The Inguinal Canal: the Aponeurosis of the Obliquus Externus Abdominis Muscle and the Superficial Inguinal Ring

Q. In Figure 5-5, identify D.

A. The conjoint tendon. It is seen through the aponeurosis of the obliquus externus abdominis muscle.

Q. In Figure 5-5, identify E.

A. The spermatic cord. It is shown as it is emerges through the superficial inguinal ring.

Q. In Figure 5-5, identify F.

A. The arcuate pubic ligament. It joins the bodies of the pubic bones inferior to the pubic symphysis.

Q. In Figure 5-5, identify G.

A. The pubic tubercle.

Q. In Figure 5-5, identify H.

A. The thickened, posteriorly curled, inferior margin of the aponeurosis of the obliquus externus abdominis muscle. It forms the inguinal ligament.

Q. In Figure 5-5, identify I.

A. The anterior superior iliac spine.

Q. In Figure 5-5, identify J.

A. The iliac crest. The obliquus externus abdominis muscle is attached to its outer lip; the obliquus internus abdominis muscle is attached to its intermediate area; and the transversus abdominis muscle is attached to its inner (medial) lip.

Q. In Figure 5-6, identify A.

A. The lateral crus of the superficial inguinal ring. It is the thicker of the two crura and is attached to the pubic tubercle.

Q. In Figure 5-6, identify B.

A. The intercrural fibers of the superficial inguinal ring. They join the two crura and prevent the superficial ring from enlarging laterally.

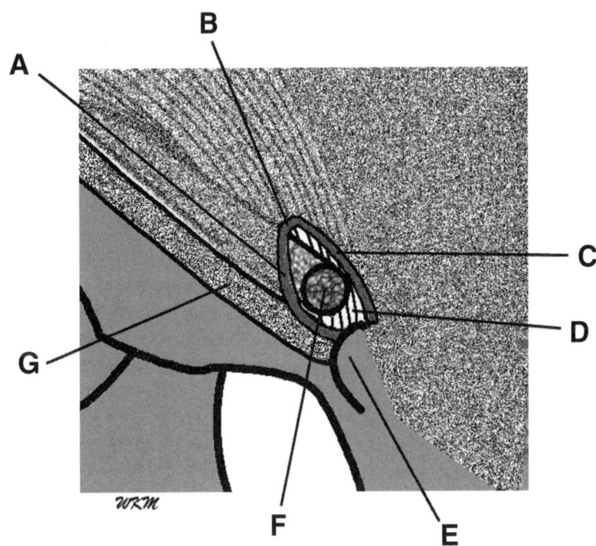

Figure 5-6 The Right Superficial Inguinal Ring

Q. In Figure 5-6, identify C.

A. The medial crus of the superficial inguinal ring. It is a flat band that is attached to the front of the pubic symphysis.

Q. In Figure 5-6, identify D.

A. The conjoint tendon. It passes posterior to the superficial ring and to the spermatic cord. It protects, strengthens, and reinforces the superficial ring and the posterior wall of the medial part of the inguinal canal.

Q. In Figure 5-6, identify E.

A. The pubic tubercle.

Q. In Figure 5-6, identify F.

A. The cut spermatic cord. It is seen as it emerges through the superficial inguinal ring.

Q. In Figure 5-6, identify G.

A. The medial end of the inguinal ligament. The thickened, posteriorly curved, upturned, inferior margin of the inguinal ligament is said to form the floor of the inguinal canal.

Q. In Figure 5-7, identify A.

A. The transversus abdominis muscle.

Q. In Figure 5-7, identify B.

A. The obliquus internus abdominis muscle. It continues, blending with the spermatic cord, as the cremaster muscle.

Q. In Figure 5-7, identify C.

A. The aponeurosis of the obliquus externus abdominis muscle. It continues as the external spermatic fascia.

Q. In Figure 5-7, identify D.

A. The fatty layer of superficial fascia (Camper's fascia).

Q. In Figure 5-7, identify E.

A. The deeper, membranous layer of superficial fascia (Scarpa's fascia).

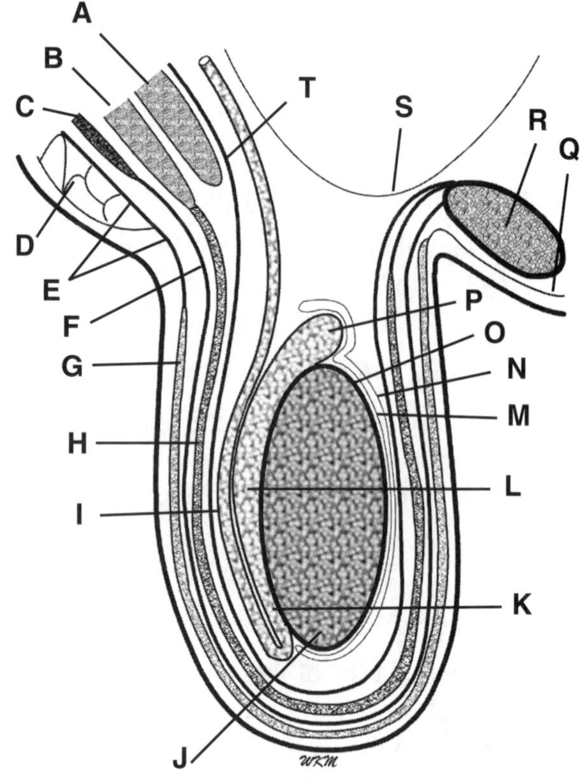

Figure 5-7 The Coverings of the Testis

Q. In Figure 5-7, identify F.

A. The external spermatic fascia. It is continuous with the aponeurosis of the obliquus externus abdominis muscle.

Q. In Figure 5-7, identify G.

A. The dartos muscle. It is continuous with the membranous layer of the superficial fascia. Composed of visceral muscle, it is responsible for keeping the testis near body temperature when external temperatures are too low for spermatogenesis.

Q. In Figure 5-7, identify H.

A. The cremaster muscle. It is a continuation of the obliquus abdominis muscle. It is supplied by the genital branch of the genitofemoral nerve.

Q. In Figure 5-7, identify I.

A. The ductus (vas) deferens.

Q. In Figure 5-7, identify J.

A. The lower pole of the testis.

Q. In Figure 5-7, identify K.

A. The tail (cauda) of the epididymis. It is formed by the coiled distal end of the duct of the epididymis.

Q. In Figure 5-7, identify L.

A. The body (corpus) of the epididymis. It is also formed by the coiled duct of the epididymis.

Q. In Figure 5-7, identify M.

A. The visceral layer of the tunica vaginalis testis. It is a thin serous layer, akin to the visceral layer of the peritoneum. Indeed, it is derived from fetal peritoneum and descends into the scrotal sac with the testis. It enables movement of the testis within the tunica vaginalis.

Q. In Figure 5-7, identify N.

A. The parietal layer of the tunica vaginalis testis. It also is derived from fetal peritoneum.

Q. In Figure 5-7, identify O.

A. The tunica albuginea of the testis. The tunica albuginea testis is a thick, tough, fibrous, white covering that forms a protective coat around the testis. The tunica albuginea oopharus, which covers the ovary, is much thinner, allowing for the monthly passage of an unfertilized ovum.

Q. In Figure 5-7, identify P.

A. The head (caput) of the epididymis. It is made up of numerous lobules, each connected to a group of efferent ductules of the testis. The lobules ultimately unite to form the duct of the epididymis.

Q. In Figure 5-7, identify Q.

A. The continuation of the membranous layer of superficial fascia into the perineum. It has been renamed Colles' fascia. Over the testis, it had become the dartos muscle.

Q. In Figure 5-7, identify R.

A. The symphysis pubis.

Q. In Figure 5-7, identify S.

A. The parietal layer of the peritoneum.

Q. In Figure 5-7, identify T.

A. The continuation of the transversalis fascia. It now forms the internal spermatic fascia, which surrounds the scrotal contents.

THE PERITONEUM

Q. The walls of the abdominal cavity are lined by a serous membrane, which allows free movements of the abdominal alimentary canal, which it contains. The membrane that lines the abdominal cavity is . . .

A. The peritoneum.

Q. The peritoneum that lines the walls of the abdominal cavity is known as . . .

A. The parietal peritoneum.

Q. The parietal peritoneum is attached to, and strengthened by, an external layer of fascia named after the appropriate region of the abdominal wall. On the posterior surface of the anterior abdominal wall muscles, this layer of fascia is named . . .

A. The transversalis fascia.

Q. The parietal peritoneum on the posterior surface of the anterior body wall is raised in three folds extending inferiorly from the diaphragm. They are . . .

A. The median, the medial, and the lateral inferior umbilical folds.

Q. The infraumbilical folds are caused by underlying structures lying in the transversalis fascia. These structures are, from the median to the lateral side, . . .

A. The remains of the urachus of the fetus, the obliterated umbilical artery, and the deep inferior epigastric vessels.

Q. The peritoneum covering the intraabdominal viscera is . . .

A. The visceral peritoneum.

Q. The visceral and the parietal layers of the peritoneum are connected by double-layered folds of peritoneum. In the case of solid organs, such as the liver and the uterus, these double layers of peritoneum are known as . . .

A. The ligaments of the organ concerned.

Q. The liver is connected anteriorly to the supraumbilical posterior surface of the anterior abdominal wall by . . .

A. The falciform ligament. It has a lower free margin.

Q. In the free edge of the falciform ligament lies . . .

A. The obliterated umbilical vein, the ligamentum teres hepaticus.

Q. The liver is attached to the diaphragm by a series of double folds of peritoneum. These layers are not necessarily in close apposition, and therefore leave several areas where the liver and diaphragm are in direct contact. These areas are known as . . .

A. The bare areas of the liver.

Q. The peritoneal ligaments (folds) that attach the liver to the diaphragm are . . .

A. The anterior and posterior layers of the left and right triangular ligaments and the superior (anterior) and inferior (posterior) layers of the hepatic coronary ligaments.

Q. The reflections of all of these hepatic ligaments from the liver are continuous. The large bare area of the liver thus lies between . . .

A. The superior (anterior) and inferior (posterior) layers of the coronary ligaments.

Q. In the bare area of the liver, between the superior and inferior coronary ligaments, a large vessel is embedded in the diaphragmatic surface of the liver. It is . . .

A. The inferior vena cava.

Q. Other peritoneal folds, the mesenteries, connect much of the alimentary canal with the posterior abdominal wall. In the mesenteries are . . .

A. The arteries, the veins, and the lymphatics that supply the intestine. Autonomic nerves and visceral afferent nerves accompany them.

Q. The autonomic nerves in the mesenteries are . . .

A. Postganglionic sympathetic fibers, which have synapsed in the celiac, the superior mesenteric and the inferior mesenteric ganglia, and preganglionic parasympathetic fibers, which will synapse in the wall of the intestines themselves.

Q. The parts of the gut that have mesenteries are . . .

A. The jejunum and ileum (the mesentery proper, the mesentery); the appendix (mesoappendix); the transverse colon (transverse mesocolon); and the sigmoid colon (sigmoid mesocolon).

Q. During early embryological development, the stomach has ventral and dorsal mesenteries. The ventral mesentery (ventral mesogastrium) of the stomach in the adult is . . .

A. The lesser omentum, the gastrohepatic ligament.

Q. In postnatal anatomy, the dorsal mesentery of the stomach is divided into three regions that are named according to their attachments. They are, from proximal to distal, . . .

A. The gastrophrenic ligament; the gastrosplenic and the lienorenal ligaments; and the greater omentum. The development of the spleen, between the layers of the dorsal mesentery of the stomach (the dorsal mesogastrium), divides the intermediate region of the dorsal mesogastrium into the gastrosplenic and lienorenal ligaments.

Q. During fetal life, the ascending and the descending colon and the rectum become adherent to . . .

A. The structures of the posterior abdominal wall. Their mesenteries are therefore obliterated. These regions of the alimentary canal are thus often described as being retroperitoneal. However, they are not true components of the posterior abdominal wall.

Q. The pancreas is described as being retroperitoneal because both the ventral and the dorsal pancreatic buds from which it develops grow into the . . .

A. The dorsal duodenal mesentery. When the dorsal duodenal mesentery is absorbed by adherence to the posterior abdominal wall, the pancreas becomes retroperitoneal.

Q. In early development, the suprarenal glands and kidneys develop in the urogenital ridge of the mesoderm of the posterior abdominal wall. Thus, they never have mesenteries. Therefore, they are. . .

A. True retroperitoneal structures.

Q. The ovaries and testes develop in the same posterior abdominal wall urogenital ridge. However, the peritoneal covering of the ovary was renamed . . .

A. The germinal epithelium of the ovary because it was originally believed that this "epithelium" gave rise to ova. Therefore, the relationship of the ovary to the peritoneal cavity is unique and semantically equivocal.

Q. During embryological development, the testis slides down the posterior wall of the peritoneal processus vaginalis. Except in the presence of a congenital inguinal hernia, the connection of the processus vaginalis to the peritoneal cavity is obliterated. This leaves the testis with its own individual "peritoneal sac." This structure is called . . .

A. The tunica vaginalis testis.

Q. The peritoneal cavity is a closed cavity only in . . .

A. The male.

Q. In the female, the peritoneal cavity communicates with the exterior through . . .

A. The uterine tubes, the uterus, and the vagina. This is a potential route of infection after around 7 years of age that can occasionally result in peritonitis, especially after forcible, contaminated vaginal "douches," as may occur in water skiing.

Q. The two communicating peritoneal cavities are . . .

A. The much larger greater sac and the smaller lesser sac. The latter is situated mainly posterior to the stomach.

Q. They communicate through . . .

A. The aditus to the lesser sac, the epiploic foramen.

Q. The posterior boundary of the epiploic foramen is . . .

A. The parietal peritoneum over the inferior vena cava.

Q. The superior boundary of the epiploic foramen is . . .

A. The visceral peritoneum over the caudate process of the liver.

Q. The inferior boundary of the epiploic foramen is . . .

A. The visceral peritoneum over the first part of the duodenum.

Q. The anterior boundary of the epiploic foramen is . . .

A. The free edge of the lesser omentum.

Q. The structures enclosed in the free edge of the lesser omentum are . . .

A. The hepatic artery anteriorly and to the left, the common bile duct anteriorly and to the right, and the portal vein posteriorly.

Q. Bleeding from the liver during surgery that cannot be controlled by compressing the portal vein and the hepatic artery between a finger in the epiploic foramen and a thumb on the free edge of the lesser omentum is most likely coming from a torn . . .

A. Hepatic vein.

Q. In Figure 5-8, identify A.

A. The right kidney.

Q. In Figure 5-8, identify B.

A. The right lobe of the liver.

Q. In Figure 5-8, identify C.

A. The inferior vena cava.

Q. In Figure 5-8, identify D.

A. The portal vein. Note that it is only separated from the inferior vena cava by the epiploic foramen.

Q. In Figure 5-8, identify E.

A. The common bile duct. It lies in the free edge of the lesser omentum.

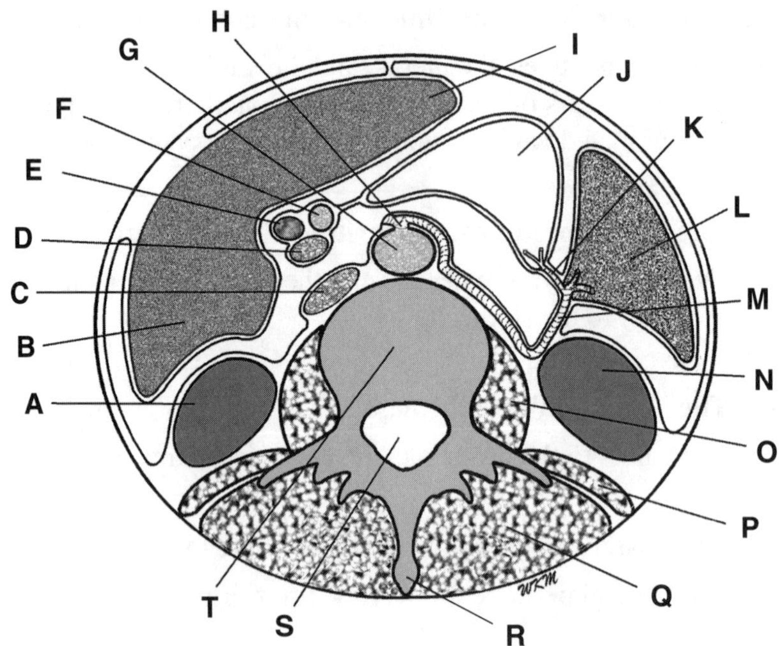

Figure 5-8 Transverse Section of the Abdomen at L1: Organs and Vessels

Q. In Figure 5-8, identify F.

A. The proper hepatic artery. It is the continuation of the common hepatic artery, which is a branch of the celiac trunk. It has traveled retroperitoneally above the first part of the duodenum to reach the free edge of the lesser omentum.

Q. In Figure 5-8, identify G.

A. The aorta.

Q. In Figure 5-8, identify H.

A. The celiac trunk. It gives rise to three branches, all of which supply embryological foregut derivatives. These branches are the common hepatic artery, the splenic artery, and the left gastric artery. The left gastric artery is not visible in this section.

Q. In Figure 5-8, identify I.

A. The left lobe of the liver.

Q. In Figure 5-8, identify J.

A. The body of the stomach.

Q. In Figure 5-8, identify K.

A. The left gastroepiploic artery. It is a branch of the splenic artery. It reaches the greater curvature of the stomach via the gastrosplenic ligament.

Q. In Figure 5-8, identify L.

A. The spleen.

Q. In Figure 5-8, identify M.

A. The splenic artery. It arises from the celiac trunk and supplies the pancreas, the greater curvature of the stomach, and the spleen.

Q. In Figure 5-8, identify N.

A. The left kidney.

Q. In Figure 5-8, identify O.

A. The left psoas major muscle.

Q. In Figure 5-8, identify P.

A. The left quadratus lumborum muscle.

Q. In Figure 5-8, identify Q.

A. The left erector spinae muscle.

Q. In Figure 5-8, identify R.

A. The spine of the 1st lumbar vertebra.

Q. In Figure 5-8, identify S.

A. The vertebral canal.

Q. In Figure 5-8, identify T.

A. The body of the 1st lumbar vertebra.

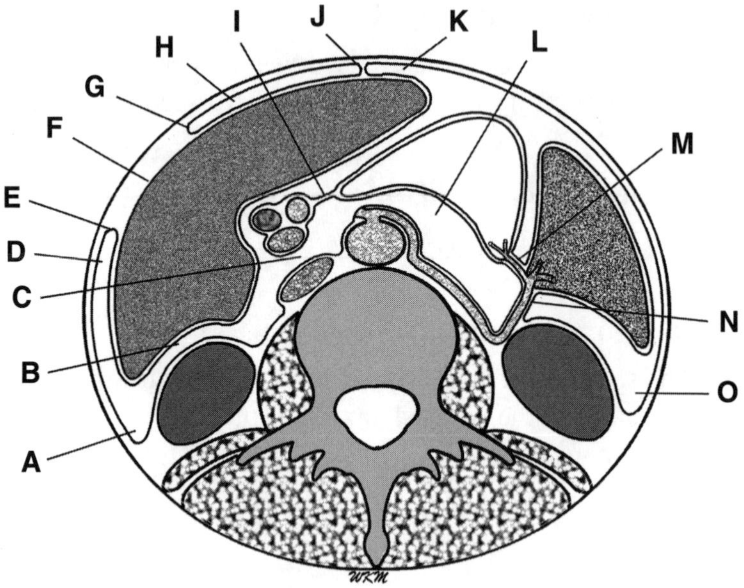

Q. In Figure 5-9, identify A.

A. The right paracolic gutter. It leads downward from the hepatorenal recess lateral to the ascending colon and the cecum into the pelvis.

Q. In Figure 5-9, identify B.

A. The hepatorenal recess, Morison's pouch. Fluid leaking from a perforated gastric or duodenal ulcer tends to collect here.

Q. In Figure 5-9, identify C.

A. The epiploic foramen, the aditus to the lesser sac. It is bounded anteriorly by the portal vein in the free edge of the lesser omentum, posteriorly by the inferior vena cava, superiorly by the caudate lobe of the liver, and inferiorly by the first part of the duodenum.

Figure 5-9 Transverse Section of the Abdomen at L1: Peritoneal Folds and Spaces

Q. In Figure 5-9, identify D.

A. The right posterior subphrenic space. An abscess in this space is difficult to diagnose and difficult to treat. Hence the saying, "Pus somewhere, pus nowhere else, pus under the diaphragm."

Q. In Figure 5-9, identify E.

A. The inferior layer of the hepatic coronary ligament.

Q. In Figure 5-9, identify F.

A. The bare area of the liver. This is the region where the liver lies in direct contact with the diaphragm.

Q. In Figure 5-9, identify G.

A. The superior layer of the hepatic coronary ligament.

Q. In Figure 5-9, identify H.

A. The right anterior subphrenic space.

Q. In Figure 5-9, identify I.

A. The lesser omentum, the gastrohepatic ligament.

Q. The arteries that run along the lesser curvature of the stomach in the lesser omentum are . . .

A. The left and right gastric arteries.

Q. In Figure 5-9, identify J.

A. The falciform ligament. Its free margin contains the ligamentum teres hepatis.

Q. The ligamentum teres hepatis is the fibrous remnant of . . .

A. The left umbilical vein of fetal life.

Q. In Figure 5-9, identify K.

A. The left anterior subphrenic space.

Q. In Figure 5-9, identify L.

A. The lesser sac of peritoneum, the bursa omentalis.

Q. In Figure 5-9, identify M.

A. The gastrosplenic ligament.

Q. The arteries in the gastrosplenic ligament are . . .

A. The left gastroepiploic artery and the short gastric arteries.

Q. In Figure 5-9, identify N.

A. The lienorenal ligament.

Q. The artery in the lienorenal ligament is . . .

A. The splenic artery.

Q. In Figure 5-9, identify O.

A. The left paracolic gutter. Clinically, it is not as important as its right counterpart because it is rarely the site of an infective process.

Q. In Figure 5-10, identify A.

A. The inferior vena cava.

Q. In Figure 5-10, identify B.

A. The superior (anterior) layer of the coronary ligament.

Q. In Figure 5-10, identify C.

A. The orifices in the inferior cava for the hepatic veins.

Q. In Figure 5-10, identify D.

A. The right lobe of the liver.

Q. In Figure 5-10, identify E.

A. The common bile duct. Inferiorly, it deviates to the right to enter the second part of the duodenum.

Q. In Figure 5-10, identify F.

A. The epiploic foramen, the aditus to the lesser sac, seen from the right.

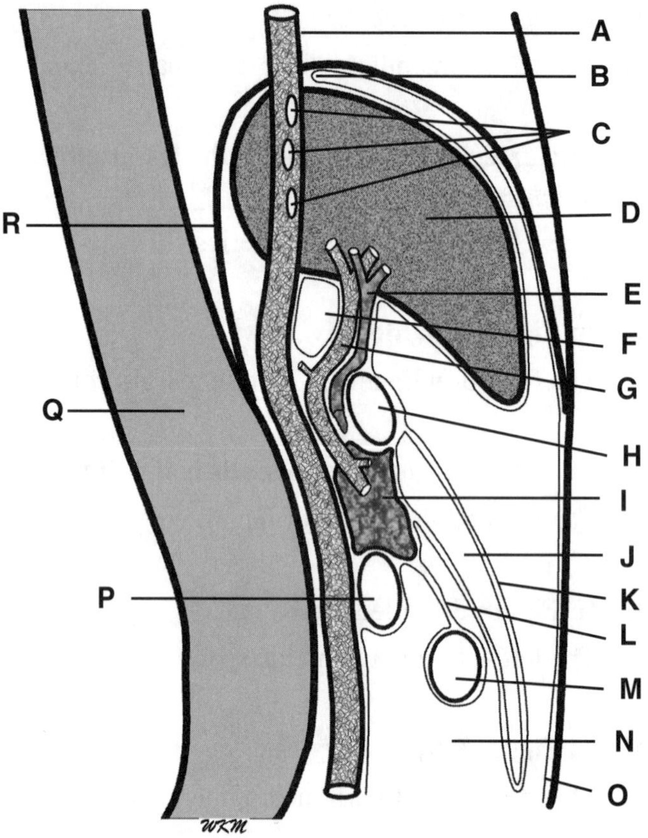

Figure 5-10 Parasagittal Section Through the Epiploic Foramen of the Abdomen

Q. In Figure 5-10, identify G.

A. The portal vein in the free edge of the lesser omentum. It forms the anterior boundary of the epiploic foramen.

Q. In Figure 5-10, identify H.

A. The lumen of the first part of the duodenum.

Q. In Figure 5-10, identify I.

A. The neck of the pancreas. It runs anteriorly and to the left to connect the head to the body of the pancreas.

Q. In Figure 5-10, identify J.

A. The cavity of the lesser sac. Here it lies between the folds of the greater omentum. In the adult, this part of the lesser sac is usually obliterated by adhesions between the adjacent surfaces of the greater omentum.

Q. In Figure 5-10, identify K.

A. The anterior two layers of the greater omentum.

Q. In Figure 5-10, identify L.

A. The transverse mesocolon. In the adult, the transverse mesocolon is usually fused with the posterior two layers of the greater omentum.

Q. The artery that runs in the transverse mesocolon is . . .

A. The middle colic artery. Its right and left branches also run in this mesentery.

Q. In Figure 5-10, identify space M.

A. The lumen of the transverse colon.

Q. In Figure 5-10, identify N.

A. The lower part of the greater sac. It lies behind the greater omentum.

Q. The major structure in the inferior part of the greater peritoneal sac is . . .

A. The small intestine.

Q. In Figure 5-10, identify O.

A. The parietal layer of the peritoneum.

Q. In Figure 5-10, identify P.

A. The lumen of the third part of the duodenum. At the level of the 3rd lumbar vertebra, it crosses the inferior vena cava and the aorta from right to left.

Q. The vessels that cross the third part of the duodenum anteriorly are . . .

A. The superior mesenteric vessels.

Q. In Figure 5-10, identify Q.

A. The vertebral column.

Q. In Figure 5-10, identify R.

A. The diaphragm.

Q. In Figure 5-11, identify A.

A. The superior (anterior) layer of the coronary ligament. It forms part of the boundary of the right anterior subphrenic space. The extent of the left triangular ligament is so limited that the division of the left subphrenic space into anterior and posterior spaces is somewhat academic.

Q. In Figure 5-11, identify B.

A. The fissure for the ligamentum venosum. More inferiorly, it encloses the hepatic attachment of the lesser omentum.

Q. In Figure 5-11, identify C.

A. The caudate lobe of the liver. It forms the anterior boundary of the superior recess of the lesser sac of the peritoneum.

Q. In Figure 5-11, identify D.

A. The right lobe of the liver.

Q. In Figure 5-11, identify E.

A. The superior recess of the lesser sac.

Q. In Figure 5-11, identify F.

A. The lesser sac of the peritoneal cavity.

Q. In Figure 5-11, identify G.

A. The lesser omentum.

Q. In Figure 5-11, identify H.

A. The right gastric artery. It lies in the gastric attachment of the lesser omentum.

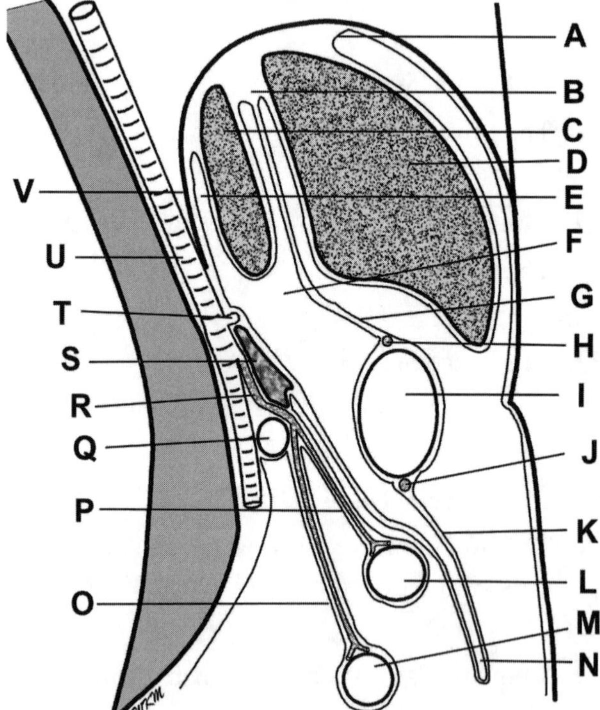

Figure 5-11 Sagittal Section of Abdomen: Peritoneal Folds

Q. The right gastric artery originates from . . .

A. The hepatic artery in the free edge of the lesser omentum. The right gastric artery anastomoses with the larger left gastric artery, one of the three branches of the celiac trunk.

Q. In Figure 5-11, identify I.

A. The stomach.

Q. In Figure 5-11, identify J.

A. The right gastroepiploic artery. It lies in the attachment of the greater omentum to the greater curvature of the stomach.

Q. The right gastroepiploic artery is a branch of . . .

A. The gastroduodenal artery. It anastomoses with the left gastroepiploic branch of the splenic artery.

Q. In Figure 5-11, identify K.

A. The anterior fold of the greater omentum. It is attached to the greater curvature of the stomach.

Q. In Figure 5-11, identify L.

A. The transverse colon. In the adult, the posterior fold of the greater omentum adheres to it. The fold of the greater omentum, connecting the stomach to the transverse colon in the adult, is therefore known as the gastrocolic ligament.

Q. In Figure 5-11, identify M.

A. A loop of small intestine.

Q. In Figure 5-11, identify N.

A. The inferior recess of the lesser sac, the omental bursa. In the adult, it is obliterated by adhesions.

Q. In Figure 5-11, identify O.

A. The mesentery of the small intestine.

Q. In Figure 5-11, identify P.

A. The transverse mesocolon. It contains the middle colic branch of the superior mesenteric artery. In the adult, it fuses with the adjacent layers of the greater omentum.

Q. In Figure 5-11, identify Q.

A. The third part of the duodenum. It crosses the aorta, which separates it from the body of the 3rd lumbar vertebra.

Q. In Figure 5-11, identify R.

A. The superior mesenteric artery.

Q. In Figure 5-11, identify S.

A. The neck of the pancreas.

Q. In Figure 5-11, identify T.

A. The celiac trunk. Behind the peritoneum of the posterior wall of the lesser sac, it divides into the hepatic, splenic, and left gastric arteries.

Q. In Figure 5-11, identify U.

A. The descending aorta.

Q. In Figure 5-11, identify V.

A. The diaphragm.

Q. In Figure 5-12, identify A.

A. The attachment of the falciform ligament.

Q. In Figure 5-12, identify B.

A. The attachment of the superior (anterior) layer of the coronary ligament.

Q. In Figure 5-12, identify C.

A. The superior recess of the lesser sac.

Q. In Figure 5-12, identify D.

A. The inferior vena cava.

Q. In Figure 5-12, identify E.

A. The attachment of the right triangular ligament.

Q. In Figure 5-12, identify F.

A. The attachment of the inferior (posterior) layer of the coronary ligament.

Q. In Figure 5-12, identify G.

A. The right kidney.

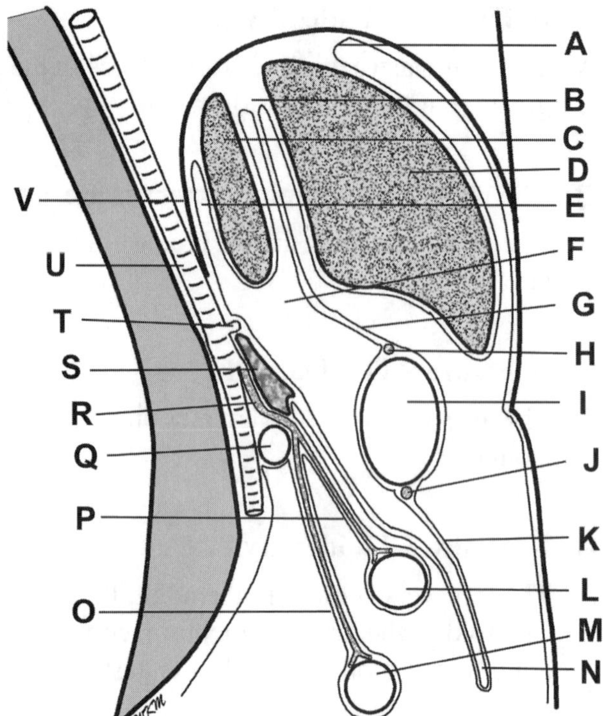

Figure 5-11 Sagittal Section of Abdomen: Peritoneal Folds

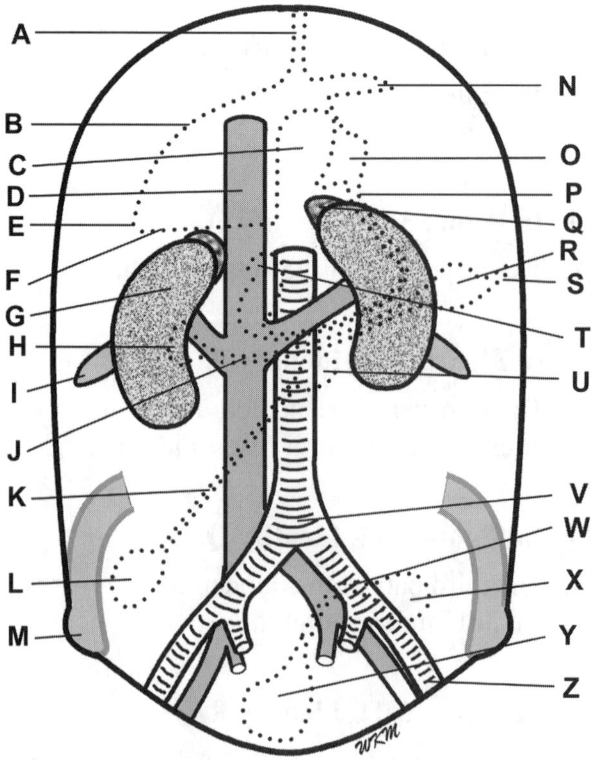

Figure 5-12 Posterior Abdominal Wall of the Abdomen: Peritoneal Reflections

Q. In Figure 5-12, identify H.

A. The "aperture" in the parietal peritoneum for the right end of the transverse colon. It is the area where the mesocolon becomes continuous with the renal parietal peritoneum.

Q. In Figure 5-12, identify I.

A. The tip of the right 12th rib.

Q. In Figure 5-12, identify J.

A. The attachment of the transverse mesocolon.

Q. In Figure 5-12, identify K.

A. The attachment of the mesentery of the small intestine, the mesentery.

Q. In Figure 5-12, identify L.

A. The "aperture" in the parietal peritoneum for the terminal ileum. It is not a true aperture, but merely the area where the visceral peritoneum over the terminal ileum becomes continuous with the parietal peritoneum on the posterior abdominal wall.

Q. In Figure 5-12, identify M.

A. The anterior superior iliac spine.

Q. In Figure 5-12, identify N.

A. The attachment of the left triangular ligament.

Q. In Figure 5-12, identify O.

A. The "aperture" for the gastric end of the esophagus. It is the area where the visceral peritoneum covering the terminal esophagus becomes continuous with the parietal peritoneum on the diaphragm. The fold of peritoneum formed by the left gastric artery also can be seen.

Q. In Figure 5-12, identify P.

A. The attachment of the gastrophrenic ligament.

Q. In Figure 5-12, identify Q.

A. The left suprarenal gland.

Q. In Figure 5-12, identify R.

A. The "aperture" for the left end of the transverse colon. It is not a true aperture, but merely the area where the visceral peritoneum over the colon becomes continuous with the parietal peritoneum on the posterior abdominal wall.

Q. In Figure 5-12, identify S.

A. The attachment of the phrenicocolic ligament, the sustentaculum lieni.

Q. In Figure 5-12, identify T.

A. The "aperture" for the first part of the duodenum. It is not a true aperture, but merely the area where the visceral peritoneum covering the duodenum becomes continuous with the parietal peritoneum on the posterior abdominal wall.

Q. In Figure 5-12, identify U.

A. The "aperture" for the duodenojejunal flexure. It is not a true aperture, but merely the area where the visceral peritoneum over the duodenum becomes continuous with the parietal peritoneum.

Q. In Figure 5-12, identify V.

A. The bifurcation of the aorta.

Q. In Figure 5-12, identify W.

A. The attachment of the sigmoid mesocolon.

Q. In Figure 5-12, identify X.

A. The "aperture" for the descending colon/sigmoid colon juncture. It is the area where the visceral peritoneum becomes continuous with the parietal peritoneum.

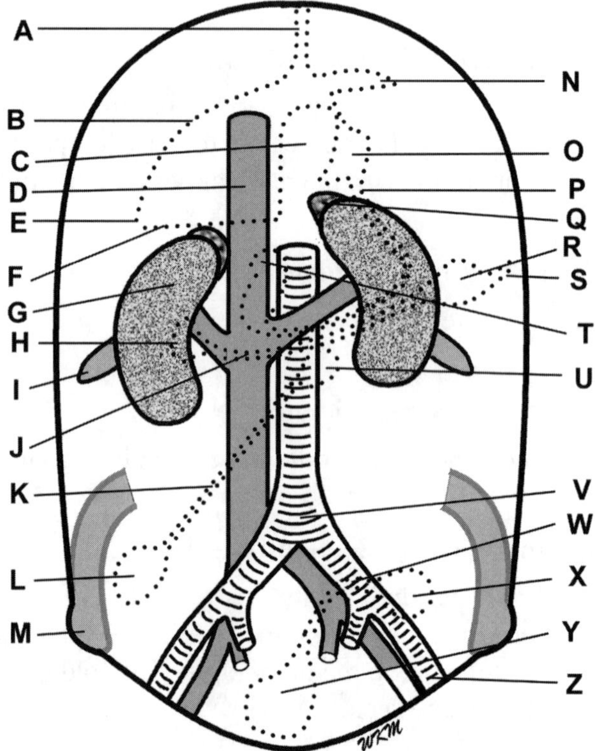

Figure 5-12 Posterior Abdominal Wall of the Abdomen: Peritoneal Reflections

Q. In Figure 5-12, identify Y.

A. The "aperture" for the rectosigmoid juncture. It is the area where the visceral peritoneum over the sigmoid colon becomes continuous with the parietal peritoneum.

Q. In Figure 5-12, identify Z.

A. The left external iliac artery.

Q. In Figure 5-13, identify A.

A. The attachment of the falciform ligament.

Q. In Figure 5-13, identify B.

A. The attachment of the left triangular ligament.

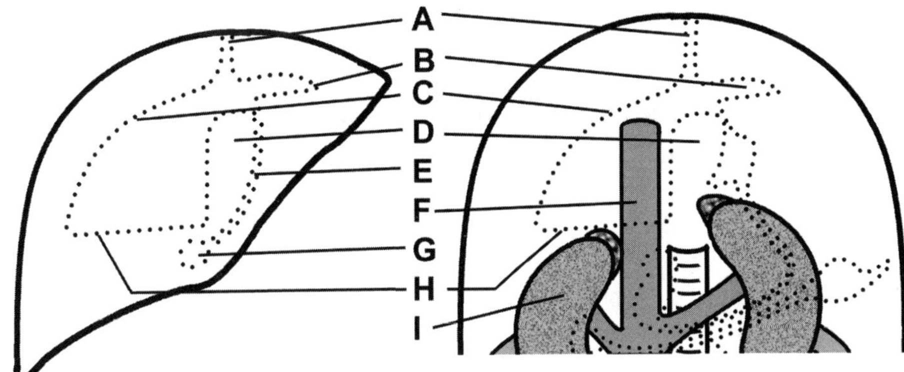

Figure 5-13 The Liver and the Subdiaphragmatic Abdominal Wall: Peritoneal Reflections
Note: The peritoneal reflections are seen through the liver.

Q. In Figure 5-13, identify C.

A. The attachment of the superior (anterior) layer of the coronary ligament.

Q. In Figure 5-13, identify D.

A. The superior recess of the lesser sac.

Q. In Figure 5-13, identify E.

A. The line of attachment of the lesser omentum in the fissure for the ligamentum venosus.

Q. In Figure 5-13, identify F.

A. The inferior vena cava. Note how it is separated from the superior recess of the lesser sac by a peritoneal reflection.

Q. In Figure 5-13, identify G.

A. The attachment of the lesser omentum around the porta hepatis.

Q. In Figure 5-13, identify H.

A. The attachment of the inferior (posterior) layer of the coronary ligament.

Q. In Figure 5-13, the peritoneal covered area labeled I forms the posterior wall of . . .

A. The hepatorenal pouch of Morison. It leads into the right paracolic gutter.

THE ARTERIAL SUPPLY TO THE ALIMENTARY CANAL

Q. The three arteries that supply the abdominal part of the alimentary canal are . . .

A. The celiac trunk, the superior mesenteric artery, and the inferior mesenteric artery.

Q. In Figure 5-14, identify A.

A. The esophageal branches of the short gastric arteries.

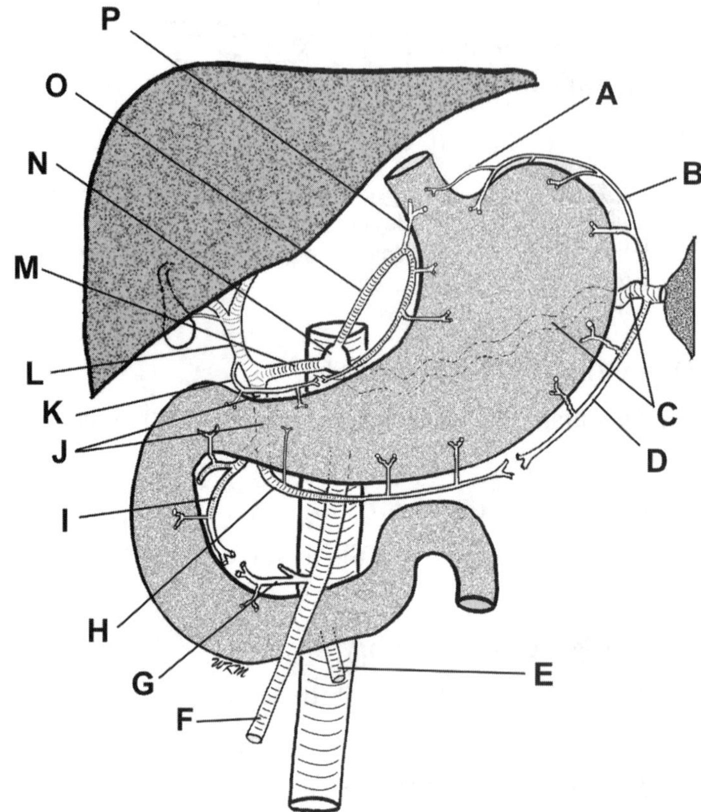

Figure 5-14 The Celiac Trunk and Its Branches

Q. In Figure 5-14, identify B.

A. The short gastric branches of the splenic artery.

Q. In Figure 5-14, identify C.

A. The tortuous splenic branch of the celiac trunk. It crosses the posterior abdominal wall behind the lesser peritoneal sac and continues to reach the hilum of the spleen in the lienorenal ligament.

Q. In Figure 5-14, identify D.

A. The left gastroepiploic branch of the splenic artery. It lies between the layers of the greater omentum, close to its attachment to the greater curvature of the stomach. It anastomoses with the right gastroepiploic artery.

Q. In Figure 5-14, identify E.

A. The inferior mesenteric artery. It arises behind the third part of the duodenum.

Q. In Figure 5-14, identify F.

A. The superior mesenteric artery. It arises from the front of the aorta at the level of L1 posterior to the body of the pancreas.

Q. In Figure 5-14, identify G.

A. The inferior pancreaticoduodenal artery. It arises from the superior mesenteric artery to supply part of the second, third, and fourth parts of the duodenum and the head of the pancreas.

Q. In Figure 5-14, identify H.

A. The right gastroepiploic branch of the gastroduodenal artery. It anastomoses with the left gastroepiploic artery in the proximal part of the greater omentum.

Q. In Figure 5-14, identify I.

A. The superior pancreaticoduodenal branch of the gastroduodenal artery.

Q. In Figure 5-14, identify J.

A. The gastroduodenal artery. Distal to its origin from the common hepatic artery, the continuation of the hepatic artery becomes the proper hepatic artery. The gastroduodenal artery divides into the superior pancreaticoduodenal artery and the right gastroepiploic artery.

Q. In Figure 5-14, identify K.

A. The right gastric artery. It arises from the proper hepatic artery in the lesser omentum. The right gastric artery runs along the lesser curvature of the stomach in the lesser omentum.

Q. In Figure 5-14, identify L.

A. The proper hepatic artery. It divides into right and left branches that supply their respective halves of the liver. The distribution of the hepatic arteries does not correspond to the standard divisions of the liver into right and left lobes. The right hepatic artery also supplies the gallbladder.

Q. In Figure 5-14, identify M.

A. The common hepatic artery. It is the second largest branch of the celiac trunk. In the fetus, due to the role the fetal liver plays in erythropoiesis, it is larger than the splenic artery.

Q. In Figure 5-14, identify N.

A. The celiac trunk. It arises from the aorta as it emerges from below the median arcuate ligament of the diaphragm at the level of the 12th thoracic vertebra.

Q. In Figure 5-14, identify O.

A. The left gastric artery. It runs across the posterior abdominal wall, posterior to the peritoneum, to reach the gastroesophageal junction immediately below the point at which the esophagus penetrates the diaphragm to enter the abdomen. It thus reaches the diaphragmatic end of the lesser omentum to pass forward and to the left between its layers along the lesser curvature of the stomach.

Q. In Figure 5-14, identify P.

A. The esophageal branches of the left gastric artery.

Q. In Figure 5-15, identify A.

A. The abdominal aorta.

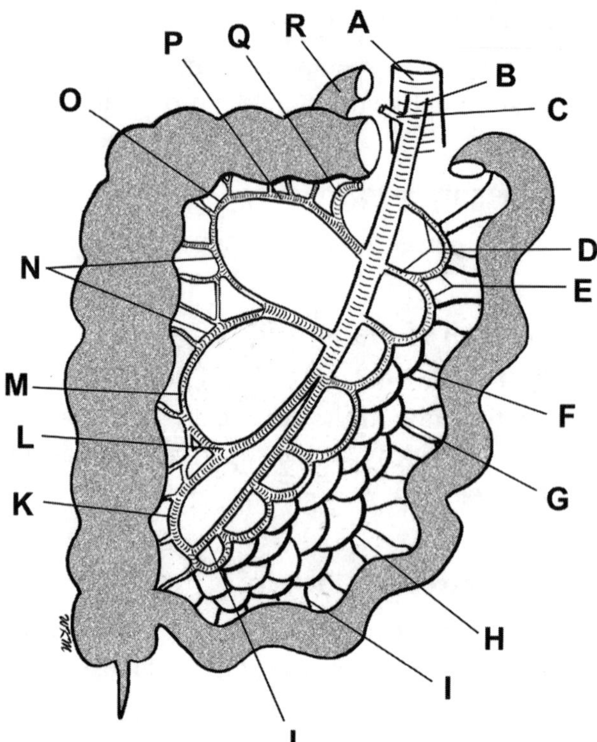

Figure 5-15 The Superior Mesenteric Artery

Q. In Figure 5-15, identify B.

A. The origin of the superior mesenteric artery.

Q. In Figure 5-15, identify C.

A. The inferior pancreaticoduodenal artery. Together with the superior pancreaticoduodenal artery, it supplies the duodenum and the head of the pancreas.

Q. In Figure 5-15, identify D.

A. The jejunal branches of the superior mesenteric artery.

Q. In Figure 5-15, identify E.

A. Single arterial arcades. The arcades provide adequate, essential, collateral circulation for the small intestine.

Q. Thrombosis of the trunk of the superior mesenteric artery results in . . .

A. Fatal ischemia of the gut distal to the clot. Even a more distal thrombosis carries a significant mortality.

Q. In Figure 5-15, identify F.

A. Double arcades. The jejunum is usually supplied only by a single or by a double arcade.

Q. In Figure 5-15, identify G.

A. A triple set of arcades. The ileum usually has three to five series of arcades.

Q. In Figure 5-15, identify H.

A. The fourth series of arcades.

Q. In Figure 5-15, identify I.

A. Terminal ileal branches. They divide to encircle the wall of the gut, as do all terminal vessels to the alimentary canal distal to the stomach.

Q. In Figure 5-15, identify J.

A. The termination of the superior mesenteric artery.

Q. A fibrous cord may be found connecting the superior mesenteric artery to the umbilicus. It is . . .

A. The vestigial remains of its embryonic vitelline (yolk sac) branch.

Q. In Figure 5-15, identify K.

A. The inferior branch of the ileocolic branch of the superior mesenteric artery. It is sometimes called the ileocecal branch. It supplies the cecum, the appendix, and the terminal ileum.

Q. In Figure 5-15, identify L.

A. The ileocolic branch of the superior mesenteric artery.

Q. In Figure 5-15, identify M.

A. The superior branch of the ileocolic artery.

Q. In Figure 5-15, identify N.

A. The superior and the inferior branches of the right colic artery.

Q. In Figure 5-15, identify O.

A. The anastomosis between the right middle colic and the superior branch of the right colic artery. The anastomoses between the various colic arteries close to the colon form the "marginal" artery. The marginal artery is important because it provides a route for collateral circulation.

Q. In Figure 5-15, identify P.

A. The right branch of the middle colic branch of the superior mesenteric artery.

Q. In Figure 5-15, identify Q.

A. The left branch of the middle colic artery. It anastomoses with the ascending branch of the left colic branch of the inferior mesenteric artery, just to the right of the splenic flexure.

Q. In Figure 5-15, identify R.

A. The first part and part of the second part of the duodenum.

Q. In Figure 5-16, identify A.

A. The terminal branch of the superior mesenteric artery. It anastomoses with the ileocecal branch of the right colic artery.

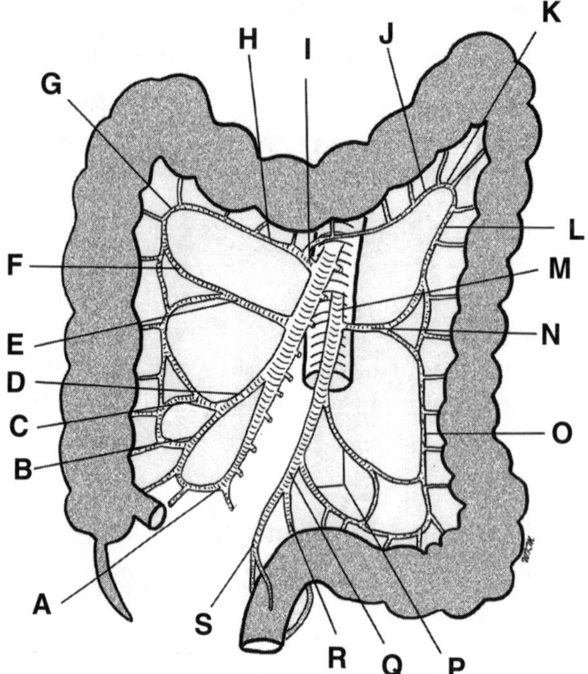

Figure 5-16 The Blood Supply to the Colon: the Superior and Mesenteric Arteries

Q. In Figure 5-16, identify B.

A. The inferior (ileocecal) branch of the ileocolic artery.

Q. In Figure 5-16, identify C.

A. The superior branch of the ileocolic artery.

Q. In Figure 5-16, identify D.

A. The ileocolic artery. It is the last colic branch of the superior mesenteric artery.

Q. In Figure 5-16, identify E.

A. The right colic artery. It divides into superior and inferior branches to contribute to the marginal artery.

Q. In Figure 5-16, identify F.

A. The superior branch of the right colic artery.

Q. In Figure 5-16, identify G.

A. The anastomosis between the middle and right colic arteries at the hepatic flexure. This diagram clearly indicates the concept of a marginal artery.

Q. In Figure 5-16, identify H.

A. The right branch of the middle colic artery.

Q. In Figure 5-16, identify I.

A. The middle colic artery. It arises from the superior mesenteric artery.

Q. In Figure 5-16, identify J.

A. The left branch of the middle colic artery.

Q. In Figure 5-16, identify K.

A. The anastomosis between the left branch of the middle colic artery and the superior branch of the left colic artery. This is sometimes called the "critical point" on the marginal artery, because it has been suggested that this anastomosis between the superior mesenteric artery and the inferior mesenteric artery may be inadequate to compensate for thrombosis of either. This anastomosis can compensate for *gradual* obstruction of the inferior mesenteric artery, for example, that due to arteriosclerosis. Alas, the inferior mesenteric artery cannot compensate for even very gradual obstruction of the superior mesenteric artery.

Q. In Figure 5-16, identify L.

A. The superior branch of the left colic artery.

Q. In Figure 5-16, identify M.

A. The inferior mesenteric artery. It arises from the aorta at the level of L3 posterior to the third part of the duodenum.

Q. In Figure 5-16, identify N.

A. The left colic artery.

Q. In Figure 5-16, identify O.

A. The superior branch of the highest sigmoid artery.

Q. In Figure 5-16, identify P.

A. The sigmoid branches of the inferior mesenteric artery.

Q. The marginal artery is said to terminate with . . .

A. The sigmoid arteries. However, the rectum can acquire collateral circulation from the middle and inferior rectal arteries if the obstruction to the superior rectal artery is gradual.

Q. In Figure 5-16, identify Q.

A. The superior rectal artery, the termination of the inferior mesenteric artery.

Q. In Figure 5-16, identify R.

A. The single left branch of the superior rectal artery.

Q. In Figure 5-16, identify S.

A. The right branch of the superior rectal artery. Note that it divides into anterior and posterior branches.

Q. The celiac trunk is the artery of the embryological foregut. As such, it supplies all of its derivatives. These derivatives are . . .

A. The stomach, the first part and part of the second part of the duodenum, the liver, the gall bladder, and part of the pancreas.

Q. The celiac trunk also supplies the spleen. The spleen is derived from . . .

A. Migrating lymphocytes. These lymphocytes "nest" in the greater omentum to form the spleen. The spleen obtains its blood supply from local foregut blood vessels.

Q. Embryologically, the first part and half of the second part of the duodenum are derived from . . .

A. The foregut.

Q. Therefore, the arterial supply of the first part and half of the second part of the duodenum is from . . .

A. The celiac trunk.

Q. The arteries involved in the supply of the first part and half of the second part of the duodenum are branches of . . .

A. The gastroduodenal branch of the common hepatic artery.

Q. The artery of the embryological midgut is . . .

A. The superior mesenteric artery.

Q. Therefore, the superior mesenteric artery will supply . . .

A. The distal half of the pancreas, the distal half of the second part of the duodenum, the third and fourth parts of the duodenum, the jejunum, the ileum, the cecum and the appendix, the ascending colon, and the transverse colon.

Q. The artery of the embryological hindgut is . . .

A. The inferior mesenteric artery.

Q. Therefore, the inferior mesenteric artery will supply . . .

A. The splenic flexure of the colon, the descending colon, the sigmoid colon, and most of the rectum.

Q. The embryological significance of the splenic flexure of the colon is that it approximates to . . .

A. The junction of the embryonic midgut and hindgut.

Q. The parasympathetic supply to the alimentary canal from the epiglottis to the splenic flexure of the colon is from . . .

A. The vagus nerve.

Q. The nerves that provide the parasympathetic supply to the colon distal to the splenic flexure are . . .

A. The pelvic splanchnic nerves (S2, S3, and S4).

Q. The parasympathetic nerves to the splenic flexure of the colon and the descending colon ascend from the pelvis following the path of . . .

A. The superior rectal artery. They then run with the inferior mesenteric artery and are distributed with its branches.

THE HEPATIC PORTAL VENOUS SYSTEM

Q. In Figure 5-17, identify A.

A. The gallbladder.

Q. In Figure 5-17, identify B.

A. The left lobe of the liver. Its left extremity has been removed to reveal the esophagus.

Q. In Figure 5-17, identify C.

A. The esophagus.

Q. In Figure 5-17, identify D.

A. The lesser curvature of the stomach. The stomach has been sectioned to reveal the duodenum and the pancreas.

Q. In Figure 5-17, identify E.

A. The fundus of the stomach.

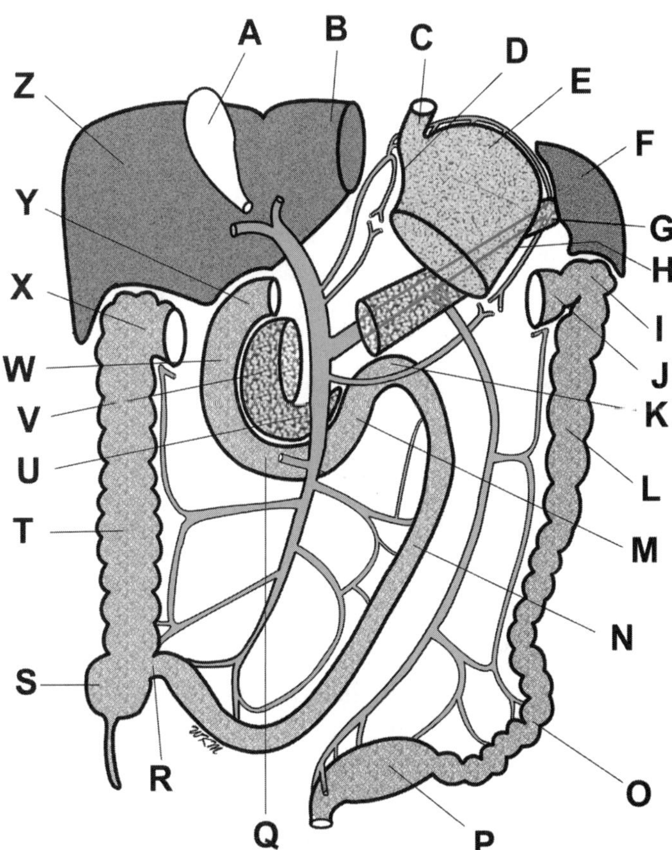

Figure 5-17 The Hepatic Portal System: Viscera
Note: This diagram reflects a view of the visceral surface of the liver.

Q. In Figure 5-17, identify F.

A. The spleen. Note that it is in contact with the stomach, the tail of the pancreas, and the splenic flexure of the colon.

Q. In Figure 5-17, identify G.

A. The tail of the pancreas. It is frequently injured when the splenic vessels are ligated during a splenectomy.

Q. In Figure 5-17, identify H.

A. The greater curvature of the stomach.

Q. In Figure 5-17, identify I.

A. The splenic flexure of the colon. A fold of parietal peritoneum the phrenicocolic ligament, the sustentaculum lieni, extends laterally to the diaphragm.

Q. In Figure 5-17, identify J.

A. The left end of the transverse colon.

Q. In Figure 5-17, identify K.

A. The duodenojejunal flexure.

Q. In Figure 5-17, identify L.

A. The descending colon.

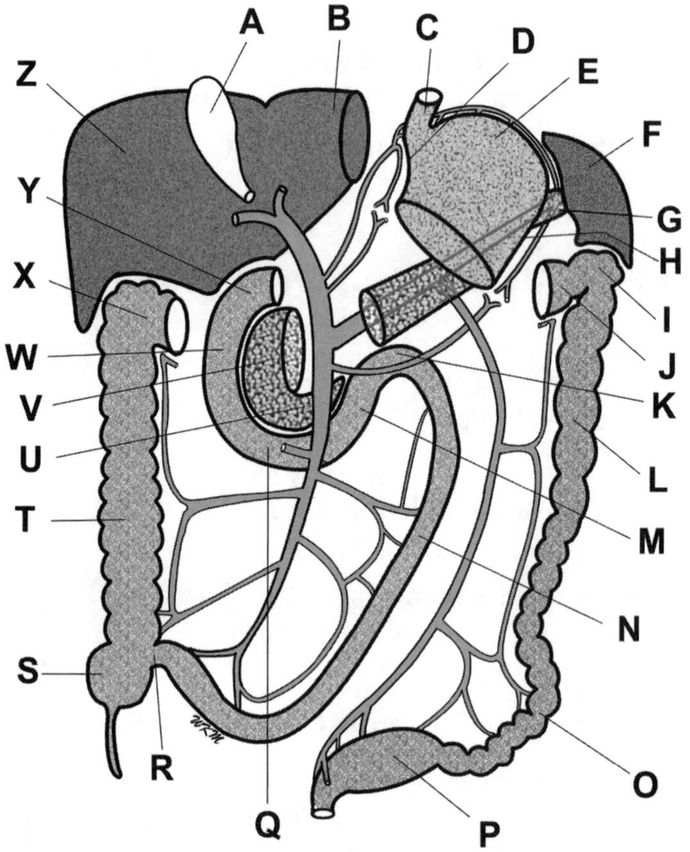

Figure 5-17 The Hepatic Portal System: Viscera
Note: This diagram reflects a view of the visceral surface of the liver.

Q. In Figure 5-17, identify M.

A. The fourth part of the duodenum. It is 1 inch long and is the shortest part of the duodenum. It ascends on the left side of the vertebral column to the duodenojejunal junction.

Q. In Figure 5-17, identify N.

A. The small intestine. The jejunum comprises the proximal two-fifths of the small intestine. The distal three-fifths consists of the ileum. There is no exact transition point.

Q. In Figure 5-17, identify O.

A. The sigmoid colon. Like the transverse colon, it has a mesentery.

Q. In Figure 5-17, identify P.

A. The rectum.

Q. In Figure 5-17, identify Q.

A. The third part of the duodenum. It is 4 inches long and crosses the aorta and the body of the 3rd lumbar vertebra. Because it is fixed in position, it is vulnerable to injury by blows to the abdomen at the level of the umbilicus.

Q. In Figure 5-17, identify R.

A. The ileocecal valve.

Q. In Figure 5-17, identify S.

A. The cecum. It is usually filled with gas. The appendix lies at its apex.

Q. In Figure 5-17, identify T.

A. The ascending colon.

Q. In Figure 5-17, identify U.

A. The uncinate process of the pancreas. It lies between the superior mesenteric vessels and the aorta.

Q. In Figure 5-17, identify V.

A. The head of the pancreas.

Q. In Figure 5-17, identify W.

A. The second part of the duodenum. It is 3 inches long and descends from the right side of the 1st lumbar vertebra to the right side of the 3rd lumbar vertebra.

Q. In Figure 5-17, identify X.

A. The hepatic flexure of the colon. It is in contact with the visceral surface of the liver.

Q. In Figure 5-17, identify Y.

A. The first part of the duodenum. Its proximal first inch is intraperitoneal. Its second inch reaches the posterior abdominal wall and is retroperitoneal, as is the rest of the duodenum.

Q. In Figure 5-17, identify Z.

A. The right lobe of the liver.

Q. In Figure 5-18, identify A.

A. The right and left branches of the portal vein.

Q. In Figure 5-18, identify B.

A. The short gastric veins. They drain the fundus of the stomach and the lower end of the esophagus.

Q. In Figure 5-18, identify C.

A. The right gastric vein. It runs along the lesser curvature of the stomach in the lesser omentum.

Q. In Figure 5-18, identify D.

A. The left gastroepiploic vein. It runs along the greater curvature of the stomach in the greater omentum to the splenic vein.

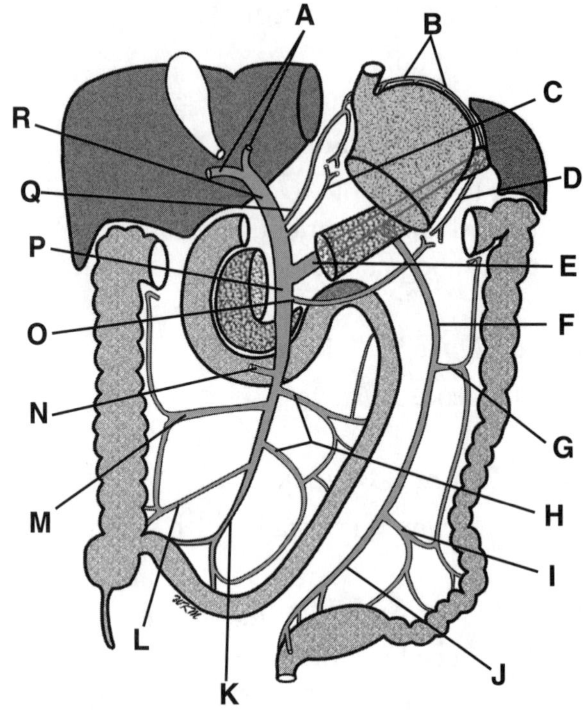

Figure 5-18 The Hepatic Portal System: Veins
Note: This diagram refects a view of the visceral surface of the liver.

Q. In Figure 5-18, identify E.

A. The splenic vein. It joins with the superior mesenteric vein to form the portal vein.

Q. In Figure 5-18, identify F.

A. The inferior mesenteric vein. It ends by joining the splenic vein.

Q. In Figure 5-18, identify G.

A. The left colic vein.

Q. In Figure 5-18, identify H.

A. The jejunal and the ileal tributaries of the superior mesenteric vein.

Q. In Figure 5-18, identify I.

A. The sigmoid colic vein. It drains the sigmoid loop of the colon.

Q. In Figure 5-18, identify J.

A. The superior rectal vein. It anastomoses with the systemic middle and inferior rectal veins. If the venous pressure in the portal system of veins increases, it may cause dilation of these anastomoses and result in the varicosities known as hemorrhoids.

Q. In Figure 5-18, identify K.

A. The beginning of the superior mesenteric vein.

Q. In Figure 5-18, identify L.

A. The ileocolic vein.

Q. In Figure 5-18, identify M.

A. The right colic vein.

Q. In Figure 5-18, identify N.

A. The middle colic vein. It drains the transverse colon.

Q. In Figure 5-18, identify O.

A. The right gastroepiploic vein. It joins the superior mesenteric vein.

Q. In Figure 5-18, identify P.

A. The superior mesenteric vein. It is joined by the splenic vein to form the portal vein.

Q. In Figure 5-18, identify Q.

A. The left gastric vein. From the plexus of veins around the gastroesophageal junction, it crosses the posterior abdominal wall to join the portal vein.

Q. In Figure 5-18, identify R.

A. The portal vein. It runs in the free edge of the lesser omentum to reach the porta hepatis.

Q. Connections between the portal and systemic system of veins become important when the portal circulation is obstructed, as occurs in cirrhosis of the liver. The two most important portosystemic connections are . . .

A. The anastomoses between the esophageal branches of the left gastric vein and the veins of the lower end of the esophagus, which drain to the hemiazygos vein and to the azygos vein; and the connections between the superior rectal veins and the middle and inferior rectal veins. Hemorrhage from rupture of the venous varicosities at the lower end of the esophagus resulting from portal hypertension is a major problem in cirrhosis of the liver. The connections between the epigastric veins and the portal vein along the ligamentum teres of the liver are less significant, although dilatation of the veins around the umbilicus may form a "Caput Medusae." Finally, there are a series of connections where abdominal organs are in contact with the abdominal wall without intervening peritoneum. These occur over the bare area of the liver and behind the ascending colon and descending colon.

LYMPHATIC DRAINAGE OF THE ABDOMINAL VISCERA

Q. The lymphatic pathways draining the abdominal viscera closely follow . . .

A. The arteries that supply them.

Q. A large number of lymph nodes drain the abdominal viscera. They can be divided conveniently into three groups. They are . . .

A. The peripheral groups, the intermediate groups, and the central groups.

Q. Each peripheral group lies . . .

A. Close along the side of or at the hilum of the viscus it drains.

Q. The peripheral groups of lymph nodes are named from . . .

A. The viscus they drain or from the peripheral artery that supplies the viscus concerned.

Q. Each group of peripheral lymph nodes drains into . . .

A. The group of intermediate lymph nodes lying along the artery supplying the viscus drained.

Q. The intermediate groups of lymph nodes are named . . .

A. Based on the artery along which they lie.

Q. The intermediate groups of lymph nodes drain into . . .

A. The central groups of preaortic lymph nodes. Each group surrounds the origin of the artery around which it lies.

Q. The peripheral lymph nodes draining the lower end of the esophagus are named . . .

A. The paraesophageal lymph nodes.

Q. The paraesophageal lymph nodes are situated . . .

A. In a ring around the lower end of the esophagus. The inferior nodes of this group are often named the paracardial nodes.

Q. The peripheral lymph nodes that drain the lesser curvature of the stomach drain to the left. They are named . . .

A. The left gastric group of peripheral lymph nodes.

Q. The left gastric peripheral lymph nodes are situated in . . .

A. The lesser omentum along the lesser curvature of the stomach.

Q. The peripheral lymph nodes that drain the greater curvature of the stomach drain to the right. They are named . . .

A. The right gastroepiploic lymph nodes.

Q. The right gastroepiploic lymph nodes lie in . . .

A. The greater omentum along the greater curvature of the stomach.

Q. The peripheral lymph nodes that drain the duodenum are named . . .

A. The superior pancreaticoduodenal and the inferior pancreaticoduodenal lymph nodes.

Q. The superior and inferior pancreaticoduodenal lymph nodes are situated in . . .

A. The groove between the head of the pancreas and the duodenum.

Q. The peripheral lymph nodes that drain the jejunum and ileum are named . . .

A. The peripheral groups of mesenteric lymph nodes.

Q. The peripheral groups of mesenteric lymph nodes are situated in . . .

A. The mesentery. They lie along the mesenteric attachment of the jejunum and the ileum.

Q. The peripheral lymph nodes that drain the colon are named . . .

A. The paracolic peripheral lymph nodes.

Q. The paracolic lymph nodes are frequently subdivided into . . .

A. The right colic, the middle colic, the left colic, and the sigmoid groups of peripheral lymph nodes.

Q. The paracolic peripheral lymph nodes are situated along . . .

A. The medial borders of the ascending and the descending colon and along the mesenteric attachments of the transverse colon and the sigmoid colon.

Q. The peripheral lymph nodes that drain the mucosal lining of the rectum and the upper two-thirds of its muscular wall are named . . .

A. The pararectal group of peripheral lymph nodes.

Q. The pararectal peripheral lymph nodes are situated along . . .

A. The left and right sides of the rectum. They are associated with the right and left terminal branches of the superior rectal artery.

Q. The lower one-third of the muscular wall of the rectum and the mucosal lining of the anal canal above the mucocutaneous junction drain into . . .

A. The middle rectal group of internal iliac lymph nodes.

Q. However, the anal canal below the mucocutaneous junction drains to . . .

A. The superficial group of inguinal lymph nodes. This is clinically important because carcinoma involving the anal canal will metastasize to these nodes. Hence the saying, "If you don't put your finger in it, you put your foot in it," which applies when examining a patient with painless enlargement of the inguinal lymph nodes.

Q. The peripheral lymph nodes draining the gallbladder and the liver are named . . .

A. The hepatic lymph nodes.

Q. The hepatic group of peripheral lymph nodes is situated . . .

A. At the porta hepatis in the lesser omentum.

Q. The peripheral lymph nodes that drain the pancreas and spleen are named . . .

A. The pancreaticosplenic lymph nodes. The pancreaticosplenic lymph nodes also act as an intermediate group of lymph nodes, because they receive lymph from that part of the stomach supplied by the left gastroepiploic and the short gastric arteries.

Q. The pancreaticosplenic lymph nodes are situated along . . .

A. The course of the splenic artery, which runs along the upper border of the pancreas.

Q. Numerous lymph nodes lie along the branches of the celiac trunk, the superior mesenteric artery, and the inferior mesenteric artery. They are . . .

A. The intermediate lymph nodes. They are named after the artery that they surround. They drain the area supplied by that artery.

Q. The intermediate groups of lymph nodes drain into three central groups of preaortic lymph nodes. They are . . .

A. The celiac group of preaortic nodes, the superior mesenteric group of preaortic lymph nodes, and the inferior mesenteric group of preaortic lymph nodes. Each of these groups provides lymphatic drainage from the area supplied by the artery after which they are named.

Q. The celiac trunk, the embryological artery of the foregut, provides arterial blood to . . .

A. The stomach, the first part and the proximal half of the second part of the duodenum, the liver, the pancreas, and the spleen.

Q. The intermediate groups of lymph nodes that drain into the celiac nodes are therefore . . .

A. The left gastric, the hepatic, the pyloric (gastroduodenal), and the pancreaticosplenic groups of intermediate lymph nodes. Each group lies along the artery of the same name.

Q. The superior mesenteric artery, the embryological artery to the midgut, provides blood to . . .

A. The second, third, and fourth parts of the duodenum; the jejunum; the ileum; the cecum; the ascending colon; and the transverse colon.

Q. The intermediate groups of lymph nodes that drain into the superior mesenteric nodes are therefore named . . .

A. The mesenteric, the ileocolic, the right colic, and the middle colic groups of intermediate lymph nodes. Each group lies along the artery of the same name.

Q. The inferior mesenteric artery supplies arterial blood to . . .

A. The descending colon, the sigmoid colon, and the rectum.

Q. Therefore, the intermediate groups of lymph nodes that drain into the inferior mesenteric nodes are named . . .

A. The left colic, the sigmoid, and the superior rectal groups of intermediate lymph nodes. Each group lies along the artery after which it is named.

Q. The superior mesenteric preaortic lymph nodes and the inferior mesenteric preaortic nodes are really preterminal lymph nodes because they drain into . . .

A. The celiac group of preaortic lymph nodes.

Q. The lymph from the celiac group (the terminal group) of preaortic lymph nodes passes into . . .

A. The right and the left intestinal lymphatic trunks.

Q. The right and the left intestinal trunks end in a lymphatic sac named . . .

A. The cisterna chyli, the abdominal confluence of lymphatic trunks. It is the inferior extremity of the thoracic duct.

PLANES USED IN EXAMINATION OF THE ABDOMEN

Q. In a supine patient, the approximate vertebral level of the plane of the xiphisternal joint is . . .

A. The upper border of the 10th thoracic vertebra. Of course, the sternum rises and falls with respiration.

Q. The transpyloric plane lies at the level of . . .

A. The midpoint between the symphysis pubis and the suprasternal notch.

Q. Other approximations that may be used to locate the transpyloric plane are . . .

A. Halfway between the xiphisternum and the umbilicus; at the level of the tip of the 9th costal cartilage; a hand's-breadth below the inferior end of the sternum; and the point where the linear semilunaris intersects the costal margin.

Q. Tenderness at the tip of the 9th right costal cartilage is usually diagnostic of . . .

A. Acute cholecystitis. The tip of the 9th right costal cartilage is an accurate surface landmark of the fundus of the gallbladder in a patient with a liver of normal size.

Q. The vertebral level of the transpyloric plane is . . .

A. The lower part of the body of the 1st lumbar vertebra.

Q. The subcostal plane marks the lowest point of the 10th costal cartilage. The vertebral level of the subcostal plane is . . .

A. The 3rd lumbar vertebra.

Q. The supracristal plane is the plane at the highest point of the iliac crests. The vertebral level of the supracristal plane is . . .

A. The 4th lumbar vertebra. More importantly, it is used to determine the level of the 4th lumbar spine. Lumbar puncture is usually performed between lumbar spines 3 and 4 or 4 and 5.

Q. The transtubercular plane is the plane indicated by the tubercles of the iliac crest. The vertebral level of the transtubercular plane is . . .

A. The body of the 5th lumbar vertebra.

Q. The position of the tubercles of the iliac crest can be confirmed by palpation except in the very obese. They are located . . .

A. On the iliac crests, 5 cm (2 inches) posterior to the easily palpable anterior superior iliac spines.

Q. The interspinous plane is the plane of the anterior superior iliac spines. The vertebral level of the interspinous plane is . . .

A. The sacral promontory or a little lower.

Q. The suprapubic plane is the plane immediately above the pubic crest. The vertebral level of the suprapubic plane is . . .

A. The tip of the coccyx or just below it, depending on the tilt of the sacrum.

Q. The cardiac plateau is . . .

A. The central tendon of the diaphragm.

Q. The surface marking of the cardiac plateau is on . . .

A. The xiphisternal plane at the level of the 10th thoracic vertebra.

Q. Both cupulae of the diaphragm extend above this plane, reaching the 9th thoracic vertebra. The higher cupula is . . .

A. The right cupula. The presence of the liver in the right side of the upper abdomen elevates the diaphragm on that side.

Q. The esophagus penetrates the diaphragm at the level of . . .

A. The xiphisternal plane at the level of the 10th thoracic vertebra.

Q. The other structures that penetrate the diaphragm at this level are . . .

A. The inferior vena cava, the right and the left phrenic nerves, and the left and right vagus nerves. By this level, the vagus nerves have formed the anterior and posterior esophageal plexuses.

Q. The nerves that penetrate the diaphragm with the esophagus are . . .

A. The vagus nerves or, more precisely, the esophageal plexuses that they form.

Q. The left vagus nerve mainly forms . . .

A. The anterior esophageal plexus.

Q. The right vagus mainly forms . . .

A. The posterior esophageal plexus.

Q. The pylorus of the stomach does not always lie on the transpyloric plane, because the level of stomach varies markedly in different subjects, in different positions, and with different degrees of filling. However, many other structures do lie on or close to this plane. These other structures that lie on or close to the transpyloric plane are . . .

A. The tip of the gallbladder, the neck of the pancreas, the origin of the superior mesenteric artery, the formation of the portal vein, the lower end of the spinal cord in the adult, and the hila of both kidneys.

Q. Although the hila of both kidneys lie on or close to the transpyloric plane, the kidney that is significantly higher is . . .

A. The left kidney. This makes it more difficult to palpate. The large right lobe of the fetal liver depresses the right kidney or perhaps prevents the ascent of the right kidney during embryological development. As a result, the right kidney lies at a lower level than the left kidney. Therefore, the right kidney is more easily palpable bimanually than is the left kidney.

Q. The renal arteries arise from the aorta approximately halfway between the transpyloric and subcostal planes at the level of . . .

A. The 2nd lumbar vertebra. This is also the level of the duodenojejunal flexure, which marks the junction of the duodenum and the jejunum.

Q. The third part of the duodenum crosses the vertebral column at the level of . . .

A. The subcostal plane, the level of the 3rd lumbar vertebra. The inferior mesenteric artery also originates from the aorta at this level.

Q. A severe blow to the abdomen at the level of the umbilicus, such as can result from the steering wheel of a car, is most likely to damage or rupture . . .

A. The third part of the duodenum. This part of the viscus is fixed in position retroperitoneally as it crosses, from right to left, the aorta and the body of the 3rd lumbar vertebra.

Q. The inferior vena cava leaves the abdomen and enters the right atrium of the heart at the level of the 10th thoracic vertebra. The inferior vena cava is formed at the level of . . .

A. The 5th lumbar vertebra on the transtubercular plane by the union of the two common iliac veins.

Q. The aorta bifurcates on the front of the body of . . .

A. The 4th lumbar vertebra. This level lies just inferior to the umbilicus, which, in the average supine subject, is situated about midway between the subcostal and transtubercular planes on the supracristal plane.

Q. The techniques used in examination of the thorax and abdomen during a physical examination include inspection, palpation, percussion, and auscultation. The best technique for determining the size of the liver during a physical examination is by . . .

A. Percussion. The upper border of the liver creates dullness in the 4th right intercostal space. Its lower border corresponds to the right costal margin as far forward as the tip of the right 9th costal cartilage. Its lower border crosses the epigastrium to reach the left costal margin between the tips of the 7th and the 8th costal cartilages.

Q. The right and the left lateral planes run on each side from the midpoint of the clavicle to the midinguinal point. The right and left lateral planes cross the costal margins at the tips of . . .

A. The 9th costal cartilages. Their abdominal extent, therefore, more or less corresponds to the upper part of the linear semilunaris.

Q. Both the ascending colon and the descending colon lie . . .

A. Lateral to their respective lateral planes and therefore lateral to the lineae semilunaris.

Q. The hepatic flexure of the colon only reaches as high as . . .

A. The transpyloric plane due to the presence of the large right lobe of the liver.

Q. The vertebra at the level of the splenic flexure of the colon is . . .

A. The 11th thoracic vertebra, well above the transpyloric plane.

Q. A fold of peritoneum extends laterally from the splenic flexure of the colon to the diaphragm. It is . . .

A. The phrenicocolic ligament, which is also called the sustentaculum lieni or the supporter of the spleen.

Q. A point one-third of the way along a line from the anterior superior iliac spine to the umbilicus is called McBurney's point. It marks the usual position of . . .

A. The base of the appendix.

Q. Tenderness and/or guarding in the right lower quadrant of the abdomen in the region of McBurney's point often indicates appendicitis. Other causes of such signs include . . .

A. A calculus in the left ureter or, in the female, salpingitis, which is an inflammation of the uterine tube. Rupture of an ovarian follicle or of an ovarian cyst, which always causes slight bleeding, also can cause pain and tenderness by irritation of the parietal peritoneum.

Q. In Figure 5-19, identify plane A and give its vertebral level.

A. The xiphisternal plane. It lies at the level of the body of the 10th thoracic vertebra.

Q. In Figure 5-19, identify plane B and give its vertebral level.

A. The transpyloric plane. It lies at the level of the body of the 1st lumbar vertebra.

Q. In Figure 5-19, identify plane C and give its vertebral level.

A. The subcostal plane. It lies at the level of the body of the 3rd lumbar vertebra.

Q. In Figure 5-19, identify plane D and give its vertebral level.

A. The supracristal plane. It lies at the level of the body of the 4th lumbar vertebra.

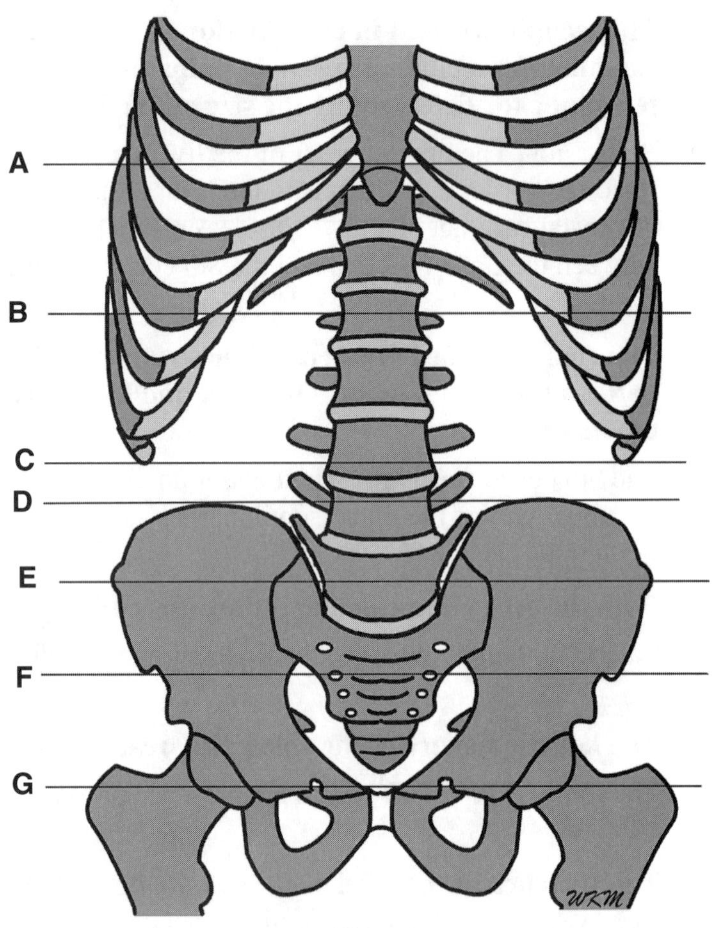

Figure 5-19 Planes of the Abdomen

Q. In Figure 5-19, identify plane E and give its vertebral level.

A. The transtubercular plane. It lies at the level of the body of the 5th lumbar vertebra.

Q. In Figure 5-19, identify plane F and give its vertebral level.

A. The interspinous plane. It lies at the level between the sacral promontory and the 2nd piece of the sacrum.

Q. In Figure 5-19, identify plane G and give its vertebral level.

A. The suprapubic plane. It lies just below the tip of the coccyx.

THE POSTERIOR ABDOMINAL WALL

Q. The posterior abdominal wall can be divided, from top to bottom, into three regions: the area above the 12th rib, the area between the 12th rib and the iliac crest, and the area below the iliac crest. The muscular wall above the 12th rib is formed by . . .

A. The diaphragm.

Q. Between the iliac crests and the diaphragm, the muscles that constitute the posterior abdominal wall are . . .

A. The quadratus lumborum muscles and the transversus abdominis muscles. The psoas major and minor muscles are a smaller medial component.

Q. Name the ligaments that separate the diaphragmatic posterior abdominal wall from the infradiaphragmatic posterior abdominal wall.

A. The lateral arcuate ligaments. They arch across the quadratus lumborum muscles.

Q. The medial arcuate ligaments arch across . . .

A. The psoas major muscles.

Q. The median arcuate ligament arches across . . .

A. The aorta.

Q. The medial and lateral arcuate ligaments give origin superiorly to . . .

A. The posterior fibers of the diaphragm.

Q. The median arcuate ligament connects . . .

A. The two crura of the diaphragm.

Q. The right crus of the diaphragm gains origin from the right side of the bodies of . . .

A. The upper three lumbar vertebrae. Superiorly, its fibers cross to the left to surround the esophageal opening in the diaphragm to form a functional sphincter.

Q. The left crus of the diaphragm gains attachment to the left side of the bodies of . . .

A. The upper two lumbar vertebrae.

Q. The posterior abdominal wall below the iliac crest consists of . . .

A. The iliacus muscle, laterally, and the psoas major muscle, medially.

Q. In Figure 5-20, identify A.

A. The anterior superior iliac spine.

Q. In Figure 5-20, identify B.

A. The right iliac fossa.

Q. In Figure 5-20, identify C.

A. The sacral promontory.

Q. In Figure 5-20, identify D.

A. The crest of the ilium.

Q. In Figure 5-20, identify E.

A. The transverse process of the 3rd lumbar vertebra. Note that it is the longest of the lumbar transverse processes.

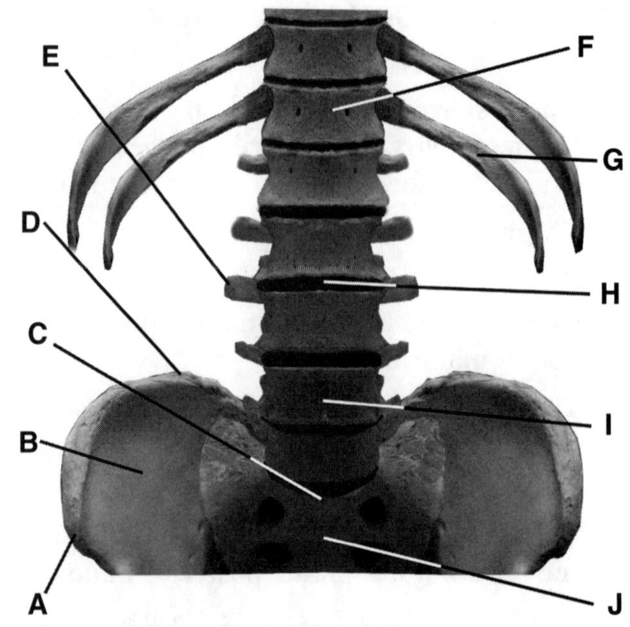

Figure 5-20 The Posterior Abdominal Wall: Bones

Q. In Figure 5-20, identify F.

A. The body of the 12th thoracic vertebra.

Q. In Figure 5-20, identify G.

A. The point of attachment of the lateral arcuate ligament to the 12th rib.

Q. In Figure 5-20, identify H.

A. The intervertebral disc between the 2nd and the 3rd lumbar vertebrae.

Q. In Figure 5-20, identify I.

A. The body of the 4th lumbar vertebra. It is at the level of the highest point of the iliac crest.

Q. In Figure 5-20, identify J.

A. The body of the 2nd sacral vertebra. The lines of fusion of the sacral vertebra are at the level of the sacral foramina.

Q. In Figure 5-21, identify A.

A. The right crus of the diaphragm.

Q. In Figure 5-21, identify B.

A. The medial arcuate ligament.

Q. In Figure 5-21, identify C.

A. The lateral arcuate ligament.

Q. In Figure 5-21, identify D.

A. The median arcuate ligament.

Q. In Figure 5-21, identify E.

A. The diaphragm.

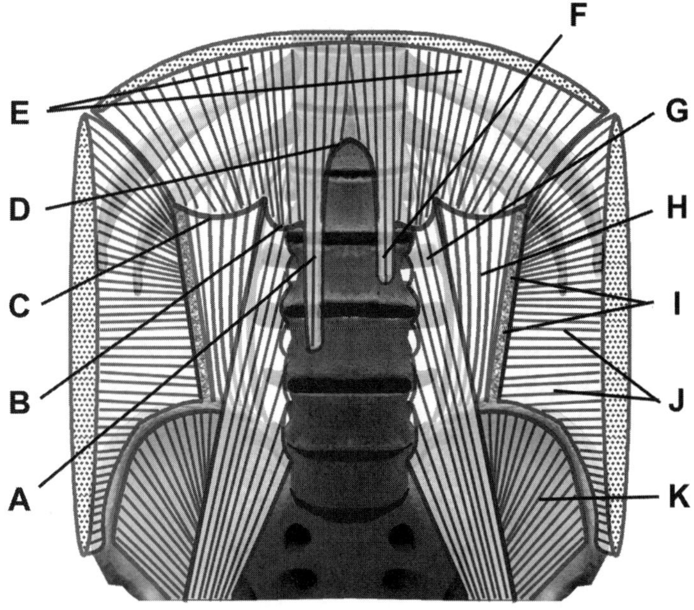

Figure 5-21 The Posterior Abdominal Wall: Muscles

Q. In Figure 5-21, identify F.

A. The left crus of the diaphragm. Note that it arises from the bodies of the upper two lumbar vertebrae. The right crus arises from the upper three lumbar vertebrae.

Q. In Figure 5-21, identify G.

A. The psoas major muscle. The highest part of this muscle is covered by the lateral arcuate ligament and the fibers of the diaphragm that arise from it. The psoas minor muscle has been omitted from this diagram.

Q. In Figure 5-21, identify H.

A. The quadratus lumborum muscle. It arises from the medial half of the 12th rib and emerges from under the lateral arcuate ligament.

Q. In Figure 5-21, identify I.

A. The thoracolumbar fascia. It gives origin to the posterior fibers of the transversus abdominis muscle.

Q. In Figure 5-21, identify J.

A. The transversus abdominis muscle.

Q. In Figure 5-21, identify K.

A. The iliacus muscle.

Q. In Figure 5-22, identify A.

A. The femoral nerve. It arises from the dorsal divisions of the anterior primary rami of the 2nd, 3rd, and 4th lumbar spinal nerves. It supplies the muscles and skin of the front of the thigh and the medial side of the leg and foot.

Q. In Figure 5-22, identify B.

A. The lateral femoral cutaneous nerve. It arises from the anterior primary rami of the 2nd and the 3rd lumbar nerves.

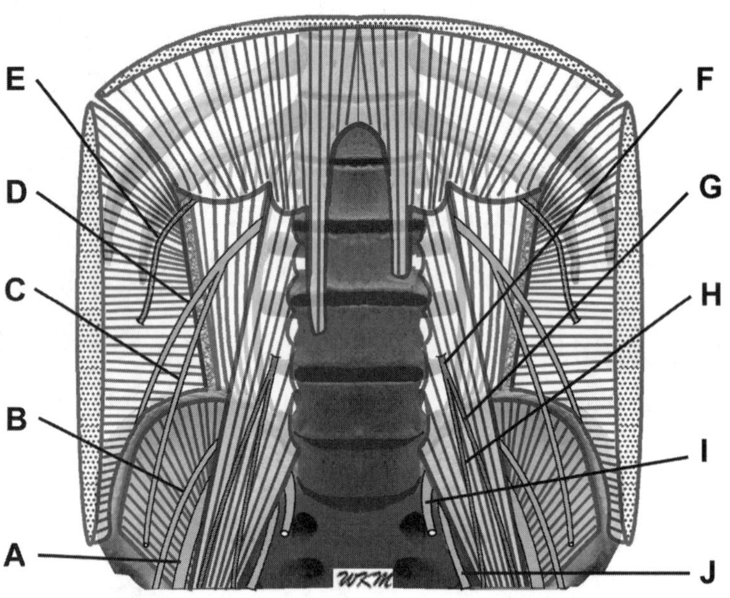

Figure 5-22 The Posterior Abdominal Wall: Nerves

Q. In Figure 5-22, identify C.

A. The ilioinguinal nerve. It passes through the superficial inguinal ring and supplies the skin of the groin and the scrotum.

Q. In Figure 5-22, identify D.

A. The iliohypogastric nerve. It supplies the skin above the pubis, the hypogastrium.

Q. In Figure 5-22, identify E.

A. The subcostal nerve. It is the anterior primary ramus of the 12th thoracic nerve.

Q. In Figure 5-22, identify F.

A. The genitofemoral nerve. It emerges onto the anterior surface of the psoas major muscle.

Q. In Figure 5-22, identify G.

A. The genital branch of the genitofemoral nerve. It will enter the inguinal canal through the deep inguinal ring and terminate by supplying the cremaster muscle.

Q. In Figure 5-22, identify H.

A. The femoral branch of the genitofemoral nerve. It leaves the anterior surface of the psoas major muscle to run with the femoral artery. It supplies the skin over the femoral triangle.

Q. In Figure 5-22, identify I.

A. The lumbosacral trunk. It carries the contribution of the 4th and 5th lumbar anterior primary rami to the sacral plexus.

Q. In Figure 5-22, identify J.

A. The obturator nerve. It arises from the ventral divisions of the anterior primary rami of the 2nd, 3rd, and 4th lumbar nerves. It supplies the adductor muscles and the skin over the medial side of the thigh.

Q. Embryologically, the viscera lying on the anterior surface of the posterior abdominal wall can be divided into two groups: those that develop as part of the abdominal wall and those that develop in association with the alimentary tract. The viscera that are closely associated with the posterior abdominal wall that develop from the urogenital ridge mesoderm are . . .

A. The suprarenal glands, the kidneys, and the ureters.

Q. Therefore, the suprarenal glands, the kidneys, and the ureters are. . .

A. Primary retroperitoneal viscera.

Q. The retroperitoneal structures on the posterior abdominal wall that develop as part of the alimentary tract are . . .

A. The duodenum and the pancreas, the ascending and the descending colon, and the vessels that supply them. Therefore, this group is anterior to primary retroperitoneal structures.

Q. The structures derived from the alimentary tract become retroperitoneal as a result of secondary adhesions during fetal life. Therefore, they are considered to be . . .

A. Secondarily retroperitoneal.

Q. Therefore, the left and right colic arteries cross their respective ureters . . .

A. Anteriorly.

Q. The alimentary-canal-derived organ that, although not primarily retroperitoneal, does come into direct contact with the posterior abdominal wall without the interposition of peritoneum is . . .

A. The liver. The posterior surface of the liver includes a bare area in contact with both the diaphragm and the inferior vena cava. The inferior vena cava travels in a deep groove in the posterior surface of the liver.

Q. Both the alimentary canal viscera and the urogenital viscera lie, posteriorly, on . . .

A. The muscles and skeletal structures of the posterior abdominal wall and the vessels and nerves that supply them. The aorta, the inferior vena cava, and the sympathetic chain belong in this group.

Q. In Figure 5-23, identify A.

A. The aorta.

Q. In Figure 5-23, identify B.

A. The inferior vena cava receiving the two renal veins.

Q. In Figure 5-23, identify C.

A. The renal pelvis of the ureter.

Q. In Figure 5-23, the structure in contact with area D is . . .

A. The diaphragm.

Q. In Figure 5-23, the structure in contact with area E is . . .

A. The psoas major muscle.

Q. In Figure 5-23, the structure in contact with area F is . . .

A. The quadratus lumborum muscle.

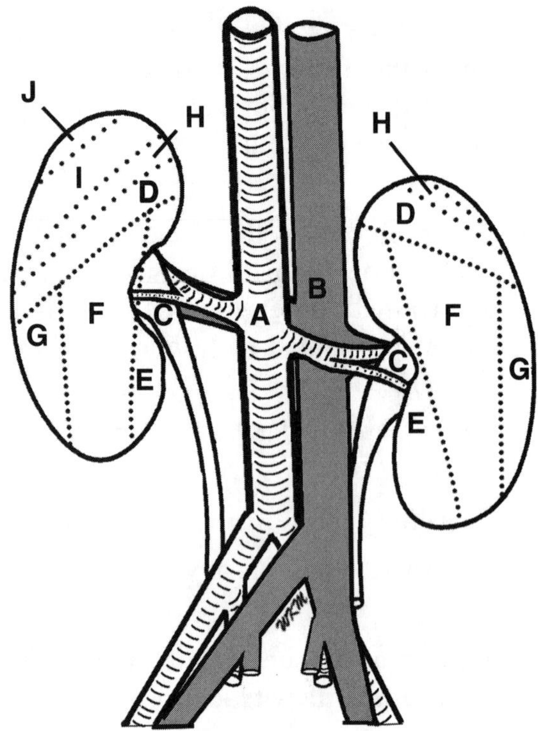

Figure 5-23 The Kidneys: Posterior Relations

Q. In Figure 5-23, the structure in contact with area G is . . .

A. The transversus abdominis muscle.

Q. In Figure 5-23, H indicates . . .

A. The 12th rib. It is separated from the kidney by the diaphragm.

Q. In Figure 5-23, I indicates . . .

A. The 11th intercostal space. It is separated from the kidney by the diaphragm.

Q. In Figure 5-23, the structure indicated by J is . . .

A. The 11th rib. It is separated from the kidney by the diaphragm.

Q. In the renal hilum, the most anterior structure is . . .

A. The renal vein. The pelvis of the ureter is posterior, separated from the renal vein by the renal artery. A small branch of the renal artery may pass posterior to the ureteric pelvis.

Q. In Figure 5-24, identify A.

A. The inferior vena cava. Here it is joined by the left and right renal veins.

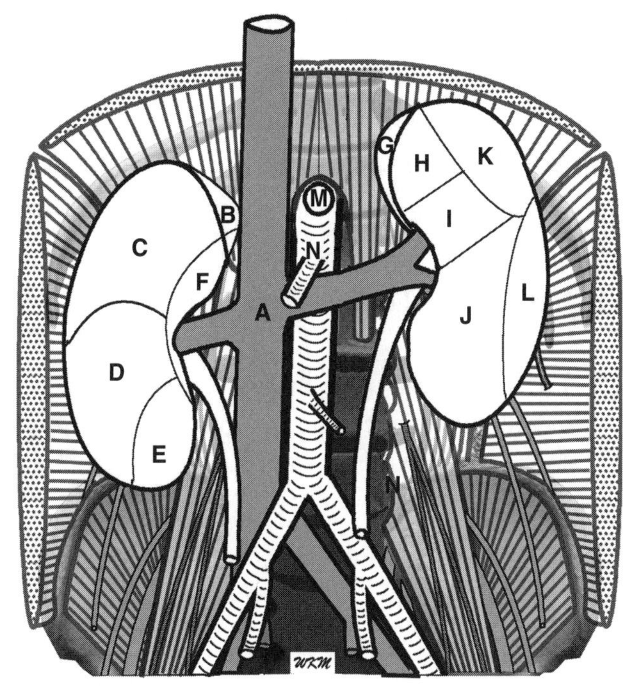

Figure 5-24 The Kidneys: Anterior Relations

Q. In Figure 5-24, identify B.

A. The right suprarenal gland.

Q. In Figure 5-24, the organ related to area C is . . .

A. The right lobe of the liver covered by peritoneum. Between the liver and the kidney is the hepatorenal pouch of the greater sac of the peritoneal cavity.

Q. Inferiorly, the hepatorenal pouch opens into . . .

A. The right paracolic gutter.

Q. In Figure 5-24, the organ related to area D is . . .

A. The hepatic flexure of the colon.

Q. In Figure 5-24, the organ related to area E is . . .

A. The small intestine. Here, the kidney is covered by a layer of parietal peritoneum. The small intestine is covered by a layer of visceral peritoneum.

Q. In Figure 5-24, the organ related to area F is . . .

A. The second part of the duodenum.

Q. In Figure 5-24, the organ related to area G is . . .

A. The left suprarenal gland.

Q. In Figure 5-24, the organ related to area H is . . .

A. The stomach, separated by the lesser sac of peritoneum. The left kidney forms part of the posterior wall of the lesser sac.

Q. In Figure 5-24, the organ related to area I is . . .

A. The tail of the pancreas before it passes into the lienorenal ligament.

Q. In Figure 5-24, the organ related to area J is . . .

A. The jejunum. Its coils are separated from the kidney by visceral and parietal peritoneum.

Q. In Figure 5-24, the organ related to area K is . . .

A. The spleen, inferior and posterior to its hilum.

Q. In Figure 5-24, the organ related to L is . . .

A. The splenic flexure of the colon and the adjacent descending colon. This area is not covered by peritoneum.

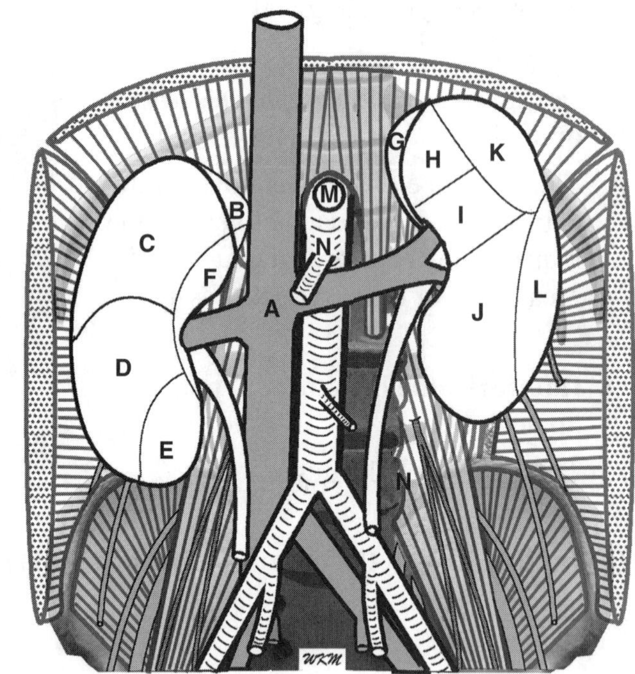

Figure 5-24 The Kidneys: Anterior Relations

Q. In Figure 5-24, identify M.

A. The origin of the celiac trunk from the aorta.

Q. In Figure 5-24, identify N.

A. The superior mesenteric artery.

Q. Separating the renal veins from the pelvis of the kidneys are . . .

A. The renal arteries.

Q. The renal arteries are not seen because . . .

A. They lie posterior to and are smaller than the renal veins.

Q. In Figure 5-25, identify A.

A. The hepatic flexure of the colon.

Q. In Figure 5-25, identify B.

A. The junction between the diaphragmatic area and the renal area of the right lobe of the liver.

Q. In Figure 5-25, identify C.

A. The tip of the gallbladder.

Q. In Figure 5-25, identify D.

A. The quadrate lobe of the liver.

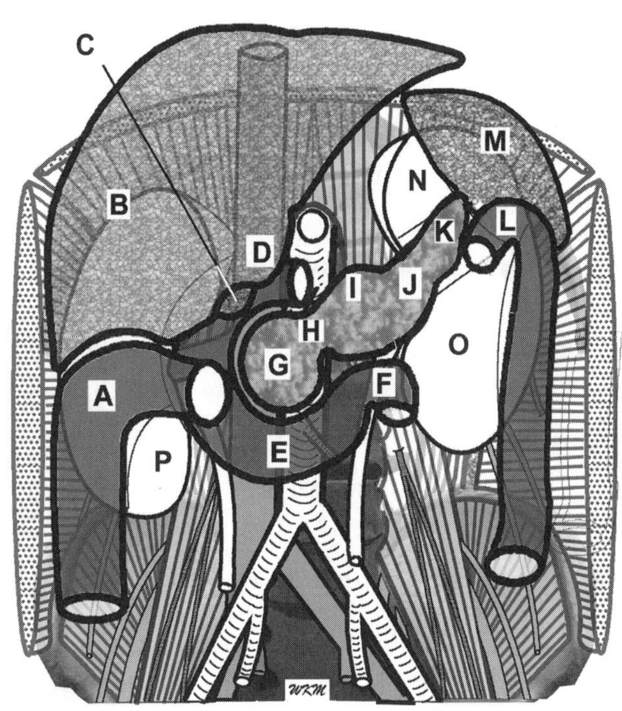

Figure 5-25 Abdominal Organ Relations

Q. In Figure 5-25, identify E.

A. The third part of the duodenum.

Q. In Figure 5-25, identify F.

A. The duodenojejunal flexure.

Q. In Figure 5-25, identify G.

A. The head of the pancreas.

Q. In Figure 5-25, identify H.

A. The neck of the pancreas.

Q. In Figure 5-25, identify I.

A. The tuber omentale of the pancreas. It is in contact with the lesser omentum superior to the lesser curvature of the stomach.

Q. In Figure 5-25, identify J.

A. The body of the pancreas.

Q. In Figure 5-25, identify K.

A. The tail of the pancreas.

Q. In Figure 5-25, identify L.

A. The splenic flexure of the colon.

Q. In Figure 5-25, identify M.

A. The spleen. Its visceral surface has an impression, posteriorly, from the left kidney, and one, anteriorly, from the stomach.

Q. In Figure 5-25, the areas N, O, and P are covered by parietal peritoneum. The peritoneal cavity separates them from . . .

A. The stomach (N), the lesser sac, and coils of small intestine (**O** and **P**), the greater sac.

RADIOLOGY OF THE ABDOMEN

Q. In Figure 5-26, identify A.

A. Gas in the fundus of the stomach.

Q. In Figure 5-26, identify B.

A. Rugae in the wall of the stomach.

Q. In Figure 5-26, identify C.

A. The body of the stomach.

Q. In Figure 5-26, identify D.

A. Coils of the jejunum.

Q. In Figure 5-26, identify E.

A. The pyloric antrum.

Q. In Figure 5-26, identify F.

A. The pyloric canal. This is the most common site for gastric ulcers.

Q. In Figure 5-26, identify G.

A. The contracted pyloric sphincter.

Q. In Figure 5-26, identify H.

A. The duodenal cap.

Q. In Figure 5-26, identify I.

A. The 1st lumbar vertebra.

Q. In Figure 5-26, identify J.

A. The right 12th rib.

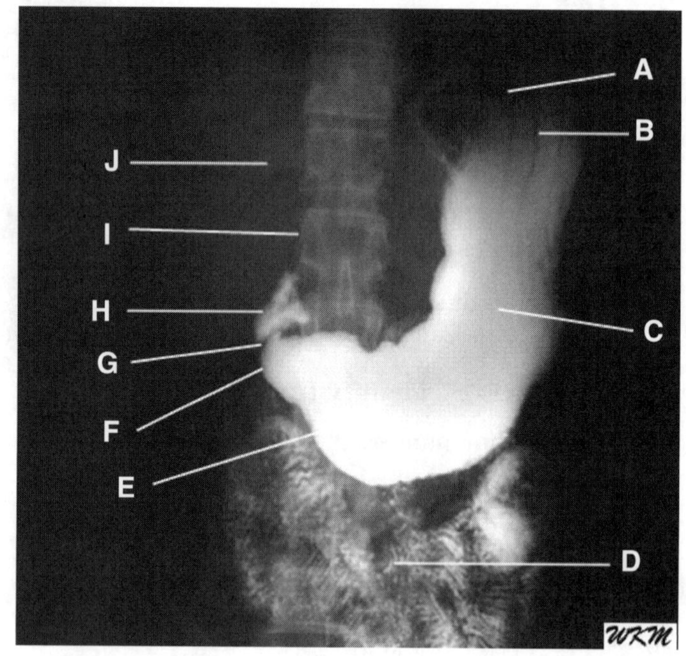

Figure 5-26 A Postbarium Meal X-Ray

Q. In Figure 5-27, identify A.

A. Coils of ileum.

Q. In Figure 5-27, identify B.

A. The appendix.

Q. In Figure 5-27, identify C.

A. The cecum.

Q. In Figure 5-27, identify D.

A. The ascending colon. The fluid level of the barium contrast indicates that the barium enema was administered and the X-ray taken with the patient lying on his or her right side.

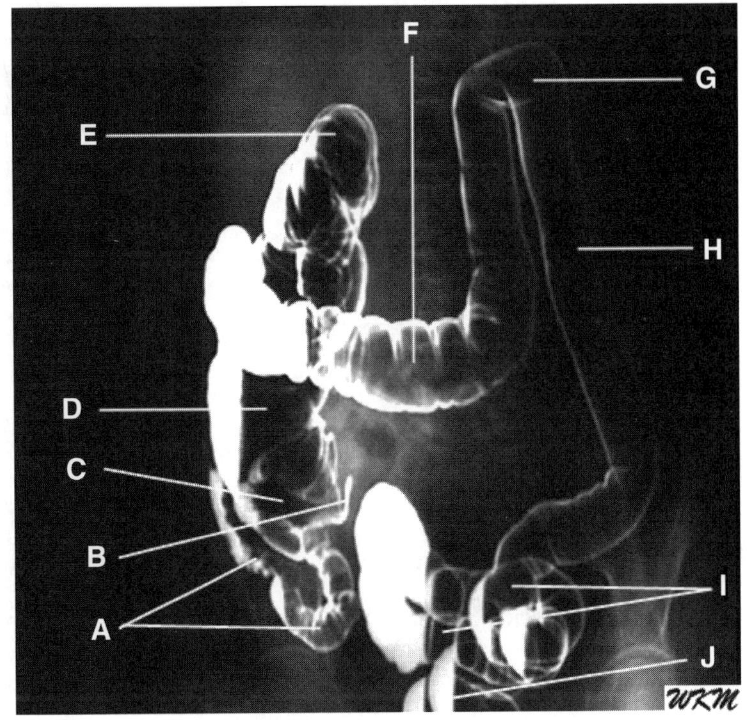

Figure 5-27 A Postbarium Enema X-Ray

Q. In Figure 5-27, identify E.

A. The hepatic flexure of the colon.

Q. In Figure 5-27, identify F.

A. The transverse colon. Note the haustrations.

Q. In Figure 5-27, identify G.

A. The splenic flexure of the colon.

Q. In Figure 5-27, identify H.

A. The descending colon.

Q. In Figure 5-27, identify I.

A. The sigmoid colon. The fluid level of the barium contrast indicates that the barium enema was administered and the X-ray taken with the patient lying on his or her right side.

Q. In Figure 5-27, identify J.

A. The rectum.

Q. In Figure 5-28, identify A.

A. The 12th rib.

Q. In Figure 5-28, identify B.

A. A catheter in the right ureter.

Q. In Figure 5-28, identify C.

A. The right sacroiliac joint.

Q. In Figure 5-28, identify D.

A. A minor calyx.

Q. In Figure 5-28, identify E.

A. The left superior major calyx.

Q. In Figure 5-28, identify F.

A. The renal pelvis.

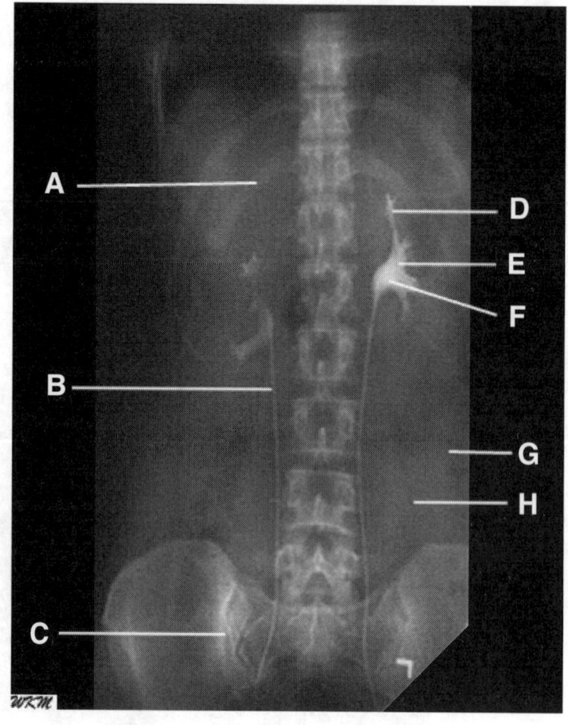

Figure 5-28 A Retrograde Pyelogram

Q. In Figure 5-28, identify G.

A. The lateral edge of the quadratus lumborum muscle.

Q. In Figure 5-28, identify H.

A. The lateral edge of the psoas major muscle.

Q. In Figure 5-29, identify A.

A. The right crus of the diaphragm.

Q. In Figure 5-29, identify B.

A. The aorta. The inferior vena cava is embedded in the liver and thus not clearly discernible.

Q. In Figure 5-29, identify C.

A. The right lobe of the liver.

Q. In Figure 5-29, identify D.

A. The celiac trunk.

Q. In Figure 5-29, identify E.

A. The ligamentum teres hepaticus, the round ligament of the liver. It is the fibrous remnant of the embryonic umbilical vein.

Q. In Figure 5-29, identify F.

A. The left lobe of the liver.

Q. In Figure 5-29, identify G.

A. Gas in the stomach. Note the fluid level in the supine patient.

Q. In Figure 5-29, identify H.

A. The stomach wall. The stomach contains contrast medium, a barium meal, and some gas.

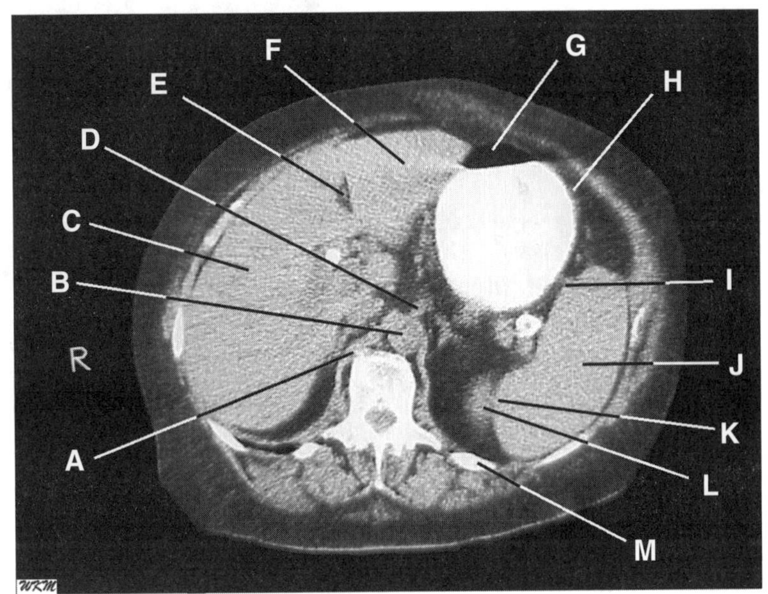

Figure 5-29 MRI of the Abdomen at T12

Q. In Figure 5-29, identify I.

A. The gastric impression on the spleen.

Q. In Figure 5-29, identify J.

A. The spleen. It is somewhat enlarged in this patient.

Q. In Figure 5-29, identify K.

A. The renal impression on the spleen.

Q. In Figure 5-29, identify L.

A. The left kidney. It is lying lower than is normal in this patient, possibly due to the enlargement of the spleen.

Q. In Figure 5-29, identify M.

A. The 12th rib.

Q. In Figure 5-30, identify A.

A. The right psoas major muscle.

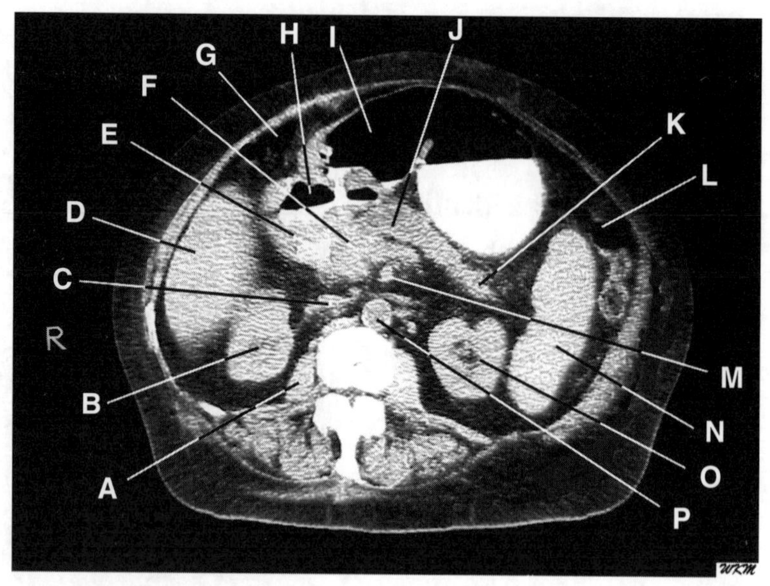

Figure 5-30 MRI of the Abdomen at L2

Q. In Figure 5-30, identify B.

A. The right kidney. It lies between the psoas major muscle and the right lobe of the liver.

Q. In Figure 5-30, identify C.

A. The inferior vena cava. It is collapsed.

Q. The inferior vena cava collapses during . . .

A. Inspiration.

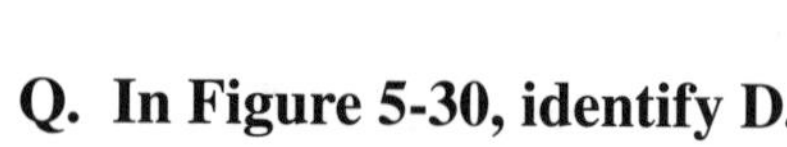

Q. In Figure 5-30, identify D.

A. The right lobe of the liver.

Q. At this level, the visceral surface of the right lobe of the liver is in contact with . . .

A. The kidney and the first part of the duodenum.

Q. The right lobe of the liver is separated from the kidney and first part of the duodenum by . . .

A. The layers of peritoneum that cover them.

Q. In Figure 5-30, identify E.

A. The second part of the duodenum.

Q. In Figure 5-30, identify F.

A. The head of the pancreas. It lies in the "C" of the duodenum. Here, it lies medial to the second part of the duodenum.

Q. In Figure 5-30, identify G.

A. Gas in the transverse colon.

Q. In Figure 5-30, identify H.

A. The pyloric antrum. It contains both gas and fluid.

Q. In Figure 5-30, identify I.

A. The body of the stomach.

Q. The stomach contains . . .

A. Both gas and fluid. Note the fluid level.

Q. In Figure 5-30, identify J.

A. The body of the pancreas.

Q. In Figure 5-30, identify K.

A. The tail of the pancreas. It lies posterior to the stomach in the posterior wall of the omental bursa. It reaches the hilum of the spleen.

Q. In Figure 5-30, identify L.

A. The splenic end of the transverse colon. It is in contact with the spleen and contains some gas. It does not usually intervene between the spleen and the abdominal wall.

Q. In Figure 5-30, identify M.

A. The superior mesenteric artery.

Q. The superior mesenteric artery arises from the aorta at the level of . . .

A. The lower margin of the 1st lumbar vertebra.

Q. In Figure 5-30, identify N.

A. The spleen. It is somewhat enlarged.

Q. In Figure 5-30, identify O.

A. The left kidney. It lies on the psoas major muscle and, more laterally, the thinner quadratus lumborum muscle. Anterolaterally, it is in contact with the visceral surface of the spleen posterior to its hilum. The pararenal body is a mass of fat posterior to the kidney.

Q. In Figure 5-30, identify P.

A. The abdominal aorta.

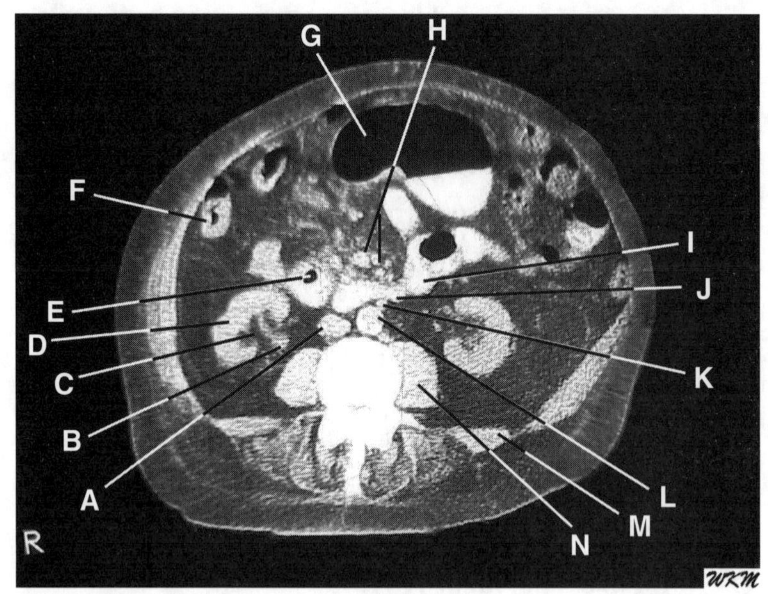

Figure 5-31 MRI of the Abdomen at L3

Q. In Figure 5-31, identify A.

A. The inferior vena cava.

Q. In Figure 5-31, identify B.

A. The right renal artery.

Q. In Figure 5-31, identify C.

A. The right renal pelvis.

Q. In Figure 5-31, identify D.

A. The right kidney.

Q. The area anterior and lateral to the right kidney is known as . . .

A. The right paracolic gutter.

Q. The clinical significance of the right paracolic gutter is that . . .

A. It can serve as a pathway for infected fluid from the gallbladder or from a perforated peptic ulcer to reach the pelvis in the region of the appendix.

Q. This can cause an erroneous diagnosis of . . .

A. Acute appendicitis.

Q. In Figure 5-31, identify E.

A. Gas in the second part of the duodenum.

Q. In Figure 5-31, identify F.

A. The ascending colon.

Q. In Figure 5-31, identify G.

A. Gas in the body of the stomach.

Q. In Figure 5-31, identify H.

A. The superior mesenteric vessels.

Q. The superior mesenteric vessels supply . . .

A. The small intestine and the ascending and transverse colon.

Q. In Figure 5-31, identify I.

A. The fourth part of the duodenum.

Q. In Figure 5-31, identify J.

A. The third part of the duodenum.

Q. In Figure 5-31, identify K.

A. The inferior mesenteric artery.

Q. The inferior mesenteric artery arises from . . .

A. The aorta, posterior to the third part of the duodenum.

Q. The inferior mesenteric artery arises from the aorta at the level of . . .

A. The body of the 3rd lumbar vertebra.

Q. In Figure 5-31, identify L.

A. The abdominal aorta.

Q. In Figure 5-31, identify M.

A. The left quadratus lumborum muscle.

Q. The most important function of the quadratus lumborum muscles is to assist in . . .

A. Inspiration. The two muscles "fix" the 12th ribs to assist the action of the diaphragm. Acting individually, they act as lateral flexors of the vertebral column.

Q. In Figure 5-31, identify N.

A. The left psoas major muscle.

Q. The most important action of the psoas major muscle is to . . .

A. Flex the thigh.

Q. In Figure 5-32, identify A.

A. The iliac crest.

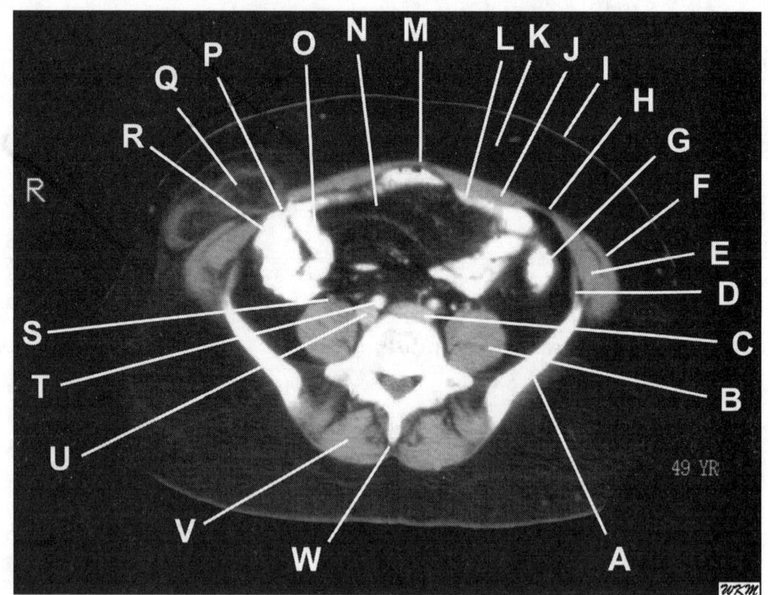

Figure 5-32 MRI of the Abdomen at L5

Q. In Figure 5-32, identify B.

A. The psoas major muscle.

Q. In Figure 5-32, identify C.

A. The left common iliac vein.

Q. In Figure 5-32, identify D.

A. The left transversus abdominis muscle.

Q. In Figure 5-32, identify E.

A. The left internal oblique muscle.

Q. In Figure 5-32, identify F.

A. The left external oblique muscle.

Q. In Figure 5-32, identify G.

A. The descending colon. The colon has been delineated by an MRI contrast enema.

Q. In Figure 5-32, identify H.

A. The left linea semilunaris at the lateral border of the rectus sheath. It was originally called the Spigelian line after a Flemish anatomist.

Q. In Figure 5-32, identify I.

A. Skin.

Q. In Figure 5-32, identify J.

A. The left rectus abdominis muscle.

Q. In Figure 5-32, identify K.

A. Subcutaneous fat.

Q. In Figure 5-32, identify L.

A. The transverse colon.

Q. In Figure 5-32, identify M.

A. The linea alba, so-called because it is avascular and aponeurotic, and therefore white.

Q. In Figure 5-32, identify N.

A. Gas in the ileum.

Q. In Figure 5-32, identify O.

A. The descending colon.

Q. In Figure 5-32, identify P.

A. The small aperture in the linea semilunaris through which some loops of terminal ileum (**Q**) have extruded to form a Spigelian hernia. Spigelian hernias are quite rare. In this case, due to the significant layer of subcutaneous fat, no obvious bulge of the anterior abdominal wall is observed.

Q. In Figure 5-32, identify R.

A. The cecum. It is usually attached to the posterior abdominal wall. Thus, it does not herniate.

Q. In Figure 5-32, identify S.

A. The right ureter lying on the front of psoas major muscle.

Q. In Figure 5-32, identify T.

A. The right common iliac artery.

Q. In Figure 5-32, identify U.

A. The right common iliac vein.

Q. In Figure 5-32, identify V.

A. The sacrospinalis muscle.

Q. In Figure 5-32, identify W.

A. The spine of the 5th lumbar vertebra.

Q. In Figure 5-33, identify A.

A. The celiac trunk. It is very short and arises from the aorta at the level of T12.

Q. The celiac trunk immediately divides into three branches. The three branches are . . .

A. The common hepatic artery, the splenic artery, and the left gastric artery.

Q. In Figure 5-33, identify B.

A. The splenic artery.

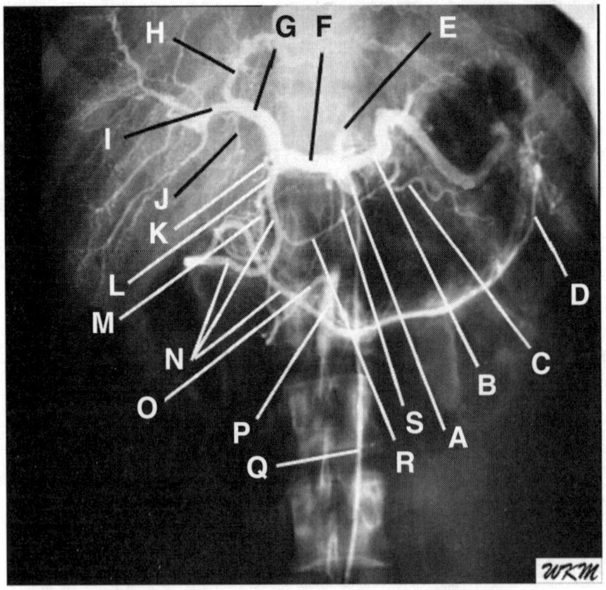

Figure 5-33 Arteriogram of the Celiac Trunk

Q. In Figure 5-33, identify C.

A. The great pancreatic artery.

Q. In Figure 5-33, identify D.

A. The left gastroepiploic artery. It arises from the splenic artery at the hilum of the spleen. In this arteriogram, it is not well filled by the contrast medium.

Q. In Figure 5-33, identify E.

A. The left gastric artery. It is the smallest of the three branches of the celiac trunk.

Q. In Figure 5-33, identify F.

A. The common hepatic artery.

Q. In Figure 5-33, identify G.

A. The proper hepatic artery.

Q. In Figure 5-33, identify H.

A. The left hepatic artery.

Q. In Figure 5-33, identify I.

A. The right hepatic artery.

Q. In Figure 5-33, identify J.

A. The cystic artery.

Q. In Figure 5-33, identify K.

A. The right gastric artery. It runs along the lesser curvature of the stomach between the layers of the lesser omentum. Here it is obscured by the shadow of the common hepatic artery.

Q. The right gastric artery arises from . . .

A. The proper hepatic artery.

Q. In Figure 5-33, identify L.

A. The gastroduodenal artery. It arises from the common hepatic artery to run inferiorly, posterior to the first part of the duodenum. The common hepatic artery is thereafter named the proper hepatic artery.

Q. In Figure 5-33, identify M.

A. The superior pancreaticoduodenal artery. It divides into anterior and posterior branches, which anastomose with corresponding branches of the inferior pancreaticoduodenal branch of the superior mesenteric artery.

Q. In Figure 5-33, identify N.

A. The right gastroepiploic artery. It is the largest branch of the gastroduodenal artery. It runs between the two layers of the greater omentum. As its name implies, it supplies the greater curvature of the stomach and the greater omentum.

Q. In Figure 5-33, identify O.

A. The inferior pancreaticoduodenal branch of the superior mesenteric artery.

Q. In Figure 5-33, identify P.

A. The stem of the superior mesenteric artery. It has been partially filled by the anastomosis between the pancreaticoduodenal arteries.

Q. In Figure 5-33, identify Q.

A. A catheter in the aorta. Its tip is in the origin of the celiac trunk.

Q. In Figure 5-33, identify R.

A. The inferior (transverse) pancreatic artery.

Q. In Figure 5-33, identify S.

A. The superior (dorsal) pancreatic branch of the splenic artery.

Q. In Figure 5-34, identify A.

A. The left hepatic artery.

Q. In Figure 5-34, identify B.

A. The right hepatic artery.

Q. In Figure 5-34, identify C.

A. The common hepatic artery. Note that it is almost symmetrical to the splenic artery.

Q. In Figure 5-34, identify D.

A. The inferior right suprarenal artery.

Q. In Figure 5-34, identify E.

A. The right renal artery.

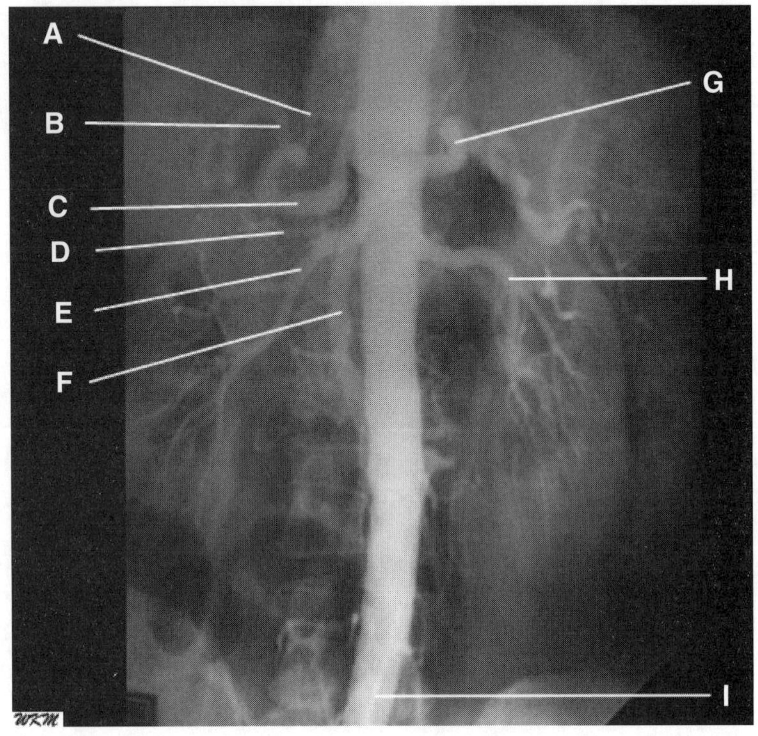

Figure 5-34 Arteriogram of the Abdominal Aorta

Q. In Figure 5-34, identify F.

A. The superior mesenteric artery. The inferior mesenteric artery is not discernible in this arteriogram.

Q. In Figure 5-34, identify G.

A. The splenic artery.

Q. In Figure 5-34, identify H.

A. The left renal artery.

Q. In Figure 5-34, identify I.

A. A catheter in the abdominal aorta. It was inserted through the right femoral artery.

Chapter 6

The Pelvis and Perineum

THE BONES OF THE PELVIS

Q. In Figure 6-1, identify A.

A. The lateral mass (ala) of the sacrum.

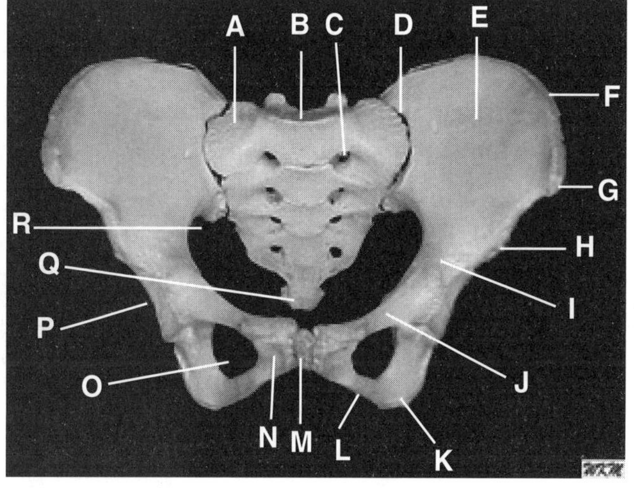

Figure 6-1 The Female Pelvis, Anterior View

Q. The lateral mass of the sacrum is formed from . . .

A. The fused transverse processes of the five sacral vertebrae.

Q. In Figure 6-1, identify B.

A. The sacral promontory.

Q. In Figure 6-1, identify C.

A. The 1st left pelvic sacral foramen. The piriformis muscle arises between and lateral to the sacral foramina.

Q. In Figure 6-1, identify D.

A. The left sacroiliac joint.

Q. In Figure 6-1, identify E.

A. The iliac fossa.

Q. The muscle that arises from the iliac fossa is . . .

A. The iliacus muscle.

Q. Together with the psoas major muscle, the iliacus muscle is inserted into . . .

A. The lesser trochanter of the femur. Together, they are the main flexors of the hip joint. When an inflamed appendix lies in association with the iliacus muscle, flexion of the hip joint becomes painful. This fact can be of importance in the diagnosis of acute appendicitis.

Q. In Figure 6-1, identify F.

A. The iliac crest.

Q. The muscles attached to the anterior segment of the iliac crest are . . .

A. The obliquus externus abdominis muscle, the obliquus internus abdominis muscle, and the transversus abdominis muscle.

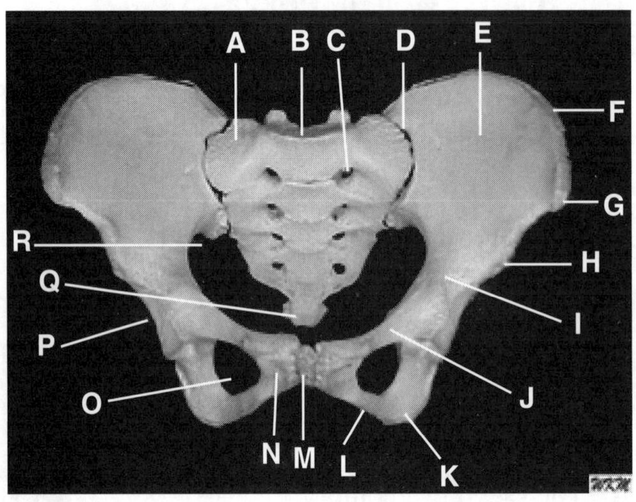

Figure 6-1 The Female Pelvis, Anterior View

Q. In Figure 6-1, identify G.

A. The anterior superior iliac spine.

Q. The muscle that arises from the anterior superior iliac spine is . . .

A. The sartorius muscle.

Q. In Figure 6-1, identify H.

A. The anterior inferior iliac spine.

Q. The muscle that arises from the anterior inferior iliac spine is . . .

A. The straight head of the rectus femoris muscle.

Q. In Figure 6-1, identify I.

A. The iliopubic eminence. At this point, the superior pubic ramus fuses with the ilium.

Q. In Figure 6-1, identify J.

A. The superior ramus of the pubis.

Q. In Figure 6-1, identify K.

A. The ischial tuberosity.

Q. In Figure 6-1, identify L.

A. The ischiopubic ramus. The inferior ramus of the pubis joins and fuses with the ramus of the ischium.

Q. In Figure 6-1, identify M.

A. The symphysis pubis. It is the fibrocartilaginous joint between the left and right pubic bones.

Q. In Figure 6-1, identify N.

A. The body of the pubis.

Q. The muscle that is attached to the anterior surface of the body of the pubis is . . .

A. The tendon of the adductor longus muscle. It is readily palpable, even in the obese. It serves as a useful locator for the pubic tubercle when differentiating an inguinal hernia from a femoral hernia.

Q. In Figure 6-1, identify O.

A. The obturator foramen. Except anterosuperiorly, it is closed by the obturator membrane.

Q. The anterosuperiorly situated aperture in the obturator membrane is named . . .

A. The obturator canal. The obturator vessels and nerve leave the pelvis through this canal.

Q. The obturator nerve supplies . . .

A. The adductor muscles of the thigh and the skin over them.

Q. Intrapelvic lesions of the obturator nerve, such as those involved in a carcinoma of the ovary, cause . . .

A. The ipsilateral limb to gradually deviate laterally when walking. This is the so-called "adductor" gait.

Q. In Figure 6-1, identify P.

A. The line points toward the acetabular fossa, which cannot be seen in this view.

Q. In Figure 6-1, identify Q.

A. The coccyx. In this specimen, it is fused with the 5th piece of the sacrum.

Q. In Figure 6-1, identify R.

A. The greater sciatic foramen. The piriformis muscle, most of the branches of the sacral plexus, the superior and the inferior gluteal vessels, and the internal pudendal vessels pass through this foramen.

Q. The structures that leave the pelvis through the greater sciatic foramen above the piriformis muscle are . . .

A. The superior gluteal vessels and the superior gluteal nerve. The superior gluteal nerve supplies the gluteus medius muscle, the gluteus minimi muscle, and the tensor fasciae latae muscle.

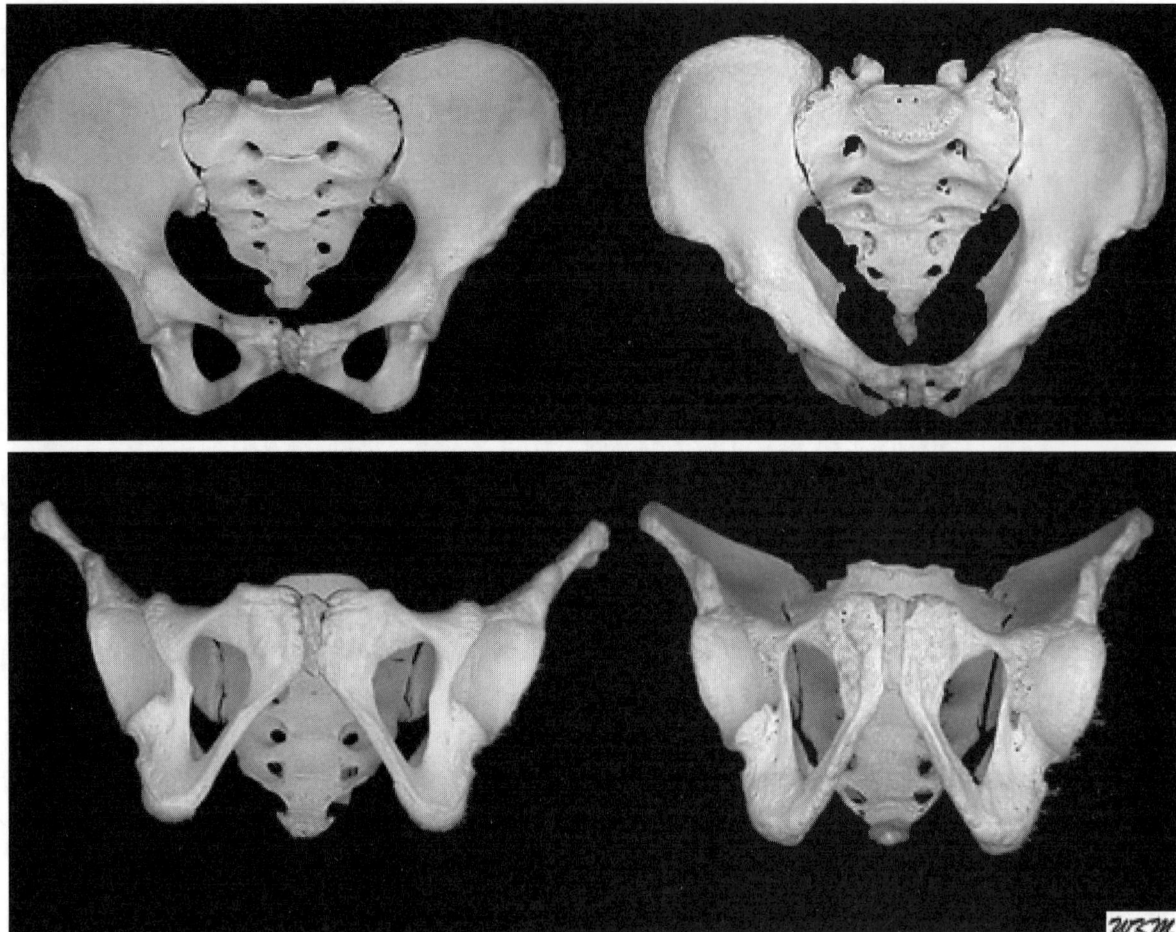

Figure 6-2 A Comparison of the Female and Male Bony Pelvis

Q. With reference to Figure 6-2, the major gender differences in the female sacrum are that . . .

A. The female sacrum is wider, shorter, and flatter than the male sacrum.

Q. With reference to Figure 6-2, the major gender differences in the body of the female pubis are that . . .

A. The pubis is much wider and the symphysis much shorter than in the male. In the male, the reverse is true, and the bone itself is much thicker and heavier.

Q. With reference to Figure 6-2, the major gender difference in the ischial spines is that in the male . . .

A. The ischial spines clearly project into the pelvic cavity. Only the tip of the left ischial spine is visible in this view of the female pelvis.

Q. With reference to Figure 6-2, the major gender difference in the iliac fossae is that in the male . . .

A. The iliac fossae are much deeper. This greater depth reflects the greater mass of the iliacus muscle in the male.

Q. With reference to Figure 6-2, the major gender differences in the iliac crests is that in the male . . .

A. The iliac crests are much heavier and more curved. This reflects the strength of the muscles attached there.

Q. With reference to Figure 6-2, the major gender difference in the anterior superior iliac spines is that in the female . . .

A. The anterior superior iliac spines are relatively farther apart.

Q. With reference to Figure 6-2, the major gender difference in the ischial tuberosities is that in the female . . .

A. The ischial tuberosities are clearly farther apart.

Q. With reference to Figure 6-2, the major gender difference in the ischiopubic rami is that in the male . . .

A. The rami are much thicker and heavier. This is necessary to support the penis.

Q. With reference to Figure 6-2, the major gender difference in the acetabular fossae is that in the male . . .

A. The acetabular fossae are much larger and face more anteriorly.

Q. With reference to Figure 6-2, the major gender difference in the subpubic angle is that in the male . . .

A. The subpubic angle is much more acute.

Q. With reference to Figure 6-2, the major gender difference in the sacroiliac joints is that in the male . . .

A. The joint surfaces are much more extensive.

Q. With reference to Figure 6-2, the major gender difference in the pelvic inlet is that in the female . . .

A. The pelvic inlet is more nearly circular and often very slightly compressed anteroposteriorly, making it a transverse oval. In the male, the large promontory of the sacrum and the lateral compression makes the inlet appear somewhat heart shaped.

Q. The pelvic cavity can be described as a short section of a long cone in . . .

A. The female. In the female, the cavity is fairly uniform in diameter throughout its length to allow for passage of the fetal head. Conversely, the male pelvis can be described as a long section of a short cone.

THE PELVIC WALLS AND FLOOR

Q. In Figure 6-3, identify A.

A. The sacral canal.

Q. In Figure 6-3, identify B.

A. The greater sciatic foramen.

Q. In Figure 6-3, identify C.

A. The sacrospinous ligament. The few remaining muscle fibers on its pelvic surface form the coccygeus muscle.

Q. In Figure 6-3, identify D.

A. The ischial spine.

Q. In Figure 6-3, identify E.

A. The lesser sciatic foramen.

Q. In Figure 6-3, identify F.

A. The sacrotuberous ligament.

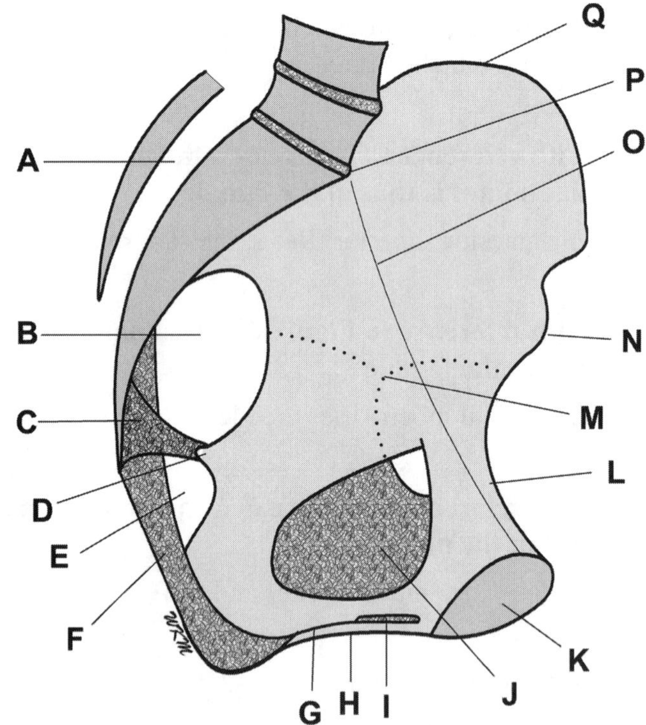

Figure 6-3 The Bones and Ligaments of the Pelvic Wall

Q. In Figure 6-3, identify G.

A. The falciform ligament. It is the continuation, anteriorly, of the sacrotuberous ligament.

Q. In Figure 6-3, identify H.

A. The ischiopubic ramus. It is formed by the union of the inferior ramus of the pubis and the ramus of the ischium.

Q. In Figure 6-3, identify I.

A. The perineal membrane. It is also called the inferior layer of the urogenital diaphragm. It forms a shelf joining the inferior rami of the pubes.

Q. In Figure 6-3, identify J.

A. The obturator membrane. It almost closes the obturator foramen. The obturator internus muscle arises from its pelvic surface. The obturator externus arises from its lateral surface.

Q. In Figure 6-3, identify K.

A. The body of the pubis. It is connected to the contralateral pubic body by the fibrocartilaginous pubic symphysis.

Q. In Figure 6-3, identify L.

A. The superior ramus of the pubis.

Q. In Figure 6-3, identify M.

A. The junction of the fused ischium, pubis, and ilium.

Q. In Figure 6-3, identify N.

A. The anterior inferior iliac spine. It gives attachment to the straight head of the rectus femoris muscle.

Q. In Figure 6-3, identify O.

A. The linea terminalis. It forms the lateral part of the pelvic inlet.

Q. In Figure 6-3, identify P.

A. The sacral promontory. It forms the posterior part of the pelvic inlet.

Q. In Figure 6-3, identify Q.

A. The iliac crest.

Q. The bony posterior wall of the true pelvis is formed by . . .

A. The five fused pieces of the sacrum and the coccyx.

Q. The only muscles on the posterior wall of the true pelvis are . . .

A. The piriformis muscles. They arise from the anterior surface of the sacrum, pass through the greater sciatic foramina, and are inserted into the greater trochanter of the appropriate femur.

Q. On the anterior surface of the piriformis muscles, but still deep to the prevertebral fascia, lie . . .

A. The right and left sciatic plexuses. They are vulnerable to pressure during passage of the fetal head in childbirth. Paresthesia and muscle weakness can occur in one or both lower limbs.

Q. The bony lateral wall of the true pelvis consists of . . .

A. The innominate bone.

Q. The innominate bone has three parts. They are . . .

A. The ilium, the ischium, and the pubis.

Q. The only muscle on the lateral wall of the pelvis is . . .

A. The obturator internus muscle.

Q. On the pelvic surface of the obturator internus muscle lie the branches of . . .

A. The internal iliac artery. The ureter and the obturator nerve also cross the pelvic surface of the obturator internus muscle.

Q. In Figure 6-4, identify A.

A. The piriformis muscle. Each piriformis muscle arises from the ipsilateral anterior surface of the sacrum between the sacral foramina. It leaves the pelvis through its respective greater sciatic foramen to be inserted into the greater trochanter of the femur. It lies mainly on the posterior wall of the pelvis, but it does contribute to the posterior part of the lateral wall.

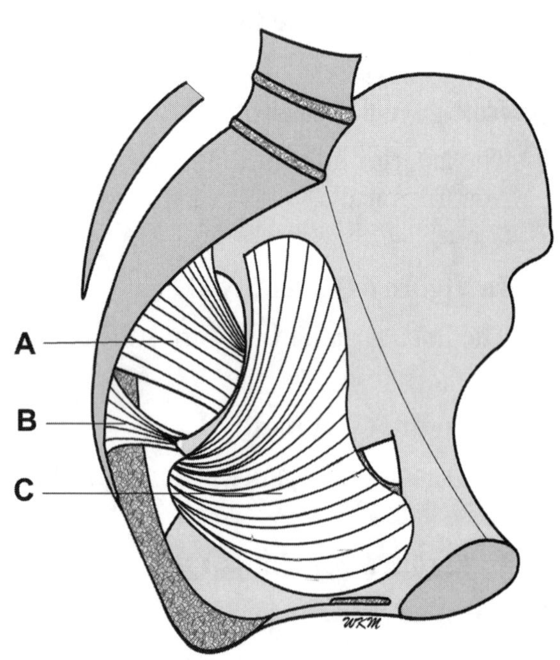

Figure 6-4 The Muscles of the Pelvic Walls

Q. In Figure 6-4, identify B.

A. The coccygeus muscle. The posterior part of each coccygeus muscle is fibrous and forms the ipsilateral sacrospinous ligament.

Q. In Figure 6-4, identify C.

A. The obturator internus muscle. Each obturator internus muscle arises from the ipsilateral obturator membrane and the surrounding areas of the ischium, ilium, and pubis. It leaves the pelvis through the lesser sciatic foramen to be inserted on the greater trochanter of the femur.

Q. In Figure 6-5, identify A.

A. The iliococcygeus muscle. It is called this because its origin was the posterior part of the linea terminalis, which, at this point, is part of the ilium. Through time, its origin has gradually slid down the fascia over the obturator internus muscle until it has reached the spine of the ischium.

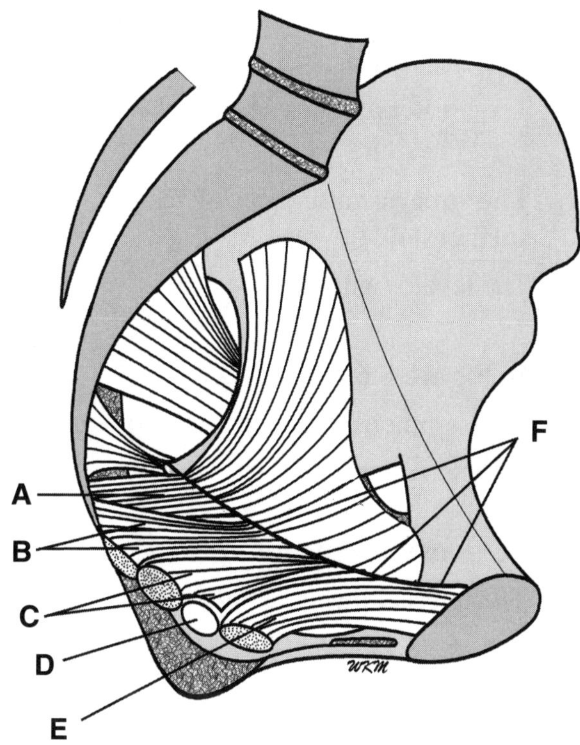

Figure 6-5 The Muscles of the Pelvic Floor

Q. In Figure 6-5, identify B.

A. The pubococcygeal part of the pubococcygeus muscle. It is attached to the coccyx and to the anococcygeal raphe, where it fuses with the contralateral muscle.

Q. In Figure 6-5, identify C.

A. The puborectalis muscle. It is the part of the puboccoccygeus that is inserted into the wall of the anorectal junction. However, most of its fibers encircle the rectum to fuse with the contralateral muscle. The puborectalis muscles cause angulation of the anorectal junction and thus help the anal sphincter to retain feces.

Q. In Figure 6-5, identify D.

A. Thc anorcctal junction.

Q. In Figure 6-5, identify E.

A. The most anterior and medial part of the pubococcygeus muscle. In the male, it is named the levator prostatae; in the female it is named the pubovaginalis muscle. In the female, it fuses with the contralateral muscle to form a fibromuscular node between the vagina and the rectum. This node is called the perineal body or the central tendon of the perineum. If it is torn or intentionally incised during childbirth, it must be repaired to prevent a subsequent uterine prolapse.

Q. In Figure 6-5, identify F.

A. The tendinous arch of the levator ani muscle. The obturator fascia between this tendinous arch and the linea terminalis is composed of a degenerate fibrous part of the levator ani muscle that is fused with the true fascia covering the obturator internus muscle.

Q. The three parts of both pubococcygeus muscles together with both iliococcygeus muscles form . . .

A. The levator ani muscle. It is also known as the pelvic diaphragm.

Q. The superior and inferior fasciae of the pelvic diaphragm cover the appropriate surfaces of . . .

A. The levator ani muscles.

Q. In Figure 6-6, identify A.

A. The common iliac artery. The common iliac arteries are formed by the bifurcation of the aorta on the anterior surface of the body of the 4th lumbar vertebra.

Q. In Figure 6-6, identify B.

A. The internal iliac artery.

Q. In Figure 6-6, identify C.

A. The posterior division of the internal iliac artery. Its branches supply only somatic structures.

Q. In Figure 6-6, identify D.

A. The anterior division of the internal iliac artery. Its branches supply both somatic and visceral structures.

Q. In Figure 6-6, identify E.

A. The external iliac artery.

Q. In Figure 6-6, identify F.

A. The obturator artery.

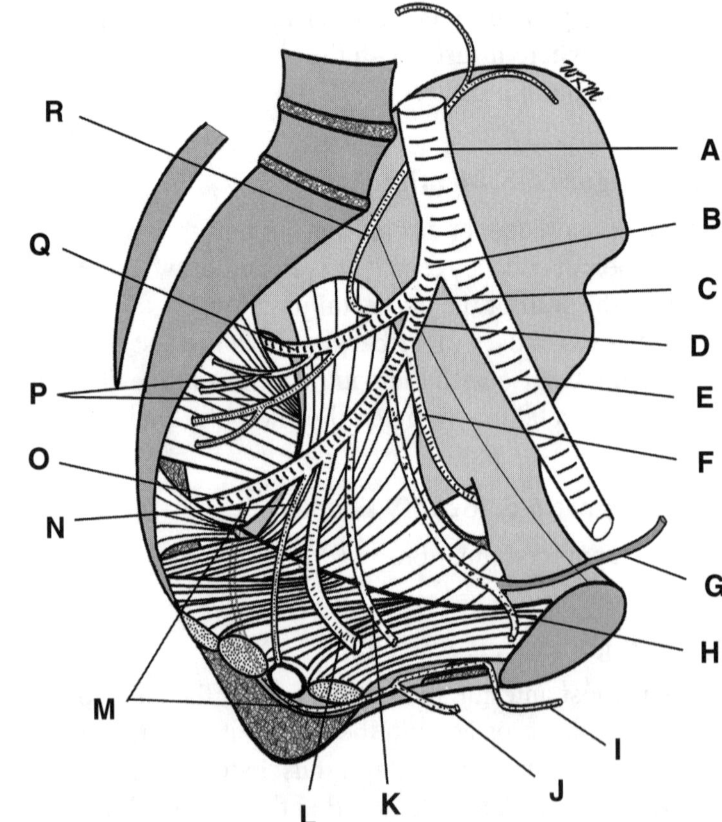

Figure 6-6 The Arteries of the Pelvis

Q. In Figure 6-6, identify G.

A. The fibrous remnant of the umbilical artery of the fetus.

Q. In Figure 6-6, identify H.

A. The superior vesical artery.

Q. In Figure 6-6, identify I.

A. The dorsal artery of the clitoris.

Q. In Figure 6-6, identify J.

A. The perineal artery.

Q. In Figure 6-6, identify K.

A. The vaginal artery. It gives off an inferior vesical artery to the bladder.

Q. In Figure 6-6, identify L.

A. The uterine artery. It increases dramatically in size during pregnancy.

Q. In Figure 6-6, identify M.

A. The internal pudendal artery. It reenters the bony pelvis through the lesser sciatic foramen.

Q. In Figure 6-6, identify N.

A. The middle rectal artery. The inferior rectal artery is a branch of the internal pudendal artery.

Q. In Figure 6-6, identify O.

A. The inferior gluteal artery. It leaves the pelvis through the greater sciatic foramen below the piriformis muscle.

Q. In Figure 6-6, identify P.

A. The lateral sacral arteries. They enter the lateral sacral foramina to supply the sacral nerve roots.

Q. In Figure 6-6, identify Q.

A. The superior gluteal artery. It leaves the pelvis through the greater sciatic foramen above the piriformis muscle.

Q. In Figure 6-6, identify R.

A. The iliolumbar artery.

THE BONES, MUSCLES, VESSELS, AND VISCERA OF THE PELVIS

Q. The bones that constitute the bony pelvis are . . .

A. The right and left innominate bones, the sacrum, and the coccyx.

Q. The three components of the innominate bone (also called the os coxa or the hip bone) are . . .

A. The ilium, the ischium, and the pubis.

Q. The pelvis is divided into a true (lesser) and a false (greater) pelvis at the pelvic brim (inlet). The pelvic brim is formed by . . .

A. The sacral promontory, the alae of the sacrum, the iliopectineal eminences, the superior rami, and the bodies and the symphysis of the pubis.

Q. The major function of the false (greater) pelvis is . . .

A. To provide attachment for the muscles of the abdomen and thigh.

Q. The gender differences that characterize the male false (greater) pelvis are that . . .

A. The bones are heavier, the muscle markings are more pronounced, and the iliac crests are more sinuous and thicker than in the female.

Q. The gender differences that characterize the shape of the pelvic inlet (brim) in the female are that . . .

A. The pelvic inlet in the female approximates a circle to allow the passage of the normal fetal head. In the male, the sacral promontory projects further forward, and the lateral margins are compressed medially, making the pelvic inlet appear heartshaped.

Q. The innominate bones consist of three developmental components. They are . . .

A. The ilium, the ischium, and the pubis.

Q. The only components of the innominate bones that take part in the formation of the greater (true) pelvis are . . .

A. The ilium and the pubis.

Q. The bones that participate in formation of the lesser (true) pelvis are . . .

A. The ilia, the ischia, and the pubes. Together with the sacrum and the coccyx, they comprise all of the bony components of the lesser (true) pelvis.

Q. The gender differences that characterize the shape of the pelvic cavity in the female are that . . .

A. The female pelvic cavity is more nearly circular, as is the female pelvic inlet, than is the case in the male. In the male, the ischial spines project further medially, thus limiting the transverse diameter of the pelvic cavity.

Q. The bones that take part in the formation of the pelvic outlet are . . .

A. The symphysis pubis, the inferior rami of the pubes, the rami of the ischia, the ischial tuberosities, and the tip of the coccyx.

Q. The ligaments that play a significant role in forming the pelvic outlet are . . .

A. The sacrotuberous ligaments.

Q. The bones that form the boundaries of the obturator foramen are . . .

A. The body and both the rami of the pubis and the body and the ramus of the ischium.

Q. The obturator membrane almost completely closes the obturator foramen. However, a small opening remains superiorly, through which pass . . .

A. The obturator nerve and the obturator vessels.

Q. The obturator nerve originates from . . .

A. The ventral divisions of L2, L3, and L4 of the lumbar plexus.

Q. The obturator nerve supplies . . .

A. The adductor muscles of the thigh and the skin over them.

Q. The obturator internus muscle arises from the inner surface of the obturator membrane and the surrounding bones, and hence provides a muscular covering for the lateral wall of the lesser (true) pelvis. Its distal attachment is to . . .

A. The greater trochanter of the femur.

Q. The obturator internus leaves the pelvis through . . .

A. The lesser sciatic foramen. It then turns laterally to reach the greater trochanter of the femur.

Q. The piriformis muscle, arising from the front of the sacrum, forms a muscular covering for the posterior pelvic wall. It exits the pelvis through . . .

A. The greater sciatic foramen.

Q. The piriformis muscle is inserted on . . .

A. The greater trochanter of the femur.

Q. The greater sciatic foramen is separated from the lesser sciatic foramina by . . .

A. The sacrospinous ligament and the spine of the ischium.

Q. The structures that lie on the anterior (pelvic) surface of piriformis are . . .

A. The lateral sacral arteries and, more importantly, the sacral plexus. The latter is occasionally traumatized during a vaginal hysterectomy.

Q. The anterior branches of the sacral plexus are . . .

A. The pelvic spanchnic nerves. They are preganglionic parasympathetic fibers from S2, S3, and S4. They supply the genitourinary system, the colon distal to the splenic flexure, and the rectum.

Q. The majority of the posterior branches of the sacral plexus leave the true pelvis through . . .

A. The greater sciatic foramen. They supply the gluteal region, the back of the thigh, and all of the muscles and most of the skin of the leg and the foot. Those branches that supply the piriformis do not leave the pelvis.

Q. The diaphragm closes the abdominal cavity superiorly. The abdominal cavity is closed inferiorly by . . .

A. The pelvic diaphragm.

Q. The part of the skeletal true pelvis above the pelvic diaphragm is clearly the lowest part of the peritoneal cavity, but it is normally referred to as the "pelvis." The area below the pelvic diaphragm constitutes . . .

A. The perineum.

Q. The muscles that constitute the pelvic diaphragm are . . .

A. The coccygeus, posteriorly, and the two parts of the levator ani, the iliococcygeus and the pubococcygeus, which are situated laterally and anteriorly, respectively.

Q. The levatores ani attach to the pelvic walls from a thickening of fascia covering . . .

A. The obturator internus muscles. This attachment follows a line from the posterior surface of the symphysis pubis to the ischial spine. This is the tendinous arch of the levator ani.

Q. The name *iliococcygeus* is used, even though the iliococcygeus muscle arises, in part, from the ischium, because . . .

A. It was originally a "tail-wagging" muscle that arose from the iliac part of the pelvic brim. However, during evolution, its origin descended down the pelvic wall. The obturator fascia superior to its attachment is somewhat thicker than that inferior to its attachment.

Q. In the female, the pubococcygeus, in addition to extending from the pubis to the coccyx, has two medial parts that encircle the rectum and the vagina. They are . . .

A. The puborectalis muscle and the pubovaginalis muscle, respectively.

Q. The male homologue of the pubovaginalis is . . .

A. The levator prostatae muscle.

Q. The most medial fibers of the pubococcygeus interdigitate with one another anterior to the rectum to join with other small perineal muscles to form . . .

A. The central tendon of the perineum, the perineal body. It is only of significance in the female.

Q. The levator ani has a layer of fascia on both its superior and inferior surfaces. They are . . .

A. The superior and inferior fascia of the pelvic diaphragm, respectively.

Q. The apertures in the pelvic diaphragm are necessary to allow passage of . . .

A. The urethra, the vagina in the female, and the rectum. The nerves and vessels originating in the pelvis and destined for the perineal region all leave the pelvis posterior to the pelvic diaphragm and below the piriformis through the greater sciatic foramen.

Q. The most posterior viscus in the pelvis is the rectum. Its relationship to the peritoneum, which lines the pelvis, is that . . .

A. The upper third of the rectum is covered by peritoneum on its anterior surface and lateral surfaces, the middle third is covered by peritoneum only on its anterior surface, and the lower third of the rectum is retroperitoneal.

Q. The blood supply to the rectum comes mainly from . . .

A. The superior rectal artery. It supplies the whole of the rectum, except for the muscular coat of its lower third, which is supplied by the middle rectal artery. However, the anastomoses between these arteries are sufficiently adequate to allow ligation of the superior rectal artery, such as during excision of a carcinoma, almost as high as its junction with the sigmoid colon without dangerously jeopardizing vascular perfusion of essentially the whole of the rectum.

Q. The lymphatic drainage of the rectum is to . . .

A. The lymph nodes that lie along the superior rectal artery.

Q. The blood supply of the anal canal is from . . .

A. The inferior rectal (inferior hemorrhoidal) artery.

Q. The lymphatic drainage of the anal canal is to . . .

A. The superficial inguinal lymph nodes. Carcinomas, stratified squamous epitheliomata, of the anus spread via the lymphatics to these nodes. Their enlargement may be the first warning sign of malignancy in the anal canal.

Q. The most anterior viscus in the pelvis is the bladder. It is covered by peritoneum only on . . .

A. The posterior surface. Hence, a distended bladder, resulting from obstruction to the urethra, which is almost always confined to the male, can be drained by a needle or catheter inserted suprapubically without entering the peritoneal cavity, thus avoiding the risk of subsequent peritonitis.

Q. Between the bladder and the rectum in the male lies . . .

A. The rectovesical peritoneal pouch. It is commonly filled with coils of small intestine, usually ileum. However, in the elderly, it may also be occupied by an elongated sigmoid colon.

Q. Between the bladder and the rectum in the female lies . . .

A. The uterus. It is covered by peritoneum on both its anterior and posterior surfaces.

Q. The rectum is separated from the uterus by . . .

A. The rectouterine pouch of peritoneum, the pouch of Douglas.

Q. The rectouterine pouch extends inferiorly to . . .

A. The posterior fornix of the vagina. Therefore, when pus has collected in the rectouterine pouch, it is relatively easy to drain it through the posterior fornix of the vagina.

Q. The peritoneal fold covering the uterus is carried to the sidewalls of the pelvic peritoneal cavity by the uterine tubes, which therefore lie in its free edge. These lateral folds of peritoneum are called . . .

A. The broad ligaments of the uterus.

Q. The broad ligaments of the uterus are roughly triangular, with the apex inferiorly and the base at the uterine tubes. However, the apex of the broad ligaments is named the base! Immediately inferior to the base of the broad ligaments are . . .

A. The cardinal (lateral or true) ligaments of the uterus. They are condensations of connective tissue connecting the cervix of the uterus to the ipsilateral lateral pelvic wall.

Q. Immediately inferior to the cardinal ligaments of the uterus are . . .

A. The two lateral fornices of the vagina.

Q. Traversing the cardinal ligaments of the uterus are . . .

A. The uterine arteries. They run from the internal iliac arteries, which lie on the lateral pelvic walls, to the sides of the cervix of the uterus.

Q. Separating the uterine arteries from the lateral fornices of the vagina are . . .

A. The ureters. They run forward to the lateral angles of the trigone of the bladder, passing inferior to the uterine arteries. They traverse the cardinal ligaments of the uterus, forming "The bridge across the river." This is an important relationship, because radiation or surgery of the cervix may damage the ureter(s).

Q. Traversing the upper part of the broad ligaments below the uterine tubes are . . .

A. The round ligaments of the uterus and the ovarian ligaments.

Q. The round ligaments are both attached to the uterus in . . .

A. The angle between the uterus and the uterine tube. They are both remnants of the female gubernacula of prenatal development.

Q. The ovary is attached to the broad ligament by . . .

A. The mesovarium.

Q. The mesovarium is continuous with the broad ligament on . . .

A. The posterior surface of the broad ligament. It lies below the uterine tube, near its pelvic attachment and upper border.

Q. The lymphatic drainage of the ovary is to . . .

A. The paraaortic lymph nodes at the origin of the ovarian artery from the aorta. The lymphatic drainage of the gonads to the paraaortic lymph nodes is more important in cases of testicular malignancy. Ovarian cancers tend to spread directly into the peritoneal cavity; thus lymphatic spread of ovarian cancer is of little significance.

Q. The ovary is usually considered to be intraperitoneal because . . .

A. Its "peritoneal" covering is germinal epithelium. Ova emerge into the peritoneal cavity through it; hence, the early peritoneal "seeding" of ovarian cancers.

Q. The ovarian arteries arise from the front of the aorta at the level of the 2nd lumbar vertebra. They descend to the ovary on the posterior abdominal wall crossing . . .

A. Anteriorly, all abdominal wall, but not gastrointestinal, structures, to reach the lateral end of the broad ligament.

Q. As they run in the broad ligament to the ovaries, the ovarian arteries are surrounded by condensations of connective tissue. These condensations are named . . .

A. The suspensory ligaments of the ovaries.

Q. At the apex of the bladder in the male, below the peritoneal pelvic floor, but superior to the pelvic diaphragm, is . . .

A. The prostate.

Q. The prostate is a fibromuscular gland that is shaped rather like a chestnut. It has a flattened base, situated at the apex of the bladder; a slightly concave posterior surface; and a convex anterior surface. It surrounds the prostatic urethra, which is itself joined on its posterior surface by the two ejaculatory ducts. The anterior surface of the prostate is in contact with . . .

A. The posterior surface of the symphysis and the body and the inferior ramus of the pubis.

Q. The vasa deferentia and the seminal vesicles pierce the base of the prostate. The most medial of these structures are . . .

A. The vasa deferentia. Their distal ends become dilated to form the ampullae, which store spermatozoa.

Q. The seminal vesicles are approximately 5 cm (2 inches) long. Their superior extremities are covered by . . .

A. Peritoneum. They bulge slightly into the pelvic peritoneal cavity, just above the prostate.

Q. The ejaculatory ducts are formed by . . .

A. The union of the ducts of the seminal vesicles with the ductus deferentes (singular, ductus deferens).

Q. The seminal vesicles can be palpated per rectum, but only with . . .

A. A long finger and some pressure. They can then just be felt above the base of the prostate.

Q. The aorta divides into the two common iliac arteries on the left anterolateral surface of the body of . . .

A. The 4th lumbar vertebra.

Q. The common iliac arteries divide into internal and external iliac branches anterior to . . .

A. The sacroiliac joint. The division occurs at the level of the lumbosacral disc, approximately on the interspinous plane.

Q. At the upper border of the piriformis, the internal iliac artery divides into . . .

A. Anterior and posterior divisions.

Q. The branches of the posterior division all pass backward and are somatic in nature. These branches are . . .

A. The iliolumbar artery, which passes upward across the alar of the sacrum, replaces the 5th lumbar artery, and then supplies iliacus; the two or three lateral sacral arteries replace the sacral arteries; and the large superior gluteal artery supplies the upper gluteal region.

Q. The iliolumbar artery and vein running anterior to the alar of the sacrum are closely related to . . .

A. The lumbosacral trunk.

Q. The superior gluteal artery, accompanied by the superior gluteal nerve and vein, leaves the pelvis through . . .

A. The greater sciatic foramen. They run through the foramen above the piriformis muscle.

Q. The anterior division of the internal iliac artery continues on the surface of the obturator fascia in the direction of the ischial spine. Here it divides into its terminal branches. They are . . .

A. The inferior gluteal artery and the internal pudendal artery.

Q. The larger of the inferior gluteal artery and the internal pudendal artery is . . .

A. The inferior gluteal artery. However, it would not be considered by many to be the more important of these two vessels.

Q. The inferior gluteal artery and the internal pudendal artery leave the pelvis by passing through . . .

A. The greater sciatic foramen below the piriformis. Six branches of the sacral plexus accompany them.

Q. In the male, one muscular branch and three visceral branches arise from the anterior aspect of the anterior division of the internal iliac artery. In the female, there is one additional visceral branch. The one muscular branch is . . .

A. The obturator artery. With the obturator vein, it passes through the obturator foramen, in company with the obturator nerve, to supply the obturator externus muscle.

Q. The visceral branches of the anterior division of the internal iliac artery are . . .

A. The superior vesical artery, the remnant of the obliterated umbilical artery, the middle rectal artery, and the inferior vesical artery. The female also has the uterine artery.

Q. The ureter crosses the commencement of the external iliac artery and follows the course of the anterior division of the internal iliac artery toward the ischial spine. The relationship of the ureter to the internal iliac artery is that it. . .

A. Lies anterior to the internal iliac artery.

Q. The branches, except the terminal ones, of the anterior division of the internal iliac artery are crossed by the ureter on their . . .

A. Medial side. The ureter separates the branches of the internal iliac artery from the pelvic peritoneum. The uterine branch of the internal iliac artery, however, passes medially, above the ureter in the base of the broad ligament, to reach the uterus.

Q. The ureter ends at . . .

A. The lateral angle of the trigone of the bladder.

Q. The structures that cross between the ureter and the peritoneum on the wall of the pelvis are . . .

A. The ductus deferens or the round ligament of the uterus. In the abdomen, the gonadal vessels also cross between the ureter and the peritoneum.

Q. The blood supply of the ureters, from top to bottom, is derived from . . .

A. The renal arteries, the aorta, the gonadal arteries, the common iliac arteries, the internal iliac arteries, the uterine arteries in the female, and the vesical arteries. Although the longitudinal anastomoses are normally good, they cannot be completely relied on following a kidney transplant.

Q. The major reason for choosing the iliac fossa as a choice site for a kidney transplant is to maintain . . .

A. The blood supply to the ureter. The transplanted ureter will then be short and thus have an adequate blood supply from the renal arteries.

THE PERINEUM

Q. In Figure 6-7, identify A.

A. The superior ramus of the pubis. It forms part of the pelvic brim.

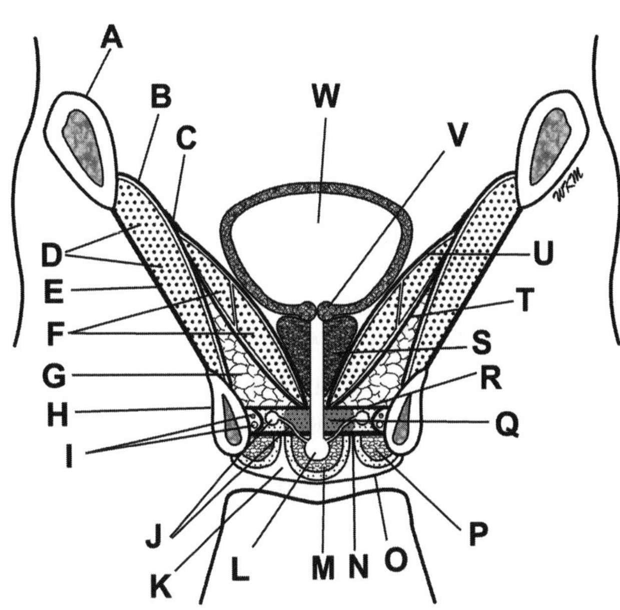

Figure 6-7 Coronal Section of the Male Pelvis and Perineum: Anterior Aspect
Note: All structures are paired, except those situated in the midline.

Q. In Figure 6-7, identify B.

A. The fascia over the obturator internus muscle. It is thickened above the attachment of the levator ani muscle, which was originally attached at the pelvic brim. During evolution, the origin descended to a line extending from the back of the pubis to the ischial spine.

Q. In Figure 6-7, identify C.

A. The tendinous arch of the levator ani muscle. It is the thickening of the obturator fascia from which the levator ani muscle arises. It essentially marks the transition from the wall to the floor of the pelvic cavity.

Q. In Figure 6-7, identify D.

A. The obturator internus muscle. Its tendon leaves the pelvis through the greater sciatic foramen, turns around the ischial spine, and is inserted into the greater trochanter of the femur.

Q. In Figure 6-7, identify E.

A. The obturator membrane. It serves for the attachment of the obturator internus muscle, medially, and of the obturator externus muscle, laterally.

Q. In Figure 6-7, identify F.

A. The levator ani muscle. It is the major component of the pelvic diaphragm. It consists of two originally distinct muscles. The superior, more posterior and lateral muscle is the iliococcygeus muscle. The inferior, more anterior and medial muscle is the pubococcygeus muscle.

Q. In Figure 6-7, identify G.

A. The forward prolongation of the ischioanal (ischiorectal) fossa. The posterosuperior surface of the pubis limits it anteriorly.

Q. In Figure 6-7, identify H.

A. The ischiopubic ramus.

Q. In Figure 6-7, identify I.

A. The anterior extremity of the pudendal canal. It is enclosed in fascia at the lateral margin of the urogenital diaphragm. It contains the dorsal artery and the dorsal nerve of the penis.

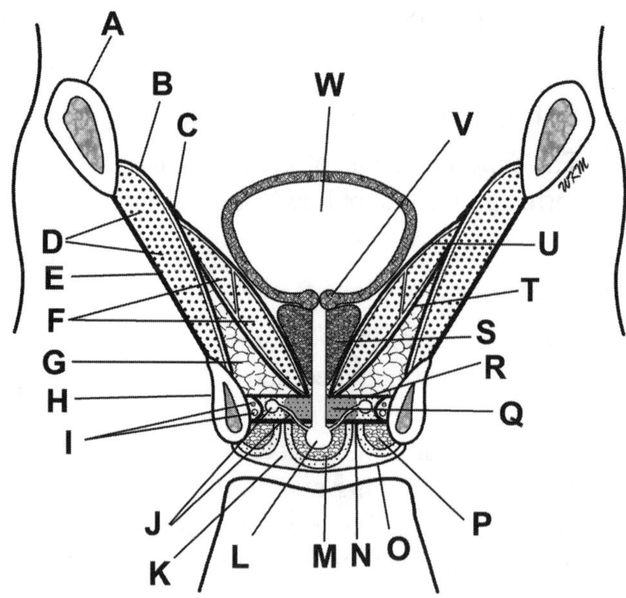

Figure 6-7 Coronal Section of the Male Pelvis and Perineum: Anterior Aspect
Note: All structures are paired, except those situated in the midline.

Q. In Figure 6-7, identify J.

A. A bulbourethral gland and its duct.
Note that the gland lies in the urogenital diaphragm and that its duct pierces the inferior layer of the urogenital diaphragm, the perineal membrane, to open into the bulb of the urethra distal to the external urethral sphincter. Its secretions lubricate the penis prior to intercourse.

Q. In Figure 6-7, identify K.

A. The superficial perineal pouch. Traumatic rupture of the bulbous urethra results in extravasation of urine deep to the membranous layer of the superficial fascia of the urogenital region (Colles' fascia).

Q. In Figure 6-7, identify L.

A. The dilated bulb of the urethra.

Q. In Figure 6-7, identify M.

A. The corpus spongiosum penis. It is covered by the thin bulbospongiosus muscle, which contracts to express the last few drops of urine or semen from the urethra. At the junction of the membranous and bulbous urethrae, the urethra turns sharply forward and becomes somewhat dilated to form the bulb of the penis.

Q. In Figure 6-7, identify N.

A. The thick inferior fascia of the urogenital diaphragm. It is often called the perineal membrane.

Q. In Figure 6-7, identify O.

A. The membranous layer of the urogenital superficial fascia (Colles' fascia). It is continuous with the membranous layer of fascia (Scarpa's fascia) on the anterior abdominal wall.

Q. In Figure 6-7, identify P.

A. The corpus cavernosum penis. It forms one crus of the penis and is covered by the thin ischiocavernosus muscle.

Q. In Figure 6-7, identify Q.

A. The external urethral sphincter. It is situated in the urogenital diaphragm; it relaxes during both micturition and ejaculation.

Q. In Figure 6-7, identify R.

A. The superior fascia of the urogenital diaphragm.

Q. In Figure 6-7, identify S.

A. The prostate. It is situated at the base of the bladder and surrounds the prostatic urethra.

Q. In Figure 6-7, identify T.

A. The inferior fascia of the pelvic diaphragm.

Q. In Figure 6-7, identify U.

A. The superior fascia of the pelvic diaphragm.

Q. In Figure 6-7, identify V.

A. The internal urethral sphincter. It is a functional sphincter. During intercourse, it contracts to prevent retrograde ejaculation of semen into the bladder.

Q. In Figure 6-7, identify W.

A. The urinary bladder.

Q. In Figure 6-8, identify A.

A. The open-ended uterine tube. It lies in the free edge of the broad ligament.

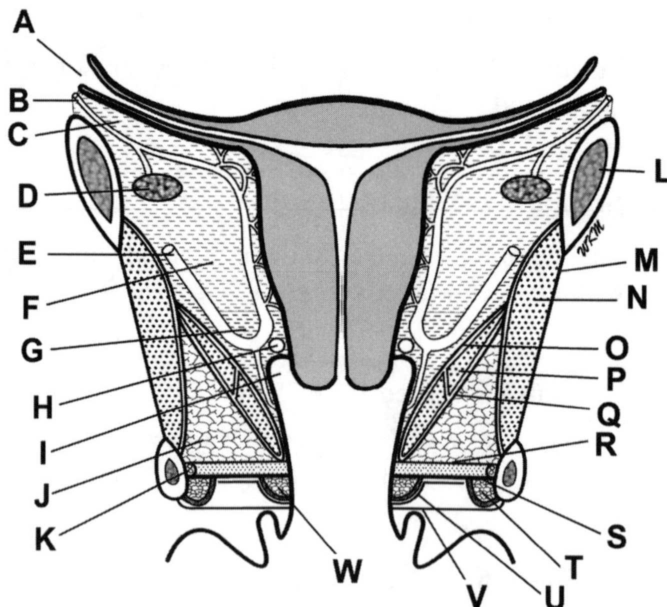

Figure 6-8 Coronal Section of the Female Pelvis and Perineum: Posterior Aspect
Note: All structures are paired, except those situated in the midline.

Q. In Figure 6-8, identify B.

A. The ovarian artery. It anastomoses with the uterine artery.

Q. In Figure 6-8, identify C.

A. The mesosalpinx. It is the part of the broad ligament that is situated just below the uterine tube.

Q. In Figure 6-8, identify D.

A. The ovary. It is suspended from the posterior surface of the broad ligament by the mesovarium and from the brim of the pelvis by the suspensory ligament of the ovary. This ligament is a condensation of the connective tissue surrounding the ovarian artery.

Q. In Figure 6-8, identify E.

A. The uterine artery. It is a branch of the anterior division of the internal iliac artery. As can be seen, it anastomoses freely with the ipsilateral ovarian artery.

Q. In Figure 6-8, identify F.

A. The broad ligament. It is a double fold of peritoneum draped over the uterine tubes. Each broad ligament extends from its own side of the uterus to the ipsilateral pelvic wall. The broad ligaments and the uterus together divide the cavity of the pelvic peritoneum into two peritoneal pouches: the very shallow, anterior, uterovesical pouch and the much deeper, posterior, rectouterine pouch.

Q. In Figure 6-8, identify G.

A. The cardinal (true or lateral) ligament of the uterus. The cardinal ligaments of the uterus are condensations of connective tissue surrounding the uterine arteries at the base of the broad ligaments. The cardinal ligaments are the main supports of the uterus.

Q. In Figure 6-8, identify H.

A. The ureter. It passes across the cardinal ligament forward to the bladder. Note its proximity to the lateral fornix of the vagina and to the uterine artery.

Q. In Figure 6-8, identify I.

A. The lateral fornix of the vagina. The four vaginal fornices—two lateral, one posterior, and one anterior—form a channel of varying depths around the uterine cervix.

Q. In Figure 6-8, identify J.

A. Fat in the forward extension of the ischioanal (ischiorectal) fossa. It fills the interval between the pelvic and the urogenital diaphragms. In the second stage of labor, during the forcible passage of the fetal head through the pelvis, this fat is displaced as the vaginal walls are pressed laterally against the pelvic walls.

Q. In Figure 6-8, identify K.

A. The forward continuation of the pudendal canal. It contains the dorsal artery and the dorsal nerve of the clitoris.

Q. In Figure 6-8, identify L.

A. The superior ramus of the pubis.

Q. In Figure 6-8, identify M.

A. The obturator membrane. It almost completely closes the obturator foramen. Its medial and lateral surfaces give rise to the obturator internus and the obturator externus muscles, respectively.

Q. In Figure 6-8, identify N.

A. The obturator internus muscle.

Q. In Figure 6-8, identify O.

A. The superior fascia of the pelvic diaphragm.

Q. In Figure 6-8, identify P.

A. The pubococcygeal segment of the pubococcygeus muscle. Medial to it, in the same compartment, the combined puborectalis and pubovaginalis muscles can be seen. They are all parts of the levator ani muscles.

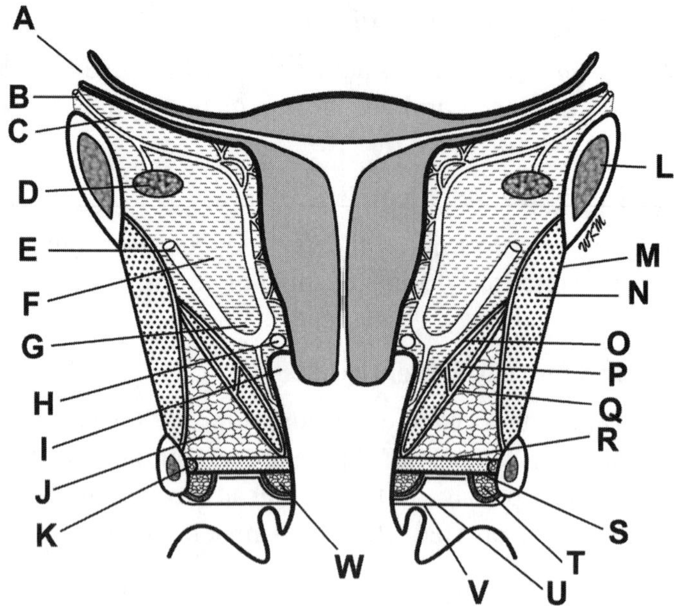

Figure 6-8 Coronal Section of the Female Pelvis and Perineum: Posterior Aspect
Note: All structures are paired, except those situated in the midline.

Q. In Figure 6-8, identify Q.

A. The inferior fascia of the pelvic diaphragm.

Q. In Figure 6-8, identify R.

A. The superior fascia of the urogenital diaphragm.

Q. In Figure 6-8, identify S.

A. The inferior fascia of the urogenital diaphragm. It is also called the perineal membrane.

Q. The space between R and S is . . .

A. The deep perineal pouch. In the female, it contains the sphincter urethra anterior to the vagina and the deep transversus perinei muscles posterior to the vagina. Although both the deep and the superficial perineal pouches are present in the female, they are not as important as their homologues in the male.

Q. In Figure 6-8, identify T.

A. The very small corpus cavernosus of the clitoris. The corpora cavernosa are composed of erectile cavernous tissue and each is surrounded by a thin layer of muscle (the ischiocavernosus muscle).

Q. In Figure 6-8, identify U.

A. The layer of deep fascia covering the bulbs of the vestibule of the vagina.

Q. In Figure 6-8, identify V.

A. The superficial fascia of the perineum.

Q. The space between U and V is . . .

A. The superficial perineal pouch. It contains the greater vestibular glands. These glands are of clinical importance because they may become infected in the presence of gonorrhea or other sexually transmitted diseases. They also are a common site of vulval carcinoma.

Q. In Figure 6-8, identify W.

A. The bulb of the vestibule. It is composed of erectile cavernous tissue and is covered by a thin layer of muscle.

Q. The muscle that covers the bulb of the vestibule is . . .

A. The bulbospongiosus muscle.

Q. The ducts of the greater vestibular glands open into . . .

A. The vestibule of the vagina.

Q. The function of the greater vestibular glands is similar to that of . . .

A. The bulbourethral glands in the male. They provide lubrication during sexual arousal and intercourse.

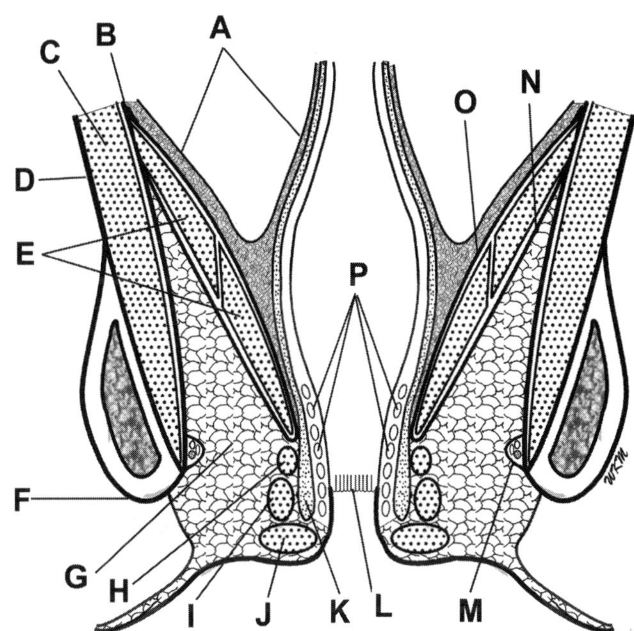

Figure 6-9 Coronal Section of the Pelvis Through the Anus
Note: All structures are paired, except those situated in the midline.

Q. In Figure 6-9, identify A.

A. The pararectal pouch of peritoneum. It extends inferiorly to cover the front and sides of the upper one-third of the rectum.

Q. In Figure 6-9, identify B.

A. The tendinous arch of the levator ani muscle.

Q. In Figure 6-9, identify C.

A. The obturator internus muscle. It is covered by the obturator fascia.

Q. In Figure 6-9, identify D.

A. The obturator membrane.

Q. In Figure 6-9, identify E.

A. The pelvic diaphragm. It is composed of the iliococcygeus muscles, posterosuperiorly, and the pubococcygeus muscles, anteroinferiorly. Together, they constitute the levator ani muscles. The levator ani muscles are covered by the superior and the inferior layers of the fascia of the pelvic diaphragm.

Q. In Figure 6-9, identify F.

A. The ischial tuberosity.

Q. In Figure 6-9, identify G.

A. The ischioanal (ischiorectal) fossa. It is bounded medially by the levator ani muscle and laterally by the fascia over the obturator internus muscle. It contains a variable amount of adipose tissue. An abscess in this fossa, an ischiorectal abscess, can contain a pint or more of pus.

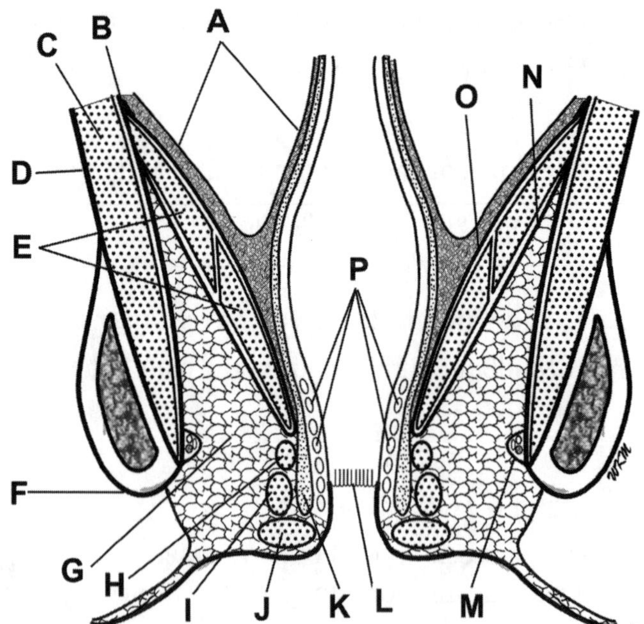

Figure 6-9 Coronal Section of the Pelvis Through the Anus
Note: All structures are paired, except those situated in the midline.

Q. In Figure 6-9, identify H.

A. The deep part of the external anal sphincter. It surrounds the lower end of the internal anal sphincter.

Q. In Figure 6-9, identify I.

A. The superficial part of the external anal sphincter.

Q. In Figure 6-9, identify J.

A. The subcutaneous part of the external ani sphincter.

Q. The external anal sphincter is a voluntary muscle. It is composed of . . .

A. Slow-twitch striated muscle fibers.

Q. The nerve supply of all of parts of the external anal sphincter is . . .

A. The inferior rectal branch of the pudendal nerve.

Q. In Figure 6-9, identify K.

A. The internal anal sphincter.

Q. The internal anal sphincter is an involuntary muscle. It is composed of . . .

A. Smooth, nonstriated, visceral muscle fibers.

Q. The nerve supply of the internal anal sphincter is . . .

A. The sacral parasympathetic nerves (S2, S3, and S4).

Q. In Figure 6-9, identify L.

A. The pectinate line. The anal columns lead down to the anal valves.

Q. Inferiorly, the anal columns are joined by crescentic mucosal folds called . . .

A. The anal valves. These are folds of the mucous membrane at the lower end of the rectal venous plexuses. They are sometimes torn by hard feces, resulting in the painful "fissure in ano." The small pouches above the valves are the anal sinuses.

Q. The sensory nerve that supplies this part of the anal canal is . . .

A. The inferior rectal branch of the pudendal nerve.

Q. In Figure 6-9, identify M.

A. The pudendal canal. It contains the pudendal nerve, the pudendal artery, and the internal pudendal vein.

Q. In Figure 6-9, identify N.

A. The inferior fascia of the pelvic diaphragm.

Q. In Figure 6-9, identify O.

A. The superior fascia of the pelvic diaphragm.

Q. In Figure 6-9, identify P.

A. The rectal venous plexus. It is drained, mainly to the portal system, by the superior rectal veins. It is also drained, via the inferior hemorrhoidal veins, into the internal pudendal veins. This dual drainage forms an important portosystemic venous connection.

Q. Varicosities of the rectal venous plexus result in . . .

A. Hemorrhoids or "piles."

Q. Possible causes of such varicosities are . . .

A. Increased rectal venous pressure or genetic abnormality of the venous walls.

Q. The most common causes of such increased venous pressure are . . .

A. Pregnancy, straining at stool, and, a distant third, portal hypertension due to cirrhosis of the liver. Surprisingly, a pregnant woman will sometimes complain of "painful piles" early in pregnancy even though the uterus has not yet significantly enlarged and pelvic venous compression is not yet evident.

Q. In Figure 6-10, identify A.

A. The lumbosacral intervertebral disc. It is much thicker anteriorly.

Q. In Figure 6-10, identify B.

A. The sacral promontory. It is much more prominent in the male.

Q. In Figure 6-10, identify C.

A. The rectum. It is usually empty, except for gas.

Q. In Figure 6-10, identify D.

A. The thin posterior vaginal fornix. Note its close relationship to the rectouterine peritoneal pouch of Douglas. This close relationship permits drainage of a pelvic abscess through the vagina without risk of contaminating the general peritoneal cavity.

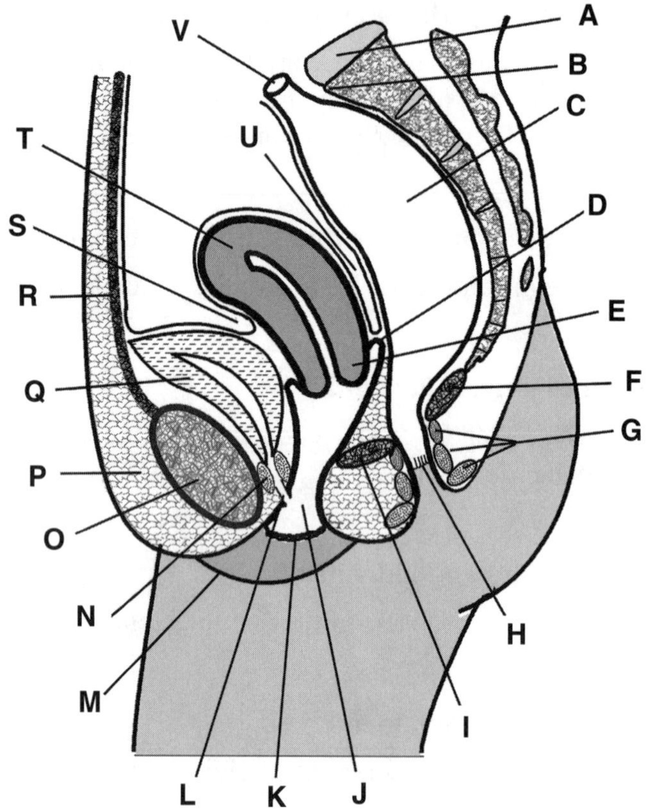

Figure 6-10 Sagittal Section of the Female Pelvis

Q. In Figure 6-10, identify E.

A. The cervix of the uterus. The external os points posteriorly to a varying degree, which varies inversely with the amount of urine in the bladder. During amateur attempts to cause an abortion, a knitting needle or a similar "instrument" is inserted into the vagina. However, it often does not enter the uterus via the cervix, but continues on into the posterior fornix. It is then likely to pierce the dome of the posterior fornix and enter the peritoneal cavity.

Q. In Figure 6-10, identify F.

A. The anococcygeal raphe. The posterior fibers of the pubococcygeus muscles and the anterior fibers of the iliococcygeus muscles contribute to its formation.

Q. In Figure 6-10, identify G.

A. The three parts of the striated external anal sphincter. They are, respectively, the deep, the superficial, and the subcutaneous anal sphincters.

Q. In Figure 6-10, identify H.

A. The anal columns and sinuses. They form the pectinate line, marking the junction of the columnar epithelium of the rectum and the stratified squamous epithelium of the anus.

Q. In Figure 6-10, identify I.

A. The perineal body, the central tendon of the perineum. Many of the muscles of the pelvic and the urogenital diaphragms come together at this point. Its integrity is essential in the female for the maintenance of the pelvic floor.

Q. In Figure 6-10, identify J.

A. The vestibule of the vagina. Note that the urethra opens through its anterior wall. The muscular urcthral sphincter can readily be felt against the pubis during a vaginal examination.

Q. In Figure 6-10, identify K.

A. The labium minus. The two labia minora meet anteriorly around the clitoris.

Q. In Figure 6-10, identify L.

A. The external urethral orifice.

Q. In Figure 6-10, identify M.

A. The labium majus.

Q. In Figure 6-10, identify N.

A. The sphincter urethrae. It lies in the urogenital diaphragm.

Q. In Figure 6-10, identify O.

A. The symphysis pubis.

Q. In Figure 6-10, identify P.

A. The mons veneris. It is a pad of fat overlying the pubis.

Q. In Figure 6-10, identify Q.

A. The wall of the bladder. It is relatively thick when the bladder is contracted and empty.

Q. In Figure 6-10, identify R.

A. The linea alba. It is the white, avascular fibrous interdigitations of the three flat muscles of the abdominal wall.

Q. In Figure 6-10, identify S.

A. The uterovesical peritoneal pouch. Note that it is quite widely separated from the anterior fornix of the vagina. Therefore, it cannot be used as a route for draining an accumulation of pus in the peritoneal cavity.

Q. In Figure 6-10, identify T.

A. The fundus of the uterus. Note that the uterus is normally anteverted and anteflexed.

Q. In Figure 6-10, identify U.

A. The rectouterine pouch of Douglas. Note its close approximation to the posterior vaginal fornix. It is the elective site for surgical peritoneal drainage in the female.

Q. In Figure 6-10, identify V.

A. The site of junction of the sigmoid colon with the dilated rectum.

Q. In Figure 6-11, identify A.

A. The symphysis pubis.

Q. In Figure 6-11, identify B.

A. The ischiopubic ramus.

Q. In Figure 6-11, identify C.

A. The ischial tuberosity. A line drawn between the ischial tuberosities arbitrarily separates the anal triangle and the urogenital triangle.

Q. In Figure 6-11, identify D.

A. The sacrotuberous ligament. The paired sacrotuberous ligaments are superficial to the sacrospinous ligaments. The coccygeus muscles, the anterior muscular part of the fibrous sacrospinous ligaments, form the posterior part of the pelvic diaphragm.

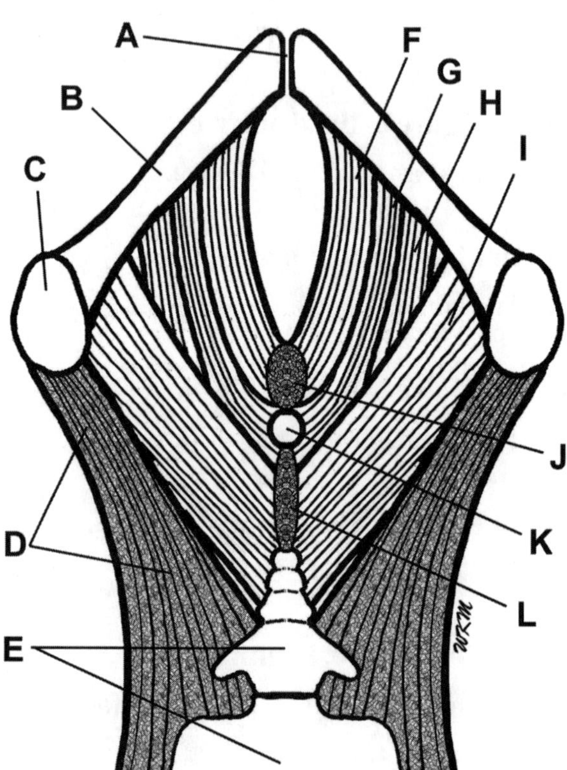

Figure 6-11 The Pelvic Diaphragm: Inferior Aspect

Q. In Figure 6-11, identify E.

A. The coccyx and sacrum.

Q. In Figure 6-11, identify F.

A. The pubovaginalis muscle in the female; the levator prostatae muscle in the male. In both sexes, it is actually the anterior and medial part of the pubococcygeus muscle.

Q. In Figure 6-11, identify G.

A. The puborectalis muscle. It is that part of the pubococcygeus muscle that encloses the rectum.

Q. In Figure 6-11, identify H.

A. The pubococcygeus segment of the pubococcygeus muscle. The entire pubococcygeus muscle is made up of three segments: the pubococcygeus muscle, the puborectalis muscle, and the anterior, pubovaginalis muscle, which in the male is the levator prostatae muscle.

Q. The main function of the pubococcygeus muscle is to . . .

A. Support the pelvic floor. Its effectiveness depends on the integrity of the central tendon of the perineum, more commonly called the perineal body. The pubovaginalis muscle acts as a "sphincter" for the vagina. The puborectalis muscle reduces the work of the anal sphincter by "kinking" the rectum. After severe weight loss, diminution of the ischioanal (ischiorectal) fat may lead to rectal prolapse in either sex.

Q. In Figure 6-11, identify I.

A. The iliococcygeus muscle. It arises from the posterior part of the tendinous arch of the pelvic fascia and from the ischium. It receives its name from its evolutionary origin from the iliac part of the pelvic brim.

Q. In Figure 6-11, identify J.

A. The perineal body. Many of the paired muscles of the pelvic floor come together at this point. They include the levator ani muscles, the superficial and transverse perinei muscles, the bulbospongiosi, and the external anal sphincter. During delivery of the fetal head, injury to the perineal body and its attached muscles can result in prolapse (descent) of the uterus; prolapse of the rectum (rectocele); and prolapse of the bladder (cystocele).

Q. In Figure 6-11, identify K.

A. The anal canal just superior to the anal sphincter.

Q. In Figure 6-11, identify L.

A. The anococcygeal raphe.

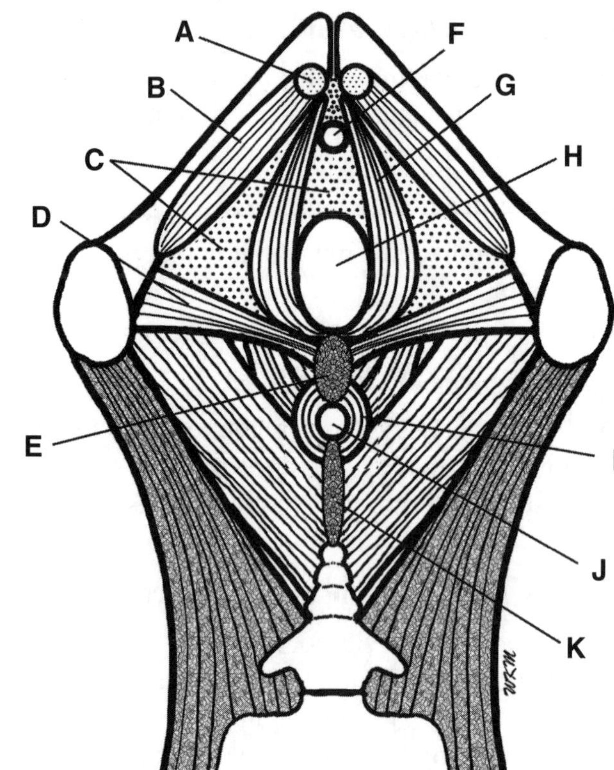

Figure 6-12 The Urogenital Diaphragm in the Female

Q. In Figure 6-12, identify A.

A. The crus of the clitoris. It is sectioned just below the pubis.

Q. In Figure 6-12, identify B.

A. The ischiocavernosus muscle. It is a thin sheet of muscle covering the corpus cavernosus clitoridis, which forms one of the two crura of the clitoris.

Q. In Figure 6-12, identify C.

A. The inferior fascia of the urogenital diaphragm. It is significantly thicker and stronger than the superior fascia of the urogenital diaphragm; thus, it is also called the perineal membrane.

Q. In Figure 6-12, identify D.

A. The superficial transversus perinei muscle. The deep transversus perinei muscle lies immediately superior to the perineal membrane, lying between the two layers of the urogenital diaphragm. The greater vestibular glands, the homologues of the male bulbourethral glands, lie in the superficial perineal pouch inferior to the perineal membrane.

Q. In Figure 6-12, identify E.

A. The central tendon of the perineum, the perineal body. It is often sectioned prior to the final stretching of the perineum by the fetal head during childbirth. This procedure is called an episiotomy.

Q. In Figure 6-12, identify F.

A. The urethra. Its sphincter lies in the substance of the urogenital diaphragm.

Q. In Figure 6-12, identify G.

A. The bulbospongiosus muscle. It is a thin layer of muscle that covers the cavernous corpus spongiosum. The right and left bulbs of the vestibule are formed from the erectile tissue of a corpus spongiosum and its covering of bulbospongiosus muscle.

Q. In Figure 6-12, identify H.

A. The vestibule of the vagina. It is encircled by the bulbospongiosus muscle.

Q. In Figure 6-12, identify I.

A. The superficial part of the sphincter ani externus muscle. The external anal sphincter is described as having deep, superficial, and subcutaneous parts. The deep part surrounds the internal anal sphincter, which is composed of visceral muscle. The superficial and the subcutaneous parts are not clearly separated.

Q. In Figure 6-12, identify J.

A. The anus.

Q. In Figure 6-12, identify K.

A. The anococcygeal raphe. It is formed largely by the iliococcygeus muscles, aided by the pubococcygeus muscles, together with some fibers of the external anal sphincter.

Q. In Figure 6-13, identify A.

A. The corpus cavernosum of the penis.

Q. In Figure 6-13, identify B.

A. The corpus spongiosum of the penis.

Q. In Figure 6-13, identify C.

A. The ischiocavernosus muscle. This is a thin layer of muscle that compresses the crus of the penis.

Q. In Figure 6-13, identify D.

A. The bulbospongiosus muscle. This is a thin muscle that compresses the corpus spongiosum, expressing any fluid remaining in the urethra.

Q. In Figure 6-13, identify E.

A. The median raphe of the two bulbospongiosus muscles.

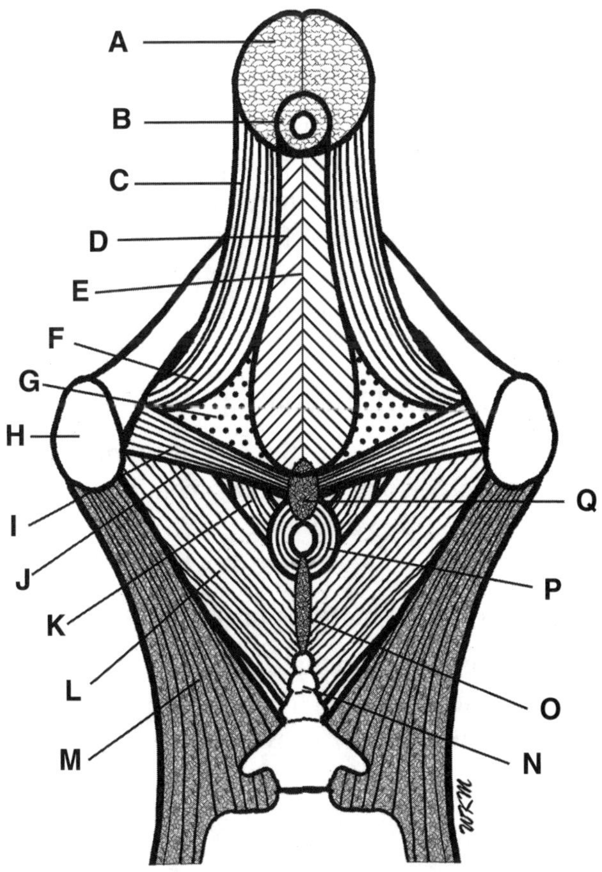

Figure 6-13 The Urogenital Diaphragm in the Male

Q. In Figure 6-13, identify F.

A. The crus of the penis. The two crura (legs), each consisting of a corpus cavernosum covered by a thin ischiocavernosus muscle, are firmly attached to the ischiopubic rami, which are thickened to support the penis.

Q. In Figure 6-13, identify G.

A. The relatively thick perineal membrane. It forms the inferior layer (inferior fascia) of the urogenital diaphragm.

Q. In Figure 6-13, identify H.

A. The ischial tuberosity.

Q. In Figure 6-13, identify I.

A. The superficial transversus perinei muscle. The two deep transversus perinei muscles lie immediately superior to the superficial transversus perinei muscles in the deep perineal pouch between the layers of the urogenital diaphragm.

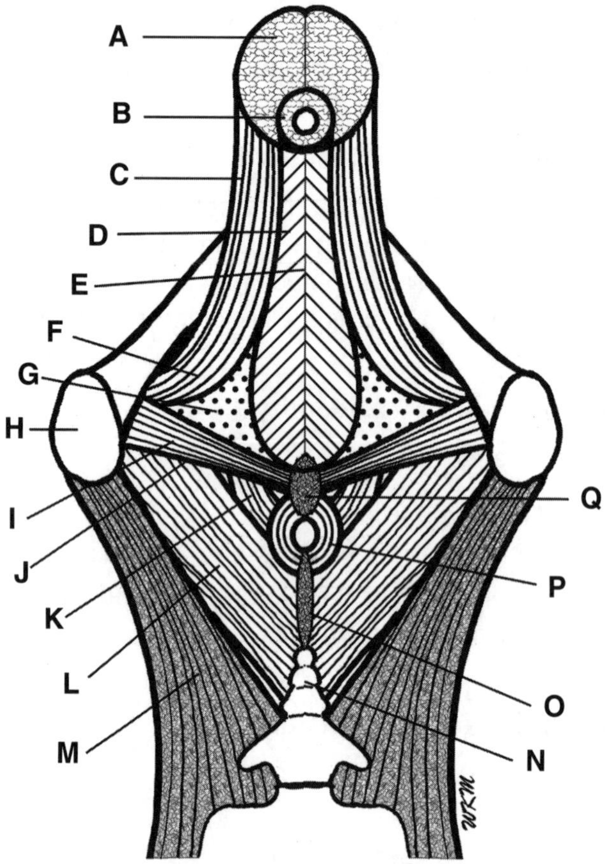

Figure 6-13 The Urogenital Diaphragm in the Male

Q. In Figure 6-13, identify J.

A. The posterior edge of the perineal membrane. The membranous layer of superficial fascia is attached to it. This attachment prevents extravasation of urine from a ruptured urethra from passing posteriorly.

Q. The other structures in the deep perineal pouch are . . .

A. The sphincter urethrae and the bulbourethral glands. The bulbourethral (Cowper's) glands can only be palpated by a finger in the rectum. They lie in the urogenital diaphragm deep to the thick inferior layer of the diaphragm.

Q. In Figure 6-13, identify K.

A. The levator prostatae muscle. In the male, it consists of the most medial and anterior fibers of the pubococcygeus muscle.

Q. In Figure 6-13, identify L.

A. The iliococcygeus muscle. Together with the pubococcygeus muscle, it constitutes the levator ani muscle.

Q. The nerve supply of the levator ani muscle is from . . .

A. The anterior primary rami of the 2nd and 3rd sacral nerves. The iliococcygeus part of the levator ani muscle receives its nerves directly from the sacral plexus. The pubococcygeus is supplied by branches from the pudendal nerve.

Q. In Figure 6-13, identify M.

A. The sacrotuberous ligament.

Q. In Figure 6-13, identify N.

A. The coccyx. It consists of three to five rudimentary vertebrae. Their degree of fusion is variable. However, the first coccygeal vertebra is usually a separate bone.

Q. In Figure 6-13, identify O.

A. The anococcygeal raphe.

Q. In Figure 6-13, identify P.

A. The sphincter ani externus muscle.

Q. In Figure 6-13, identify Q.

A. The perineal body, the central tendon of the perineum. It is of little significance in the male due to the strength of the male urogenital diaphragm.

Q. The pudendal nerve and the internal pudendal artery leave the pelvis through . . .

A. The greater sciatic foramen. They emerge into the gluteal region inferior to the piriformis muscle.

Q. After passing behind the ischial spine, the pudendal nerve and the internal pudendal artery enter the perineum through . . .

A. The lesser sciatic foramen.

Refer to Figure 6-14 for the remaining questions in this section.

Q. The pudendal nerve and the internal pudendal artery give off their first branches, the inferior hemorrhoidal nerves and the inferior hemorrhoidal arteries, in . . .

A. The pudendal canal. The pudendal canal lies in the obturator fascia in the lateral wall of the ischiorectal fossa.

Q. The perineal artery and the perineal nerve both originate . . .

A. Immediately posterior to the urogenital diaphragm.

Q. The differences between the structures supplied by the transverse perineal artery and the muscular branches of the perineal nerve are . . .

A. Insignificant. Both the artery and the nerve supply the muscles of the perineum. However, the nerve to bulbospongiosus gives off a urethral branch, whereas the arteries to the bulbous and the spongy urethra arise in the urogenital diaphragm from the continuation of the internal pudendal artery, the artery to the penis.

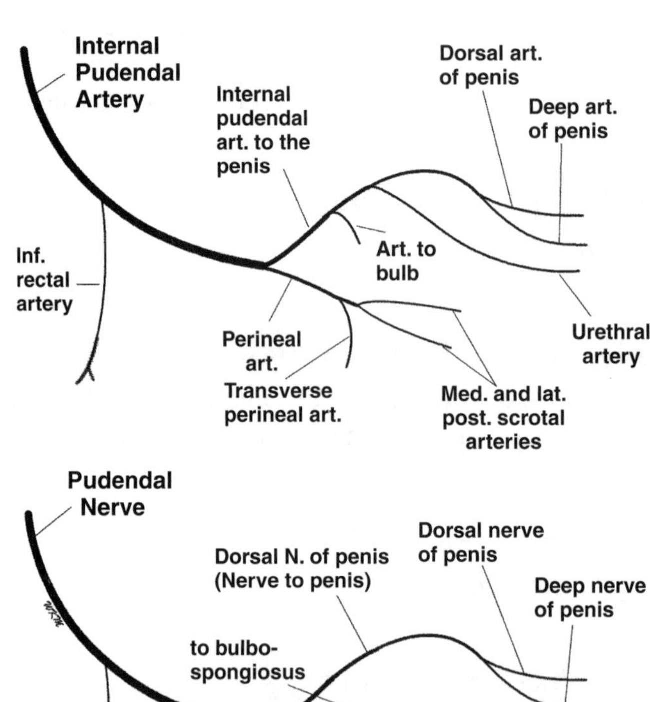

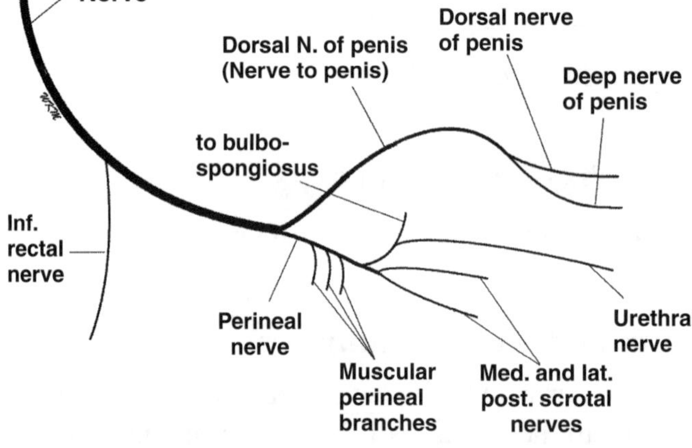

Figure 6-14 A Comparison of the Pudendal Nerve and the Internal Pudendal Artery in the Male

Q. The perineal artery and nerve divide into their terminal branches immediately after giving off the branches to the perineal muscles. These terminal branches are . . .

A. The medial and the lateral posterior scrotal arteries and nerves.

RADIOLOGY OF THE PELVIS

Q. In Figure 6-15, identify A.

A. The transverse processes of the 5th lumbar vertebra.

Q. In Figure 6-15, identify B.

A. The sacroiliac joints. Note that in the female it is smaller, extending only over two and one-half pieces of the sacrum. This allows greater mobility of the sacrum during childbirth.

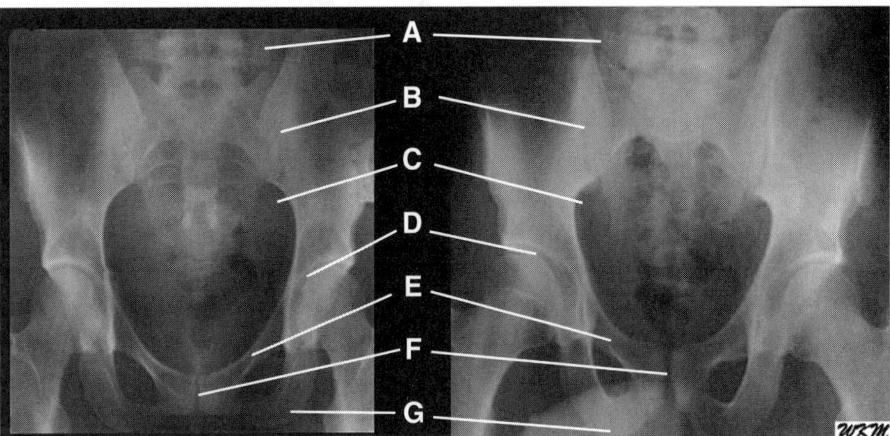

Figure 6-15 A Radiological Comparison of the Female and the Male Pelvis

Q. In Figure 6-15, identify C.

A. The greater sciatic foramina. The curvature of the ilium is less marked in the female, allowing an increase in the transverse diameter of the pelvic cavity.

Q. In Figure 6-15, identify D.

A. The cavity of the hip joints. Note the increased width of the pelvis at this point in the female and the larger and heavier head and neck of the femur in the male. The thinner femoral neck in females may partially account for the increased incidence of fractures of the femoral neck in elderly women.

Q. In Figure 6-15, identify E.

A. The superior rami of the pubis. Again, note the difference in the density and thickness of the male and female pelvises.

Q. In Figure 6-15, identify F.

A. The fibrocartilaginous pubic symphysis. The joint is much smaller and narrower in the female; the pubis is wider than its vertical height. The bones are clearly heavier and stronger in the male. Section of the pubic symphysis has been used, rarely, to increase the pelvic diameter during childbirth. However, this procedure causes a permanently unstable joint, which results in pain when walking over hard surfaces, such as concrete.

Q. In Figure 6-15, identify G.

A. The ischial tuberosities. In this X-ray of the male, the right ischial tuberosity is obscured by the penis. Again, note the thicker and heavier bones in the male and the greater separation of the tuberosities in the female.

Q. In Figure 6-16, identify A.

A. The fetal vertebral column.

Q. In Figure 6-16, identify B.

A. The maternal pelvic brim.

Q. In Figure 6-16, identify C.

A. The fetal occiput.

Q. In Figure 6-16, identify D.

A. The superior ramus of the pubis.

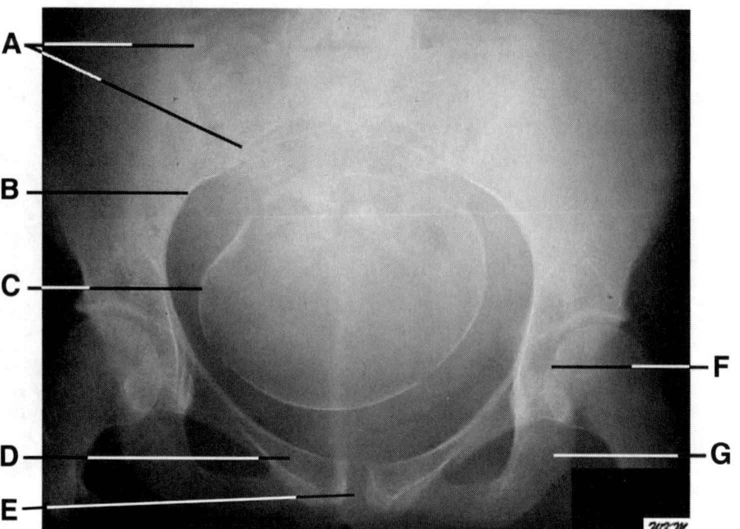

Figure 6-16 Vertex Presentation: Last Trimester
Note: Radiological pelvimetry has fallen into disuse due to the danger of radiation to the fetus. It has been replaced by MRI and ultrasound imaging.

Q. In Figure 6-16, identify E.

A. The symphysis pubis. Note the increased separation of the pubes that occurs in late pregnancy. This separation, following stretching of the pelvic ligaments due to the action of the pregnancy hormone relaxin, may make the pelvis feel unstable to the patient. The hormone disappears postpartum, and the ligaments return to the prepregnant condition.

Q. In Figure 6-16, identify F.

A. The fovea capitis femoris. This is the site of attachment of the ligament of the head of the femur.

Q. In Figure 6-16, identify G.

A. The ischial tuberosity.

Q. In Figure 6-17, identify A.

A. The bladder filled with contrast medium. Note that the full bladder rises significantly above the pubic symphysis.

Q. Immediately above the pubic symphysis, the full bladder is separated from the anterior abdominal wall by . . .

A. Loose connective tissue. The peritoneum is lifted upward by the expanding bladder.

Q. In Figure 6-17, identify B.

A. The neck of the bladder, the site of the functional internal urethral sphincter.

Q. In Figure 6-17, identify C.

A. The ischial tuberosity.

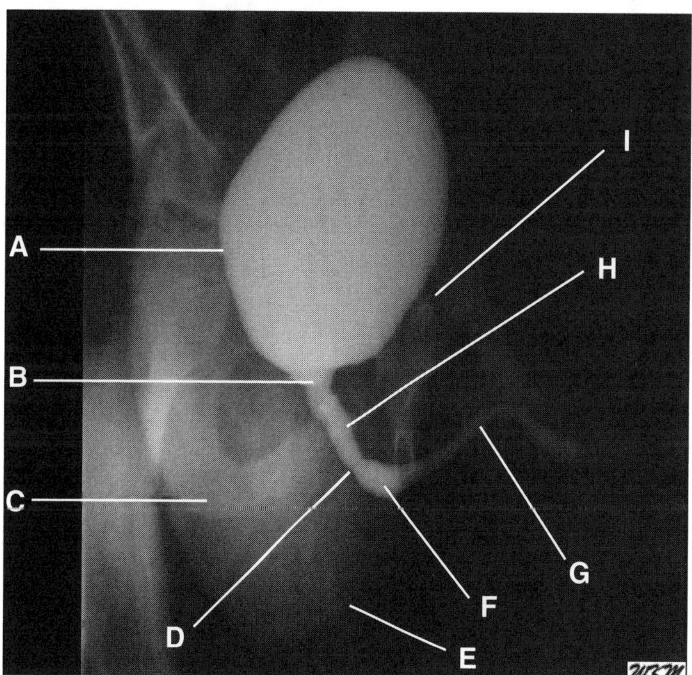

Figure 6-17 A Voiding Urethrogram

Q. In Figure 6-17, identify D.

A. The external urethral sphincter. It is relaxed during micturition.

Q. In Figure 6-17, identify E.

A. The scrotal outline. It obscures the ischial tuberosity.

Q. In Figure 6-17, identify F.

A. The bulb of the penis.

Q. In Figure 6-17, identify G.

A. The penile urethra.

Q. In Figure 6-17, identify H.

A. The prostatic urethra.

Q. In Figure 6-17, identify I.

A. The pubic symphysis.

Q. In Figure 6-18, identify A.

A. The abdominal aorta.

Q. In Figure 6-18, identify B.

A. The 4th lumbar artery.

Q. In Figure 6-18, identify C.

A. The common iliac artery.

Q. In Figure 6-18, identify D.

A. The iliolumbar artery.

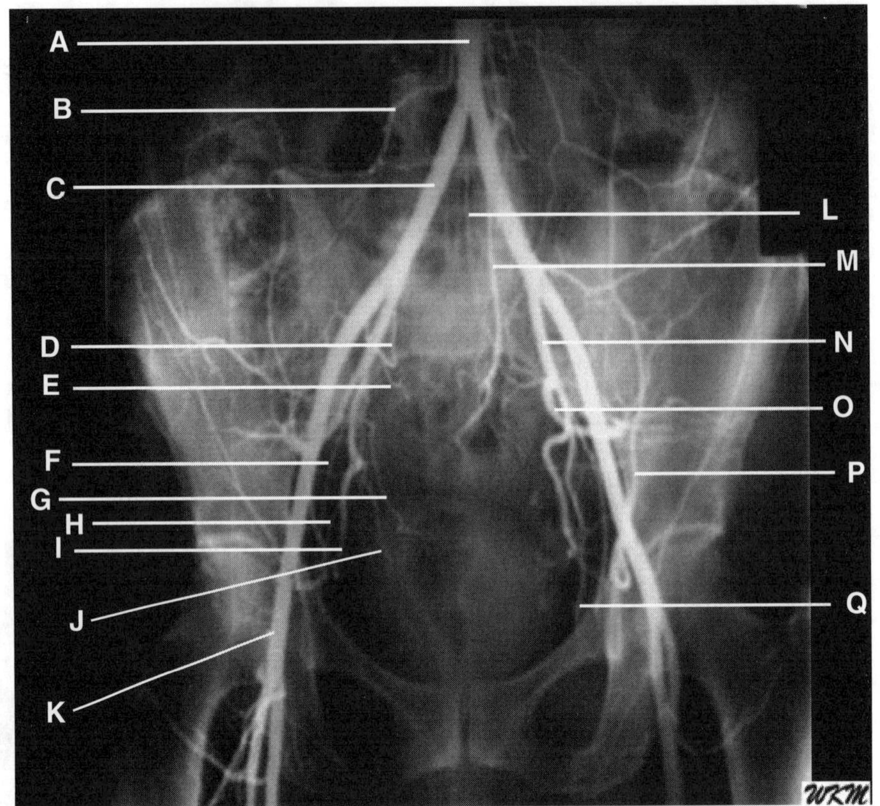

Figure 6-18 Arteriogram of the Iliac System of Arteries

Q. In Figure 6-18, identify E.

A. A lateral sacral artery.

Q. In Figure 6-18, identify F.

A. The obturator artery.

Q. In Figure 6-18, identify G.

A. The middle rectal artery. It supplies the lower third of the rectum, which in this case is filled with gas.

Q. In Figure 6-18, identify H.

A. The internal pudendal artery.

Q. In Figure 6-18, identify I.

A. The inferior gluteal artery. It is the terminal branch of the anterior division of the internal iliac artery.

Q. In Figure 6-18, identify J.

A. The inferior vesical artery.

Q. In Figure 6-18, identify K.

A. The femoral artery.

Q. In Figure 6-18, identify L.

A. The median sacral artery.

Q. In Figure 6-18, identify M.

A. The superior rectal artery.

Q. In Figure 6-18, identify N.

A. The internal iliac artery.

Q. In Figure 6-18, identify O.

A. The superior gluteal artery.

Q. In Figure 6-18, identify P.

A. The inferior epigastric artery.

Q. In Figure 6-18, identify Q.

A. The superior vesical artery.

Q. In Figure 6-19, identify A.

A. The ampulla of the uterine tube.

Q. In Figure 6-19, identify B.

A. The uterine tube. Its lumen is quite small, and it contains very little contrast medium. It cannot be visualized easily.

Q. In Figure 6-19, identify C.

A. The canula in the vagina.

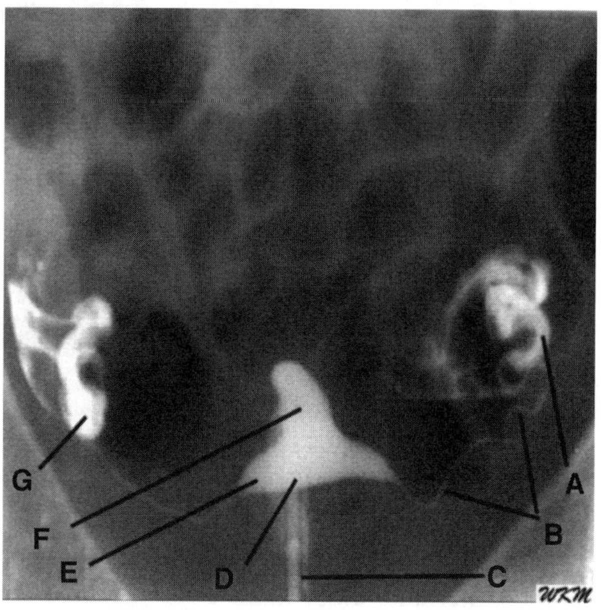

Figure 6-19 A Uterosalpingogram

Q. In Figure 6-19, identify D.

A. The fundus of the uterus. The extreme anteversion of the uterus shows that the bladder is empty. The bladder is always emptied prior to an uterosalpingogram.

Q. In Figure 6-19, identify E.

A. The cornu of the uterus.

Q. In Figure 6-19, identify F.

A. The body of the uterus.

Q. In Figure 6-19, identify G.

A. Contrast medium spilled into the peritoneal cavity through the normal open-ended uterine tube.

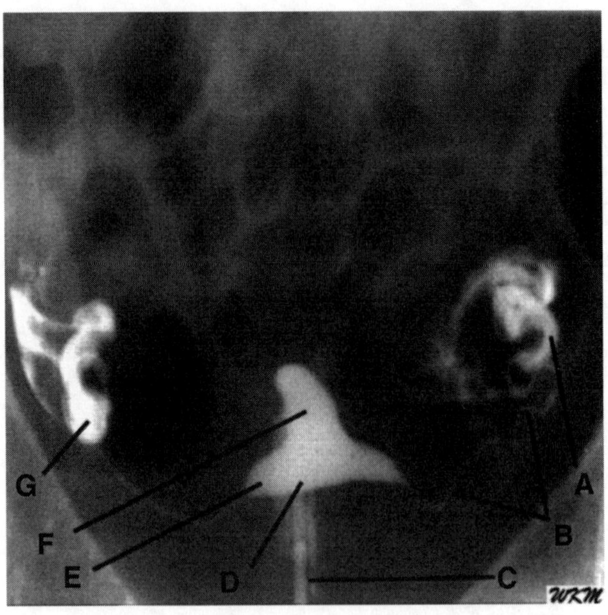

Figure 6-19 A Uterosalpingogram

Q. In Figure 6-20, identify A.

A. The third piece of the sacrum.

Q. In Figure 6-20, identify B.

A. The right sacroiliac joint.

Q. In Figure 6-20, identify C.

A. The ilium.

Q. In Figure 6-20, identify D.

A. The psoas major muscle.

Q. In Figure 6-20, identify E.

A. The iliacus muscle.

Q. In Figure 6-20, identify F.

A. The internal oblique muscle.

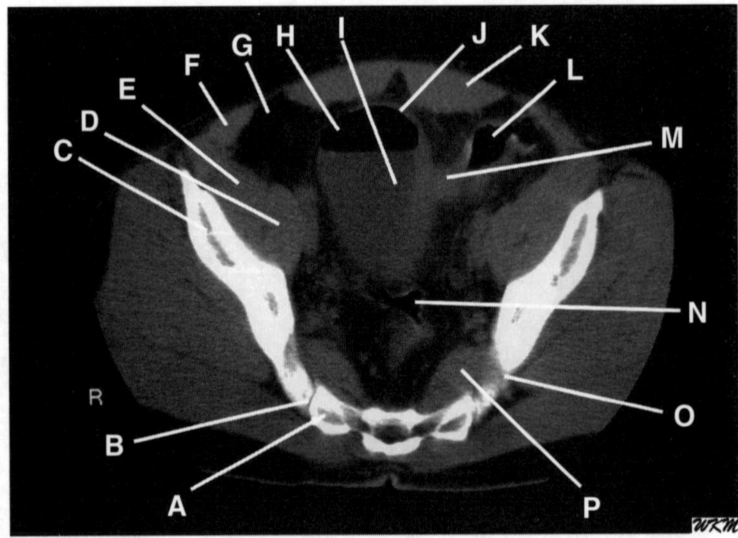

Figure 6-20 CT Scan of Pelvis at S3 Showing a Colovesical Fistula

Q. In Figure 6-20, identify G.

A. Gas in the cecum.

Q. In Figure 6-20, identify H.

A. Gas in the bladder.

Q. In Figure 6-20, identify I.

A. Urine in the bladder.

Q. In Figure 6-20, identify J.

A. The bladder wall.

Q. In Figure 6-20, identify K.

A. The rectus abdominis muscle.

Q. In Figure 6-20, identify L.

A. Gas in the sigmoid colon.

Q. In Figure 6-20, identify M.

A. Inflammatory tissue surrounding the fistula between the sigmoid colon and the bladder. An inflamed diverticulum of the sigmoid colon was the cause of the pathology.

Q. In Figure 6-20, identify N.

A. Gas in the rectum.

Q. In Figure 6-20, identify O.

A. The greater sciatic foramen.

Q. In Figure 6-20, identify P.

A. The piriformis muscle.

Chapter 7

The Lower Limb

AN OVERVIEW OF THE NERVE SUPPLY OF THE LOWER LIMB

Q. The lower extremity can be divided into three areas. They are . . .

A. The thigh, the leg, and the foot.

Q. The nerve supply of the lower extremity is from the anterior primary rami of the L2 through S2 spinal nerves. They are distributed by . . .

A. The lumbar and sacral plexuses.

Q. The two major branches of the lumbar plexus to the lower extremity are . . .

A. The femoral nerve and the obturator nerve.

Q. The femoral nerve supplies . . .

A. The muscles and skin of the front of the thigh and the skin of the medial side of the leg and foot.

Q. The obturator nerve supplies . . .

A. The skin and the muscles of the medial side of the thigh.

Q. The major branches of the sacral plexus to the lower extremity are . . .

A. The superior gluteal nerve, the inferior gluteal nerve, the posterior femoral cutaneous nerve, and the sciatic nerve.

Q. The superior gluteal nerve and the inferior gluteal nerve supply . . .

A. The muscles of the gluteal region. They have no cutaneous sensory branches.

Q. The posterior femoral cutaneous nerve supplies . . .

A. The skin of the back of the thigh.

Q. The sciatic nerve divides into tibial and common fibular branches. They supply . . .

A. The muscles of the back of the thigh, all of the muscles of the leg and foot, and most of the skin of the leg and foot. Note that the skin on the medial side of the leg and foot is supplied by the saphenous branch of the femoral nerve.

Q. The tibial nerve supplies . . .

A. The skin and muscles of the back of the leg and the sole of the foot.

Q. The common fibular (common peroneal) nerve supplies . . .

A. The skin and muscles of the front and lateral side of the leg and of the dorsum of the foot.

THE LUMBAR PLEXUS

Q. The lumbar plexus is formed from . . .

A. The anterior primary rami of the first four lumbar nerves and a contribution from the 12th thoracic anterior primary ramus.

Q. In Figure 7-1, identify A.

A. The subcostal nerve. The remainder of the anterior primary ramus of the 12th thoracic nerve joins the lumbar plexus.

Q. In Figure 7-1, identify B.

A. The iliohypogastric nerve. It supplies an iliac branch and then continues to the hypogastrium.

Q. In Figure 7-1, identify C.

A. The ilioinguinal nerve. It supplies branches to the iliac region. It continues through the superficial inguinal ring to supply the inguinal region.

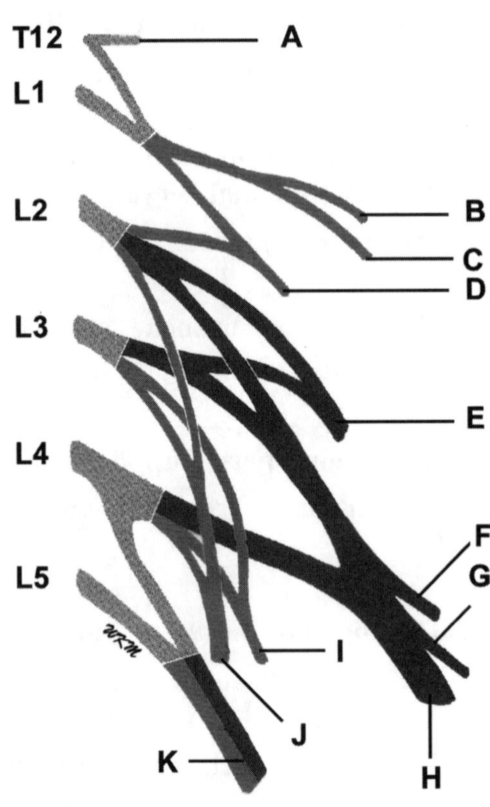

Figure 7-1 The Lumbar Plexus

Q. In Figure 7-1, identify D.

A. The genitofemoral nerve. It arises from the anterior divisions of L1 and L2. It emerges through the substance of the psoas major muscle to divide into a lateral genital and a medial femoral branch. The lateral genital branch passes through the deep inguinal ring. In the male, the lateral genital branch supplies the cremaster muscle and the skin of the scrotum. In the female, the lateral genital branch supplies the skin of the labia. In both sexes, the medial femoral branch runs with the femoral artery to supply the skin of the femoral triangle.

Q. In Figure 7-1, identify E.

A. The lateral femoral cutaneous nerve. It arises from the posterior divisions of the anterior primary rami of L2 and L3 and emerges from the lateral border of the psoas major muscle.

Q. The lateral femoral cutaneous nerve reaches the thigh by passing deep to . . .

A. The lateral end of the inguinal ligament. Here it sometimes becomes entrapped by tight jeans, causing paresthesia over the trouser-pocket region (Meralgia paresthetica).

Q. In Figure 7-1, identify F.

A. A branch, from L2 and L3, to the iliacus muscle.

Q. In Figure 7-1, identify G.

A. A branch, from L2 and L3, to the psoas major muscle.

Q. In Figure 7-1, identify H.

A. The femoral nerve. It arises from the posterior divisions of the anterior primary rami of L2, L3, and L4. It emerges from beneath the lateral border of the psoas major muscle onto the anterior surface of the iliacus muscle, just superior to the inguinal ligament. It then enters the thigh by passing deep to the inguinal ligament on the lateral side of the femoral artery.

Q. In Figure 7-1, identify I.

A. The accessory obturator nerve. When present, it arises from the ventral divisions of the anterior primary rami of L3 and L4. It then emerges from the medial border of the psoas major muscle and crosses the superior ramus of the pubis to reach the pectineus muscle.

Q. In Figure 7-1, identify J.

A. The obturator nerve. It arises from the ventral divisions of the anterior primary rami of L2, L3, and L4. It then emerges from the medial border of the psoas major muscle, crosses the pelvic brim, and then enters the adductor region via the obturator foramen. It supplies the adductor muscles of the thigh and the skin over them.

Q. In Figure 7-1, identify K.

A. The lumbosacral trunk. It arises from the ventral divisions of the anterior primary rami of L4 and L5. It crosses the ala of the sacrum, deep to the obturator nerve, to join with the anterior primary ramus of S1 to contribute to the sacral plexus.

Q. As the lumbosacral trunk crosses the ala of the sacrum, it is accompanied by . . .

A. The obturator nerve and the iliolumbar vessels.

THE ANTERIOR AND MEDIAL SIDES OF THE THIGH

Q. In Figure 7-2, identify A.

A. The iliac fossa, the origin of the iliacus muscle.

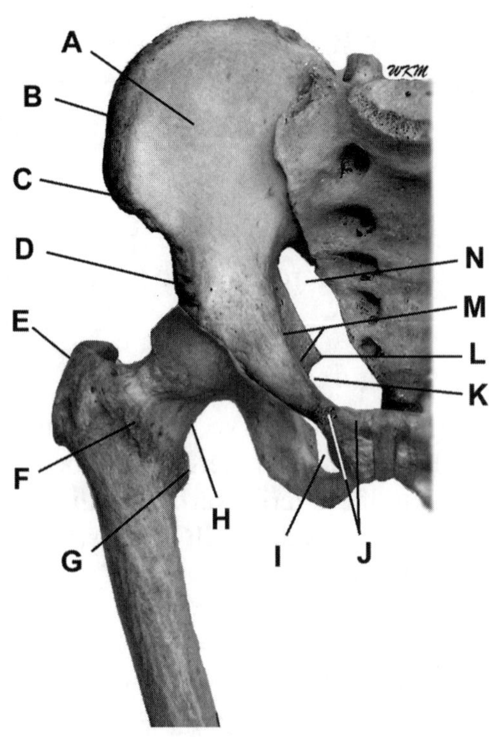

Figure 7-2 Skeleton of the Hip, Anterior Aspect

Q. In Figure 7-2, identify B.

A. The crest of the ilium. It provides attachment to the obliquus externus abdominis muscle, the obliquus internus abdominis muscle, the transversus abdominis muscle, and the tensor fasciae latae muscle.

Q. In Figure 7-2, identify C.

A. The anterior superior iliac spine. It gives origin to the sartorius muscle.

Q. In Figure 7-2, identify D.

A. The anterior inferior iliac spine. It gives origin to the straight head of the rectus femoris muscle.

Q. In Figure 7-2, identify E.

A. The greater trochanter of the femur. The gluteus medius and the gluteus minimus muscles are inserted into its lateral surface.

Q. The trochanteric fossa lies on the medial side of the greater trochanter. Into it is inserted the tendon of . . .

A. The obturator externus muscle.

Q. In Figure 7-2, identify F.

A. The intertrochanteric line of the femur.

Q. The intertrochanteric line marks the superior ends of the linear origins of . . .

A. The vastus medialis and the vastus lateralis muscles. Their linear attachments continue around the femur to the appropriate margin of the linear aspera.

Q. In Figure 7-2, identify G.

A. The lesser trochanter of the femur. It is the insertion of the iliopsoas tendon.

Q. In Figure 7-2, identify H.

A. The neck of the femur.

Q. In Figure 7-2, identify I.

A. The obturator foramen.

Q. In Figure 7-2, identify J.

A. The pubic crest and the pubic tubercle at its lateral extremity.

Q. In Figure 7-2, identify K.

A. The impression for the tendon of the obturator internus muscle.

Q. In Figure 7-2, identify L.

A. The ischial spine. The sacrospinous ligament is attached to it, forming the ligamentous boundary of the lesser sciatic foramen.

Q. In Figure 7-2, identify M.

A. The pectineal line of the superior ramus of the pubis.

Q. In Figure 7-2, identify N.

A. The greater sciatic notch. It is converted into the greater sciatic foramen by the sacrotuberous ligament.

Q. The front of the thigh consists of a medial, femoral region (the femoral triangle) and a lateral, quadriceps region. They are separated by . . .

A. The sartorius muscle.

Q. Both the skin and muscles of the quadriceps region are supplied by branches of . . .

A. The femoral nerve. The femoral nerve also supplies the sartorius muscle and gives off the saphenous nerve to the skin of the medial side of the leg and the foot.

Q. The attachments of the sartorius muscle are to . . .

A. The anterior superior iliac spine, proximally, and to a linear area on the medial surface of the medial condyle of the tibia, distally, anterior to the insertions of the gracilis muscle and of the semitendinosus muscle. Together, the insertions of the sartorius muscle, the gracilis muscle, and the semitendinosus muscle are often called the pes anserinus, "the foot of the duck."

Q. In Figure 7-3, identify A.

A. The inguinal ligament, the thickened, curled margin of the external oblique aponeurosis. It extends from the anterior superior iliac spine to the pubic tubercle.

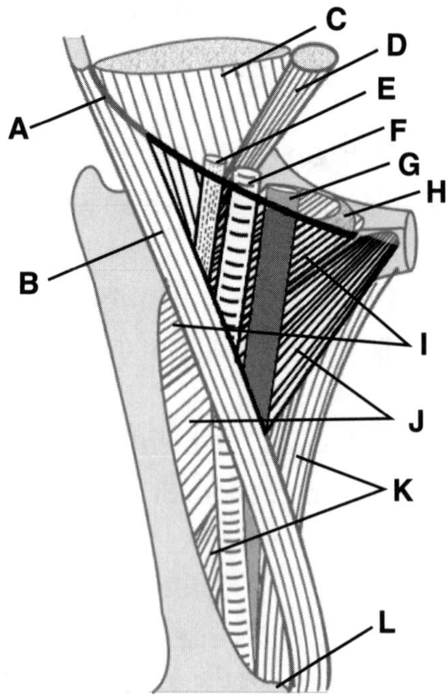

Figure 7-3 The Femoral Triangle

Q. In Figure 7-3, identify B.

A. The sartorius muscle. It arises from the anterior superior iliac spine. Its medial border forms the lateral border of the femoral triangle.

Q. In Figure 7-3, identify C.

A. The iliacus muscle. The iliacus muscle arises from the iliac fossa and is inserted into the tendon of the psoas major muscle.

Q. In Figure 7-3, identify D.

A. The psoas major muscle. The psoas major muscle is inserted into the lesser trochanter of the femur. Together with the iliacus muscle, it forms the lateral part of the floor of the femoral triangle.

Q. In Figure 7-3, identify E.

A. The femoral nerve.

Q. The posterior division of the femoral nerve supplies the quadriceps femoris muscle and continues as the saphenous nerve, passing through the adductor canal. The anterior division of the femoral nerve supplies . . .

A. The sartorius muscle and the skin of the front and medial sides of the thigh. It does so through its intermediate femoral cutaneous and medial femoral cutaneous branches.

Q. In Figure 7-3, identify F.

A. The femoral artery. It separates the femoral vein from the femoral nerve.

Q. The branches of the femoral artery in the femoral triangle are . . .

A. Three small superficial branches and two deep branches. The small superficial branches are the superficial circumflex iliac artery, the superficial inferior epigastric artery, and the superficial external pudendal artery. The two deep branches are the small deep external pudendal artery and the large deep artery of the thigh, the profunda femora artery.

Q. In Figure 7-3, identify G.

A. The femoral vein.

Q. In Figure 7-3, identify H.

A. The lacunar part of the inguinal ligament. The femoral ring is the space between the sharp lateral margin of the firm lacunar ligament and the femoral vein. It is the site of femoral herniae. Due to the shape of the female pelvis, and the smaller size of the pectineus muscles and the iliopsoas muscles, femoral herniae are more common in the female.

Q. In Figure 7-3, identify I.

A. The pectineus muscle. The pectineus muscle forms the intermediate area in the floor of the femoral triangle.

Q. The proximal attachment (origin) of the pectineus muscle is to . . .

A. The superior ramus of the pubis anterior to the pectinate line.

Q. The distal attachment (insertion) of the pectineus muscle is to . . .

A. The posterior surface of the femur lateral to the lesser trochanter.

Q. The action of the pectineus muscle is to . . .

A. Assist iliopsoas in flexing the hip joint. It is also an adductor of this joint.

Q. In Figure 7-3, identify J.

A. The adductor longus muscle. Its medial border forms the medial boundary of the femoral triangle.

Q. In Figure 7-3, identify K.

A. The "hamstring" portion of the adductor magnus muscle and the "adductor" part of the adductor magnus muscle. The hamstring part of the adductor magnus muscle is supplied by the popliteal branch of the sciatic nerve. It is inserted into the adductor tubercle on the medial condyle of the femur.

Q. In Figure 7-3, identify L.

A. The adductor tubercle of the femur. The hamstring portion of the adductor magnus muscle is inserted into it.

Q. The origin of the adductor longus muscle is from . . .

A. The body of the pubis, in the angle between the symphysis pubis and the pubic tubercle. The tendon of the adductor longus muscle is a useful guide to locate the pubic tubercle during an examination for a possible inguinal or femoral hernia.

Q. The adductor longus muscle is inserted into . . .

A. The linea aspera on the back of the femur. It lies between the origin of the vastus medialis muscle and the insertion of the adductor brevis muscle.

Q. The individual muscle fibers of the sartorius muscle are the longest in the body. Three reasons for this are that . . .

A. (1) The muscle itself is long. (2) Its muscle fibers are continuous from its origin to its insertion without a significant tendon. (3) It crosses two mobile joints, the hip joint and the knee joint.

Q. The actions of the sartorius muscle are to . . .

A. Flex both the hip joint and the knee joint. It also assists in lateral rotation of the thigh. These actions together result in the traditional sewing position used by tailors. Hence, the muscle's name, which translates to "the tailor's muscle."

Q. The sartorius muscle is supplied by . . .

A. The lateral branch of the intermediate femoral cutaneous nerve.

Q. As its name implies, the quadriceps femoris muscle has four heads. The head of the muscle that acts on two joints is . . .

A. The rectus femoris muscle.

Q. The straight head of the rectus femoris muscle arises from . . .

A. The anterior inferior iliac spine.

Q. The oblique head of the rectus femoris muscle arises from . . .

A. The ilium, superior to the acetabulum. It is in line with the remainder of the quadriceps femoris muscle when the hip is flexed.

Q. The three other heads of the quadriceps femoris muscle are the vasti muscles. The vastus medialis muscle and the vastus lateralis muscle arise from the appropriate margins of the linear aspera on the posterior aspect of the femur. Their linear origins wind around the upper part of the shaft of the femur below their respective trochanters to almost meet anteriorly. The origin of the vastus intermedius muscle is from . . .

A. The greater part of the anterior and the lateral surfaces of the shaft of the femur.

Q. The medial surface of the shaft of the femur is . . .

A. Devoid of muscle attachments. It would seem to be an ideal situation for plating in the treatment of a fractured femur. However, the proximity of the femoral artery is a problem.

Q. All four heads of the quadriceps femoris muscle blend into an aponeurosis, which is inserted into the base of the patella. The patella is attached to the tubercle of the tibia by the ligamentum patellae. The head of the quadriceps muscle that has its lower fibers running almost horizontally is . . .

A. The vastus medialis muscle. This part of the muscle is sometimes called the vastus medialis obliquus muscle.

Q. The significance of the vastus medialis obliquus muscle is that . . .

A. It prevents lateral dislocation of the patella. This dislocation occurs more frequently in women, due to their relatively wider hips and relatively shorter femora. This results in greater angulation at the knee, and thus a greater tendency to lateral patellar dislocation. Treatment consists of strengthening the vastus medialis muscle by appropriate exercises or of partial severance of the lower fibers of the vastus lateralis muscle.

Q. All the bellies of the quadriceps femoris muscle become aponeurotic toward their inferior attachment. The aponeurosis that forms on the anterior surface of its muscle belly is that of . . .

A. The vastus intermedius muscle. The aponeurosis on the posterior surface of the rectus femoris muscle fuses with the aponeurosis on the anterior surface of the vastus intermedius muscle.

Q. The nerve supply of the quadriceps femoris muscle is . . .

A. The posterior (deep) division of the femoral nerve. This division of the femoral nerve also gives off the saphenous nerve, which follows the long saphenous vein to the medial side of the foot.

Q. The segmental innervation of the quadriceps femoris muscle is . . .

A. L2, L3, and L4. A patient with spina bifida involving the spinal cord at L4 or below can still walk, albeit with much effort and great difficulty, using the iliofemoral ligaments, the quadriceps muscles, and the iliopsoas muscles. The center of gravity is kept posterior to the hip joint by leaning backward. Overextension of the hip is prevented by the taut iliofemoral ligaments.

Q. Extension of the knee joint is accomplished by the action of . . .

A. The quadriceps femoris muscle. It is the only extensor muscle of the knee. Recovery from injuries of the knee joint depends primarily on the maintenance of the strength of the quadriceps femoris muscle.

Q. The quadriceps femoris muscle also contributes to . . .

A. Flexion of the hip. This is due to the action of the rectus femoris muscle. The main flexor of the hip is, of course, the iliopsoas muscle.

Q. The femoral triangle lies medial to the sartorius on the front of the thigh. Its apex is directed inferiorly. The boundaries of the femoral triangle are . . .

A. The inguinal ligament, superiorly; the medial border of the sartorius muscle, laterally; and the medial border of the adductor longus muscle, medially.

Q. The muscles that form the floor of the femoral triangle are . . .

A. The iliopsoas muscle, laterally; the pectineus muscle and the anterior surface of adductor longus muscle, medially.

Q. The superior attachment (origin) of the iliacus part of the iliopsoas muscle is from . . .

A. The iliac fossa. The psoas major segment of the iliopsoas muscle arises from the sides and transverse processes of the lumbar vertebra.

Q. The inferior attachment (insertion) of the iliopsoas muscle is to . . .

A. The lesser trochanter of the femur.

Q. The major flexor of the thigh is . . .

A. The iliopsoas muscle. It also acts as a medial or lateral rotator of the thigh, depending on the degree of flexion of the hip.

Q. Following a nonimpacted fracture of the neck of the femur, the position of the limb is . . .

A. Laterally rotated and extended.

Q. The cause of the lateral rotation and extension of the leg following a nonimpacted fracture of the neck of the femur is that . . .

A. The fracture of the femoral neck results in a shift of the axis of rotation from a longitudinal axis through the femoral head medial to the lesser trochanter to a more lateral longitudinal axis along the shaft of the femur. This transfers the line of pull of the psoas major muscle from the lateral to the medial side of the axis of rotation. The psoas major muscle now becomes a powerful lateral rotator, rather than a weak medial rotator, of the shaft of the femur. The loss of integrity of the femoral neck clearly prevents the psoas major muscle from flexing the thigh.

Q. In its actions on the hip joint, the psoas major muscle receives considerable assistance from . . .

A. The iliacus muscle. It is inserted into the side of the tendon of the psoas major muscle.

Q. The adductor part of the adductor magnus muscle is inserted into . . .

A. The linea aspera on the posterior surface of the femur.

Q. The adductor part of the adductor magnus muscle is supplied by . . .

A. The obturator nerve.

Q. The adductor hiatus lies between . . .

A. The adductor and hamstring parts of the adductor magnus muscle.

Q. The structures that run through the adductor hiatus are . . .

A. The femoral artery and the femoral vein.

Q. When the femoral artery and the femoral vein reach the popliteal fossa on the posterior side of the adductor hiatus, they are renamed . . .

A. The popliteal artery and the popliteal vein.

Q. The medial border of the adductor longus muscle conveniently separates the anterior and medial regions of the thigh. The five muscles classified as being in the medial compartment of the thigh are . . .

A. The pectineus muscle, the adductor longus muscle, the adductor brevis muscle, the gracilis muscle, and the adductor magnus muscle.

Q. The muscles in the medial compartment of the thigh receive a nerve supply, in whole or in part, from . . .

A. The obturator nerve.

Q. The muscle of this group that may be supplied, in whole or in part, by the femoral nerve is . . .

A. The pectineus muscle.

Q. The nerve that supplies that part of the adductor magnus muscle that inserts into the adductor tubercle on the back of the medial condyle of the femur is . . .

A. The tibial part of the sciatic nerve. This part of the adductor magnus muscle originally crossed the knee joint to the tibia; it belongs to the hamstring group of muscles.

Q. The features that characterize hamstring muscles are that . . .

A. They arise from the body of the ischium lateral to the ischial tuberosity and cross both the hip joint and the knee joint. They extend the hip joint and flex the knee joint.

Q. The adductor muscle that arises from the body of the ischium is . . .

A. The adductor magnus. It also arises from the ischial ramus.

Q. The other muscles in the adductor group originate from . . .

A. The pubis. The pectineus muscle arises from the superior ramus of the pubis; the adductor longus muscle arises from the pubic body; the adductor brevis and the gracilis muscles arise from the inferior ramus of the pubis. The origin of the gracilis extends to the ramus of the ischium.

Q. The nerve supply of the pectineus muscle, the adductor longus muscle, the adductor brevis muscle, and the gracilis muscle is . . .

A. The anterior division of the obturator nerve. The pectineus muscle also receives a branch from the femoral nerve.

Q. The adductor muscle supplied by the posterior division of the obturator nerve consists of . . .

A. The adductor portion of adductor magnus muscle.

Q. The other muscle supplied by the obturator nerve is . . .

A. The obturator externus muscle. It receives a branch from the trunk of the obturator nerve as that nerve leaves the pelvis through the obturator foramen.

Q. The other structures supplied by the obturator nerve are . . .

A. The hip joint and the knee joint. It must do so because it supplies a muscle, the gracilis muscle, that acts on both of these joints. Finally, the obturator nerve supplies the skin on the medial side of the thigh via its participation in the subsartorial plexus of nerves.

Q. The adductor group of muscles is divided into three layers by . . .

A. The anterior and the posterior branches of the obturator nerve.

Q. The muscles in the anterior of the three layers are . . .

A. The pectineus muscle and the adductor longus muscle.

Q. The muscles in the middle layer of the adductor region of the thigh are . . .

A. The adductor brevis muscle and the gracilis muscle.

Q. The muscle that forms the posterior layer of the adductor region of the thigh is . . .

A. The adductor magnus muscle. This muscle is described as having both an adductor and a hamstring portion.

Q. The attachments of the gracilis muscle are as follows . . .

A. Superiorly, it originates from the body and inferior ramus of the pubis and the ramus of the ischium by a continuous, superficial tendinous origin. Inferiorly, it inserts on the medial surface of thc medial condyle of the tibia between the sartorius and the semitendinosus muscles.

Q. A lesion of the obturator nerve causes . . .

A. The lower limb on the affected side to deviate laterally on walking. The gait then becomes wide stance, the so-called "adductor gait."

Q. The most likely nontraumatic lesion that might affect the obturator nerve is . . .

A. Carcinoma of the ovary. In the pelvis, the ovary lies in the ovarian fossa, between the ureter and the obliterated umbilical artery, posterior to the broad ligament. The obturator nerve lies deep to the peritoneum in the lateral wall of that fossa.

Q. The major artery to the medial side of the thigh is . . .

A. The deep artery of the thigh, the profunda femoris artery. It is a branch of the femoral artery.

Q. The deep artery of the thigh, the profunda femoris artery, reaches the medial side of the thigh by passing posteriorly between . . .

A. The pectineus muscle and the adductor longus muscle.

Q. In the adductor compartment of the thigh, the deep artery of the thigh, the profunda femoris artery, runs between . . .

A. The adductor longus muscle and the adductor brevis muscle.

Q. The branches of the deep artery of the thigh arising in the femoral triangle are . . .

A. The medial and the lateral circumflex femoral arteries.

Q. The medial circumflex femoral artery leaves the femoral triangle by passing posteriorly through the floor of the triangle between . . .

A. The iliopsoas muscle and the pectineus muscle. The medial circumflex femoral artery ends, as it lies between the quadratus femoris muscle and the obturator externus muscle, by dividing into ascending and transverse branches.

Q. The lateral circumflex femoral artery leaves the femoral triangle by passing laterally between . . .

A. The sartorius muscle and the rectus femoris muscle, superficially, and the vastus intermedius muscle, posteriorly. The lateral femoral circumflex artery ends by dividing into ascending, transverse, and descending branches.

Q. The branches given off by the deep artery of the thigh as it descends between the adductor longus muscle and the adductor brevis muscle are . . .

A. The 2nd and 3rd perforating arteries, which penetrate the adductor brevis muscle, and the 1st and the 4th perforating arteries, which run above and below the adductor brevis muscle, respectively. All four perforating arteries penetrate the adductor magnus muscle to reach the posterior compartment of the thigh.

Q. The cruciate anastomosis on the back of the thigh is formed by . . .

A. The anastomosis between the inferior gluteal artery, the transverse branches of the medial and the lateral circumflex femoral arteries, and the first perforating artery.

Q. This anastomosis provides collateral circulation when the femoral artery is interrupted above . . .

A. The origin of the deep artery of the thigh.

Q. The femoral artery descends from the femoral triangle to the hiatus in the adductor magnus muscle via . . .

A. The adductor canal.

Q. The boundaries of the adductor canal are . . .

A. The adductor longus muscle and the adductor magnus muscle, posteriorly; the vastus medialis muscle, laterally; and the sartorius muscle, anteromedially.

Q. After it passes through the hiatus in the adductor magnus, the femoral artery becomes . . .

A. The popliteal artery on entering the popliteal fossa.

THE LUMBOSACRAL PLEXUS

Q. In Figure 7-4, identify A.

A. The contribution of L4 to the lumbar plexus. The anterior division, shown in gray, will help form the obturator nerve; the posterior division, shown in black, will join the femoral nerve.

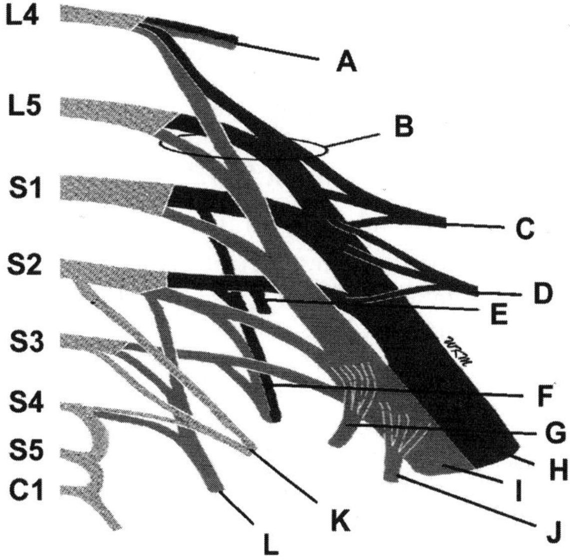

Figure 7-4 The Lumbosacral Plexus

Q. In Figure 7-4, identify B.

A. The lumbosacral trunk. It crosses the ala of the sacrum to join the sacral plexus.

Q. In Figure 7-4, identify C.

A. The superior gluteal nerve. It is the only nerve to leave the pelvis above the piriformis muscle.

Q. In Figure 7-4, identify D.

A. The inferior gluteal nerve. It leaves the pelvis below the piriformis muscle and supplies the gluteus maximus muscle.

Q. In Figure 7-4, identify E.

A. The nerve to the piriformis muscle. It is one of the few branches of the sacral plexus that does not leave the pelvis through the greater sciatic foramen.

Q. In Figure 7-4, identify F.

A. The posterior femoral cutaneous nerve. It is formed from both the ventral and the dorsal divisions of the anterior primary rami of the sacral nerves, S1, S2, and S3.

Q. In Figure 7-4, identify G.

A. The nerve to the obturator internus muscle and the superior gemellus muscle. Note that it is arising from L5, S1, and S2.

Q. In Figure 7-4, identify H.

A. The common fibular (the common peroneal) part of the sciatic nerve. It arises from the dorsal divisions of the anterior primary rami, L4, L5, S1, and S2.

Q. In Figure 7-4, identify I.

A. The tibial portion of the sciatic nerve. It arises from the anterior divisions of the anterior primary rami, L4, L5, S1, S2, and S3.

Q. In Figure 7-4, identify J.

A. The nerve to the quadratus femoris muscle and to the inferior gemellus muscle. Note that it arises from L4, L5, and S1.

Q. In Figure 7-4, identify K.

A. The parasympathetic pelvic splanchnic nerves. They arise from the anterior primary rami of S2, S3, and S4.

Q. In Figure 7-4, identify L.

A. The pudendal nerve, S2, S3, and S4.

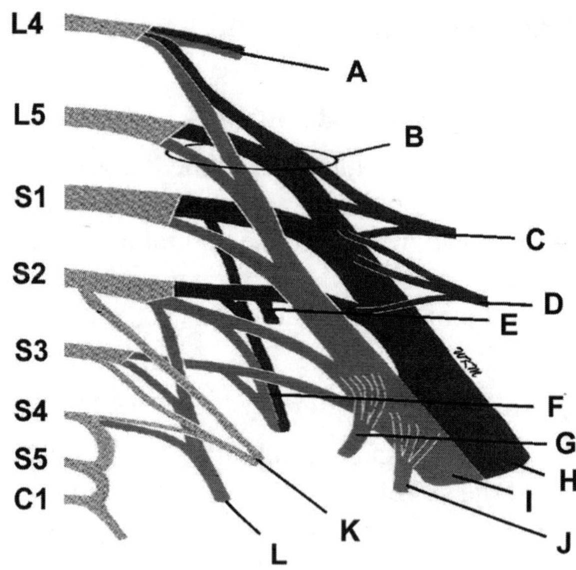

Figure 7-4 The Lumbosacral Plexus

THE GLUTEAL REGION

Q. In Figure 7-5, identify A.

A. The greater sciatic foramen.

Q. In Figure 7-5, identify B.

A. The area on the tip of the greater trochanter for the insertion of the piriformis muscle. It is just superior and posterior to the insertion of the obturator internus muscle.

Q. In Figure 7-5, identify C.

A. The quadrate tubercle. The quadratus femoris muscle is inserted into it. It lies on the upper part of the intertrochanteric crest.

Q. In Figure 7-5, identify D.

A. The gluteal line, the gluteal trochanter. The upper, deep one-quarter of the gluteus maximus muscle is inserted here.

Q. In Figure 7-5, identify E.

A. The lesser trochanter of the femur.

Q. In Figure 7-5, identify F.

A. The trochanteric fossa, the insertion of the obturator externus muscle.

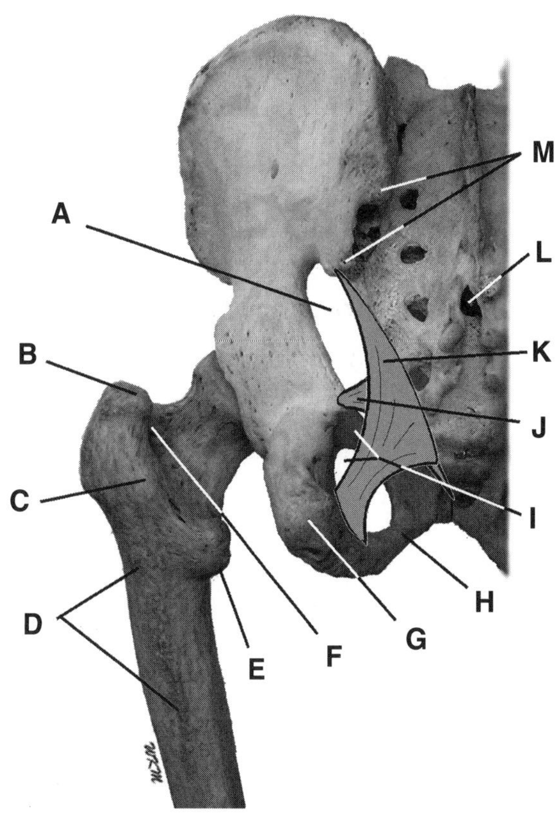

Figure 7-5 Skeleton of the Hip, Posterior Aspect

Q. In Figure 7-5, identify G.

A. The ischial tuberosity. All of the hamstring muscles—the biceps femoris muscle, the semitendinosus muscle, and the semimembranosus muscle—and the hamstring portion of the adductor magnus muscle arise from it.

Q. In Figure 7-5, identify H.

A. The ischiopubic ramus. It provides attachment on its lateral surface for all of the adductor muscles of the thigh.

Q. In Figure 7-5, identify I.

A. The lesser sciatic foramen. It is bounded by the sacrotuberous ligament, the sacrospinous ligament, and the ischium.

Q. In Figure 7-5, identify J.

A. The sacrospinous ligament. It is attached to the apex of the ischial spine, which is crossed by the internal pudendal vessels, the pudendal nerve, and the nerve to the obturator internus muscle.

Q. In Figure 7-5, identify K.

A. The sacrotuberous ligament.

Q. In Figure 7-5, identify L.

A. The sacral hiatus. It is where local anesthetic for an epidural anesthesia is injected.

Q. In Figure 7-5, identify M.

A. The posterior superior iliac spine and the posterior inferior iliac spine.

Q. In Figure 7-6, name the muscle attached at A.

A. The gluteus maximus muscle.

Q. In Figure 7-6, name the muscle attached at B.

A. The gluteus medius muscle.

Q. In Figure 7-6, name the muscle attached at C.

A. The gluteus minimus muscle.

Q. In Figure 7-6, name the muscle attached at D.

A. The tensor fasciae latae muscle.

Q. In Figure 7-6, name the muscle attached at E.

A. The superior gemellus muscle.

Q. In Figure 7-6, name the muscle attached at F.

A. The inferior gemellus muscle.

Q. In Figure 7-6, name the muscle attached at G.

A. The piriformis muscle.

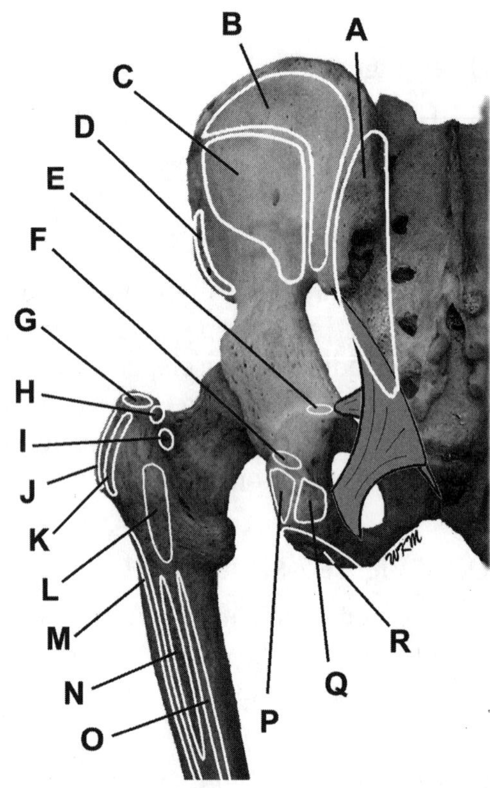

Figure 7-6 The Gluteal Region: Muscle Attachments

Q. The piriformis muscle arises from . . .

A. The anterior surface of the lateral mass of the sacrum.

Q. In Figure 7-6, name the muscle attached at H.

A. The obturator internus muscle. The superior gemellus muscle and the inferior gemellus muscle are both inserted into its tendon.

Q. The obturator internus muscle arises from . . .

A. The pelvic surface of the obturator membrane and the surrounding areas of the ilium and ischium.

Q. In Figure 7-6, name the muscle attached at I.

A. The obturator externus muscle. It arises from the lateral surface of the obturator membrane and the surrounding bone.

Q. In Figure 7-6, name the muscle attached at J.

A. The gluteus minimus muscle. It is an abductor and weak medial rotator of the thigh.

Q. In Figure 7-6, name the muscle attached at K.

A. The gluteus medius muscle. It is an abductor and weak medial rotator of the thigh.

Q. In Figure 7-6, name the muscle attached at L.

A. The quadratus femoris muscle. It is a lateral rotator of the thigh.

Q. In Figure 7-6, name the muscle attached at M.

A. The vastus lateralis muscle.

Q. In Figure 7-6, name the muscle attached at N.

A. The gluteus maximus muscle. Only the deep fibers of the inferior part of the muscle are inserted into this area, the remainder of the muscle is inserted between the layers of the fascia lata, which continues to the lateral condyle of the tibia as the iliotibial tract.

Q. Inferiorly, the fascia lata becomes a thick band named . . .

A. The iliotibial tract.

Q. The iliotibial tract gains attachment to . . .

A. The lateral condyle of the tibia, close to the knee joint.

Q. In Figure 7-6, name the muscle attached at O.

A. The adductor part of the adductor magnus muscle. This part of the muscle arises from the ischiopubic ramus. The hamstring part of the muscle, which arises from the lateral surface of the ischial tuberosity, is inserted into the adductor tubercle on the medial condyle of the femur.

Q. In Figure 7-6, name the muscle attached at P.

A. The semimembranosus muscle.

Q. In Figure 7-6, name the muscles attached at Q.

A. The semitendinosus muscle and the biceps femoris muscle.

Q. In Figure 7-6, name the muscle attached at R.

A. The hamstring portion of the adductor magnus muscle.

Q. In Figure 7-7, identify A.

A. The origin of the gluteus maximus muscle. It arises from the superior and inferior posterior iliac spines, the aponeurosis of the erector spinae, the dorsal surface of the sacrum, and the dorsal surface of the sacrotuberous ligament.

Q. The structures that can be used to identify the planes of separation of the three muscle layers are . . .

A. The superficial and deep branches of the superior gluteal artery. It supplies branches to all three layers.

Q. In Figure 7-7, identify B.

A. The upper part of the gluteus medius muscle. It arises from the ilium between the anterior and superior gluteal lines.

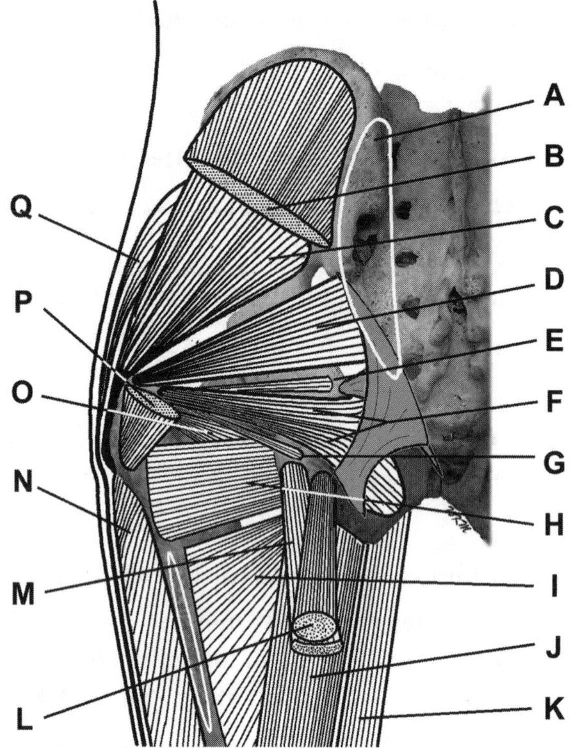

Figure 7-7 The Gluteal Region: Muscles

Q. In Figure 7-7, identify C.

A. The gluteus minimus muscle. It arises from the lateral surface of the ilium between the anterior and inferior gluteal lines. It is inserted anterior to the gluteus medius on the lateral surface of the greater trochanter.

Q. In Figure 7-7, identify D.

A. The piriformis muscle. It originates from the anterior surface of the sacrum, emerges through the greater sciatic foramen, and is inserted into the greater trochanter of the femur.

Q. In Figure 7-7, identify E.

A. The superior gemellus muscle. It is inserted into the tendon of the obturator internus muscle and is supplied by the nerve to that muscle.

Q. In Figure 7-7, identify F.

A. The obturator internus muscle. It leaves the pelvis through the lesser sciatic foramen, turning laterally around the ischial spine to reach the greater trochanter.

Q. In Figure 7-7, identify G.

A. The inferior gemellus muscle. It is inserted into the tendon of the obturator internus muscle.

Q. In Figure 7-7, identify H.

A. The quadratus femoris muscle. Its nerve, the nerve to the quadratus femoris muscle, emerging through the greater sciatic foramen, lies on the ischium deep to the sciatic nerve. This nerve also supplies the inferior gemellus muscle.

Q. In Figure 7-7, identify I.

A. The adductor portion of the adductor magnus muscle. It is inserted into the medial lip of the linea aspera and is supplied by the posterior branch of the obturator nerve.

Q. In Figure 7-7, identify J.

A. The hamstring part of the adductor magnus muscle. It is inserted into the adductor tubercle on the femur and is supplied by a branch of the tibial nerve.

Q. In Figure 7-7, identify K.

A. The gracilis muscle. It is supplied by the anterior division of the obturator nerve.

Q. In Figure 7-7, identify L.

A. The combined origin of the semitendinosus muscle and the biceps femoris muscle.

Q. In Figure 7-7, identify M.

A. The semimembranosus muscle.

Q. In Figure 7-7, identify N.

A. The vastus lateralis muscle. It arises from the intertrochanteric line, the lateral surface of the greater trochanter, and the lateral lip of the linea aspera of the femur.

Q. In Figure 7-7, identify O.

A. The obturator externus muscle. It arises from the lateral surface of the obturator membrane and the surrounding ischium. It lies in a deeper plane than the other muscles shown.

Q. In Figure 7-7, identify P.

A. The insertion of the gluteus medius muscle.

Q. In Figure 7-7, identify Q.

A. The tensor fasciae latae muscle. It is inserted into the fascia lata, as is most of the gluteus maximus muscle. The fascia lata forms a thickened band, the iliotibial tract, which is inserted into the lateral condyle of the tibia. It stabilizes the lateral side of the knee joint.

Q. In Figure 7-8, identify A.

A. The inferior gluteal nerve. It supplies only the gluteus maximus muscle.

Q. In Figure 7-8, identify B.

A. The superior gluteal nerve. As can be seen, it leaves the pelvis through the greater sciatic foramen above the piriformis muscle with the superior gluteal vessels. It runs across the gluteal region in the plane between the gluteus medius and the gluteus minimus muscles. It supplies the gluteus medius muscle, the gluteus minimus muscle, and the tensor fasciae latae muscle.

Q. In addition to sending branches to accompany the branches of the superior gluteal nerve, the superior gluteal artery gives off a superficial branch, which runs across the gluteal region in the plane between . . .

A. The gluteus maximus muscle and the gluteus medius muscle.

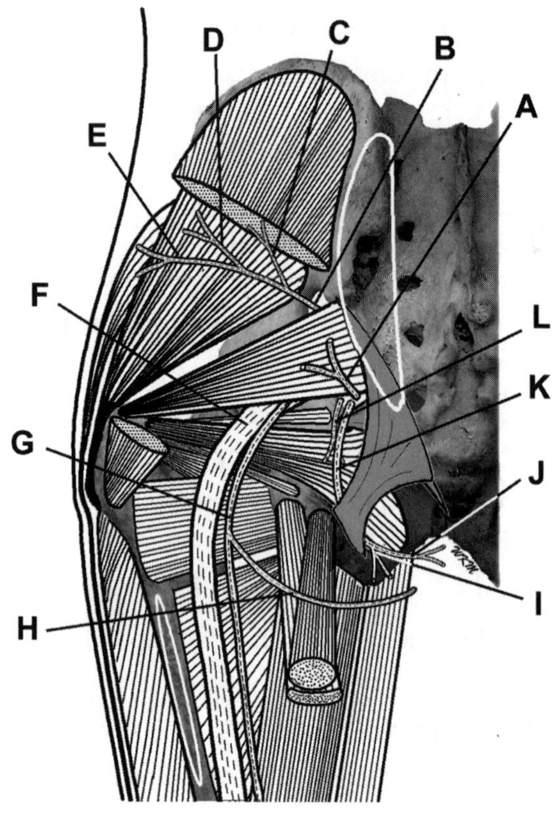

Figure 7-8 The Gluteal Region: Nerves

Q. In Figure 7-8, identify C.

A. The superior branch of the superior gluteal nerve to the gluteus medius muscle.

Q. In Figure 7-8, identify D.

A. The branch of the inferior division of the superior gluteal nerve to the gluteus minimus muscle.

Q. In Figure 7-8, identify E.

A. The branch of the inferior division of the superior gluteal nerve to the tensor fasciae latae muscle.

Q. In Figure 7-8, identify F.

A. The sciatic nerve. It receives its blood supply from a branch of the inferior gluteal artery. Interruption of this blood supply by pressure, as a result of prolonged sitting, may result in temporary paralysis of this nerve.

Q. In Figure 7-8, identify G.

A. The posterior femoral cutaneous nerve. It supplies the skin on the posterior surface of the thigh. It also supplies branches to the skin of the inferior part of the gluteal region.

Q. In Figure 7-8, identify H.

A. The perineal branch of the posterior femoral cutaneous nerve. It supplies the skin on the lateral part the labium majorum or scrotum and the upper part of the medial side of the thigh.

Q. In Figure 7-8, identify I.

A. The inferior hemorrhoidal nerve. It is a branch of the pudendal nerve.

Q. In Figure 7-8, identify J.

A. The continuation of the pudendal nerve. It divides into the dorsal nerve of the penis or clitoris and the perineal nerve.

Q. In Figure 7-8, identify K.

A. The pudendal nerve. It leaves the pelvis through the lower part of the greater sciatic foramen and crosses posterior to the iliac spine to enter the lesser sciatic foramen deep to the sacrotuberous ligament. It is accompanied by the internal pudendal vessels.

Q. In Figure 7-8, identify L.

A. The nerve to the obturator internus. Here it is separated from the pudendal nerve by the internal pudendal vessels, which are not shown in this diagram.

Q. The sacral plexus is formed from . . .

A. The anterior primary rami of the 4th and 5th lumbar nerves and of all of the sacral nerves.

Q. The gluteus maximus muscle is the largest muscle in the body. It has an extensive origin from . . .

A. The posterior gluteal line of the ilium, extending medially, almost to the midline, and extending inferiorly to include the sacrotuberous ligament and the corresponding part of the sacrum.

Q. The gluteus maximus muscle is inserted into . . .

A. The gluteal tuberosity on the upper part of the posterior surface of the femur. However, most of the muscle is inserted into the iliotibial tract, by which it gains attachment to the lateral condyle of the tibia.

Q. The nerve supply of the gluteus maximus muscle is from . . .

A. The inferior gluteal nerve (L5, S1, and S2). It is the only muscle supplied by this nerve.

Q. The gluteal region has three muscle layers. The gluteus maximus muscle is one of the two superficial muscles. The other superficial muscle is . . .

A. The tensor fasciae latae muscle.

Q. The tensor fasciae latae muscle arises from . . .

A. The anterior 5 cm (2 inches) of the outer lip of the iliac crest.

Q. The tensor fasciae latae muscle is inserted between . . .

A. The layers of the iliotibial tract. The major part of the gluteus maximus muscle also is inserted between these two layers.

Q. The nerve supply of the tensor fasciae latae muscle is from . . .

A. The inferior division of the superior gluteal nerve.

Q. The action of both the gluteus maximus muscle and the tensor fasciae latae muscle is to . . .

A. Stabilize the lateral side of the knee joint. In addition, and more importantly, the gluteus maximus muscle is a powerful extensor and abductor of the thigh from the anatomical position.

Q. The muscle that lies immediately deep to the gluteus maximus muscle, and hence constitutes the second layer of muscle in the gluteal region, is . . .

A. The gluteus medius muscle.

Q. The gluteus medius muscle arises from . . .

A. The outer surface of the ilium between the anterior and the posterior gluteal lines. It is inserted into the posterior of the two ridges on the lateral surface of the greater trochanter.

Q. The nerve supply of the gluteus medius muscle is from . . .

A. The superior gluteal nerve (L4, L5, and S1).

Q. The primary action of the gluteus medius muscle is to . . .

A. Abduct the hip. During walking, acting together with gluteus minimus muscle, it serves to raise the pelvis on the contralateral side, allowing the foot to clear the ground during the swing phase of locomotion. Its anterior fibers also serve as a medial rotator of the hip.

Q. The primary action of the gluteus minimus muscle is to . . .

A. Abduct the hip. During walking, acting together with gluteus medius muscle, it serves to raise the pelvis on the contralateral side, allowing the foot to clear the ground during the swing phase of locomotion. It also serves as a medial rotator of the hip.

Q. The nerve supply of the gluteus minimus muscle is from . . .

A. The superior gluteal nerve (L4, L5, and S1).

Q. The skin over the gluteal region is supplied by cutaneous branches from . . .

A. The dorsal primary rami of L1, L2, L3, S1, S2, and S3 and, inferiorly, by gluteal branches from the posterior cutaneous nerve of the thigh.

TRANSVERSE SECTIONS OF THE THIGH

Q. In Figure 7-9, identify A.

A. The vastus intermedius muscle. It arises from most of the anterior and lateral surfaces of the shaft of the femur.

Q. In Figure 7-9, identify B.

A. The vastus lateralis muscle. It arises from the lateral part of the intertrochanteric line, the base of the greater trochanter, and the lateral lip of the linea aspera of the femur.

Q. In Figure 7-9, identify C.

A. The vastus medialis muscle. It arises from the intertrochanteric line, the upper part of the medial surface of the femur, and the whole length of the linear aspera.

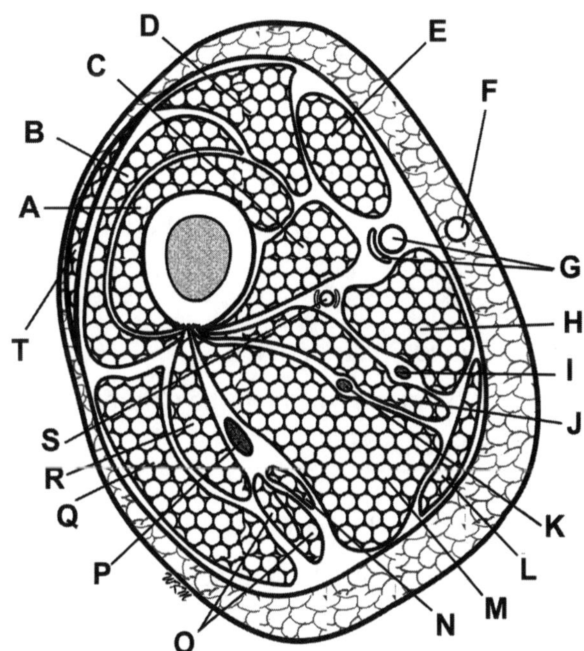

Figure 7-9 Transverse Section of the Upper Thigh

Q. In Figure 7-9, identify D.

A. The rectus femoris muscle. It arises by two heads from the ilium.

Q. In Figure 7-9, identify E.

A. The sartorius muscle. It arises from the anterior superior iliac spine. It is inserted into the medial surface of the tibia, anterior to the gracilis muscle and to the semitendinosus muscle.

Q. In Figure 7-9, identify F.

A. The great, long, saphenous vein.

Q. In Figure 7-9, identify G.

A. The femoral artery in company with the femoral vein.

Q. In Figure 7-9, identify H.

A. The adductor longus muscle. It forms the floor of the adductor (subsartorial) canal.

Q. In Figure 7-9, identify I.

A. The anterior division of the obturator nerve. It supplies all of the adductor muscles except the adductor magnus muscle.

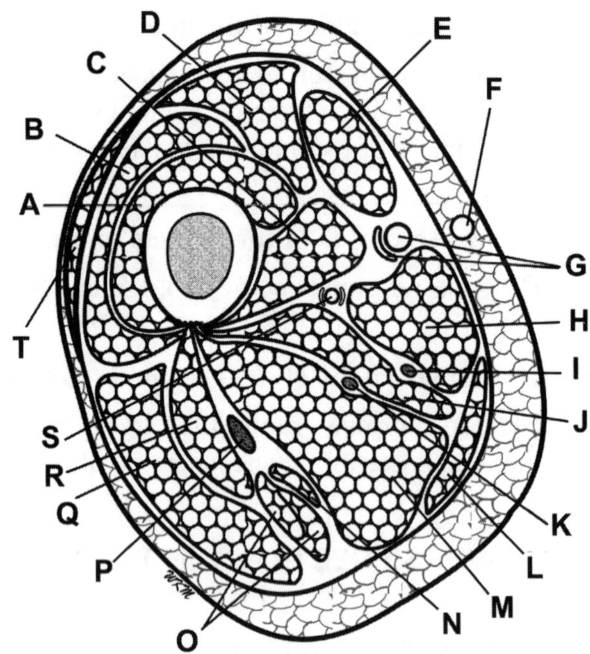

Figure 7-9 Transverse Section of the Upper Thigh

Q. In Figure 7-9, identify J.

A. The adductor brevis muscle. It arises from the ischiopubic ramus and is inserted into the linear aspera.

Q. In Figure 7-9, identify K.

A. The posterior division of the obturator nerve. It supplies most of the adductor magnus muscle.

Q. In Figure 7-9, identify L.

A. The gracilis muscle. It arises from the ischiopubic ramus and is inserted into the medial tibial condyle between the sartorius muscle and the semitendinosus muscle.

Q. In Figure 7-9, identify M.

A. The adductor magnus muscle. The adductor and hamstring parts of the muscle cannot be distinguished.

Q. In Figure 7-9, identify N.

A. The semimembranosus muscle. It is one of the three true hamstring muscles. It lies deep to the combined tendon of origin of the semitendinosus muscle and the long head of the biceps femoris muscle.

Q. In Figure 7-9, identify O.

A. The combined tendinous origin of the semitendinosus muscle and the long head of the biceps femoris muscle. All true hamstring muscles cross and act on the hip and knee joints.

Q. In Figure 7-9, identify P.

A. The sciatic nerve. At this point, it lies deep to the gluteus maximus muscle.

Q. In Figure 7-9, identify Q.

A. The superficial part of the gluteus maximus muscle. It is inserted, together with the tensor fasciae latae muscle, into the fascia lata of the thigh.

Q. In Figure 7-9, identify R.

A. The deeper part of the gluteus maximus muscle. It is inserted into the gluteal trochanter (tuberosity) on the upper part of the posterior surface of the shaft of the femur.

Q. In Figure 7-9, identify S.

A. The deep artery of the thigh, the profunda femoris artery, with its accompanying venae comitantes.

Q. The cruciate anastomosis, lying in the posterior compartment of the thigh, is formed from . . .

A. The perforating branches of the deep artery of the thigh, the medial circumflex femoral artery, the lateral circumflex femoral artery, and the inferior gluteal artery. It forms a useful collateral circulation if the femoral artery is obstructed above the origin of the deep artery of the thigh, the profunda femoris artery.

Q. In Figure 7-9, identify T.

A. The tensor fasciae latae muscle. It is inserted into the investing layer of deep fascia. This thickens inferiorly to form the iliotibial band. The iliotibial band also provides insertion for most of the gluteus maximus muscle. The iliotibial band, or tract, is inserted inferiorly into the lateral condyle of the tibia. This attachment reinforces the rather weak lateral collateral ligament of the knee joint.

Q. In Figure 7-10, identify A.

A. The vastus lateralis muscle.

Q. In Figure 7-10, identify B.

A. The vastus intermedius muscle. Its muscle fibers form a tendon on the anterior surface of the muscle. This tendon fuses with the tendon of the rectus femoris muscle.

Q. In Figure 7-10, identify C.

A. The rectus femoris muscle. It is the only part of the quadriceps femoris muscle that arises from the ilium; hence, it also acts on the hip joint.

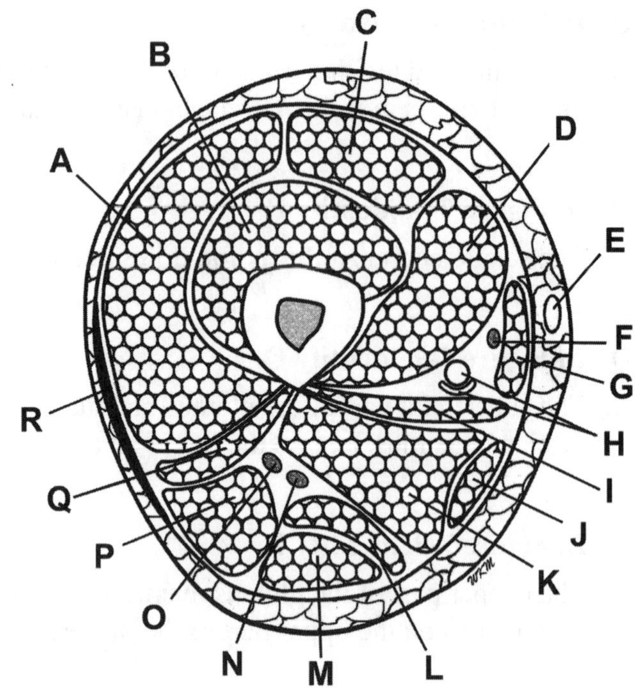

Figure 7-10 Transverse Section of the Midthigh

Q. In Figure 7-10, identify D.

A. The vastus medialis muscle. It forms the lateral wall of the adductor canal.
The roof (medial wall) of the adductor canal is formed by the sartorius muscle. The floor is formed by the adductor longus muscle, proximally, and the adductor magnus muscle, distally. It is traversed by the femoral vessels and the saphenous nerve.

Q. In Figure 7-10, identify E.

A. The great, long, saphenous vein.

Q. In Figure 7-10, identify F.

A. The saphenous nerve. It traverses the adductor canal en route to the medial side of the leg and foot.

Q. In Figure 7-10, identify G.

A. The sartorius muscle. It forms the roof of the adductor canal.

Q. In Figure 7-10, identify H.

A. The femoral artery and the femoral vein. They travel in the adductor canal.

Q. In Figure 7-10, identify I.

A. The adductor longus muscle. It forms the floor of the adductor canal. The section is below the level of the adductor brevis.

Q. In Figure 7-10, identify J.

A. The gracilis muscle. In this section, it is beginning to move posteriorly. It is inserted into the medial surface of the tibia between the sartorius muscle and the semitendinosus muscle.

Q. In Figure 7-10, identify K.

A. The adductor magnus muscle. It forms the floor of the adductor canal below the adductor longus muscle. The femoral artery and femoral vein pass through its hiatus, which is situated immediately above the adductor tubercle, to become the popliteal vessels.

Q. In Figure 7-10, identify L.

A. The semimembranosus muscle. It is already beginning to flatten prior to its insertion into the medial condyle of the tibia.

Q. In Figure 7-10, identify M.

A. The semitendinosus muscle. It lies superficial to the semimembranosus muscle.

Q. In Figure 7-10, identify N.

A. The tibial nerve.

Q. In Figure 7-10, identify O.

A. The common fibular (common peroneal) nerve.

Q. In Figure 7-10, identify P.

A. The long head of the biceps femoris muscle. This is the only muscle distal to the gluteus maximus muscle that crosses superficially to the sciatic nerve.

Q. In Figure 7-10, identify Q.

A. The short head of the biceps femoris muscle. This is the only muscle on the back of the thigh that is supplied by the common fibular nerve.

Q. In Figure 7-10, identify R.

A. The iliotibial tract. Both the tensor fasciae latae muscle and the lower three-quarters of the gluteus maximus muscle are inserted into it.

THE POSTERIOR THIGH AND THE POPLITEAL FOSSA

Q: The back of the thigh may be called the hamstring compartment. The hamstring muscles are:

A. The semitendinosus muscle, the semimembranosus muscle, and the biceps femoris muscle.

Q. All three muscles arise, under cover of the gluteus maximus, from . . .

A. The ischial tuberosity.

Q. Two nerves emerge from deep to the gluteus maximus muscle lateral to the hamstrings. They are . . .

A. The posterior femoral cutaneous nerve and the sciatic nerve.

Q. The posterior femoral cutaneous nerve crosses superficially . . .

A. The long head of the biceps femoris muscle.

Q. The muscle that crosses the sciatic nerve superficially is . . .

A. The long head of the biceps femoris muscle.

Q. A fourth muscle arises from the ischial tuberosity close to the hamstrings. It is . . .

A. The hamstring portion of the adductor magnus muscle. It is not a true hamstring muscle because it is attached inferiorly to the adductor tubercle on the femur. Therefore, it plays no part in flexing the knee joint.

Q. Two of the hamstring muscles arise from a common impression on the inferomedial aspect of the posterior surface of the ischial tuberosity. They are . . .

A. The semitendinosus muscle and the biceps femoris muscle.

Q. The three true hamstring muscles—the semimembranosus, the semitendinosus, and the biceps femoris—all . . .

A. Extend the hip and flex the knee.

Q. When the knee is flexed, the actions of the hamstring muscles differ because . . .

A. The semimembranosus muscle and the semitendinosus muscle are medial rotators of the tibia, whereas the biceps femoris muscle is a lateral rotator of the leg.

Q. The semitendinosus muscle is inserted . . .

A. Below the medial condyle of the tibia and posterior to the sartorius muscle and the gracilis muscle.

Q. The semimembranosus muscle is inserted into . . .

A. The posterior margin of the medial tibial condyle, close to the knee joint.

Q. The biceps femoris muscle is inserted into . . .

A. The head of the fibula, on either side of the fibular collateral ligament of the knee joint.

Q. Branches from the tibial part of the sciatic nerve supply all three of the hamstring muscles. The hamstring muscle that also receives a branch from the common fibular (common peroneal) nerve component of the sciatic nerve is . . .

A. The biceps femoris muscle. The common fibular nerve supplies the short head of the biceps femoris muscle. It arises from most of the linea aspera on the back of the femur between the adductor magnus muscle and the vastus lateralis muscle.

Q. The sciatic nerve emerges from the pelvis through the greater sciatic foramen. Its anterior (deep) relations are . . .

A. The nerve to the quadratus femoris muscle initially separates it from the ischium. It then crosses, in turn, the obturator internus muscle and the two gemelli muscles and the quadratus femoris muscle. It then lies on the posterior surface of the adductor magnus muscle until it reaches the adductor hiatus. There it divides into its terminal branches, the tibial nerve and the common fibular nerve.

Q. The hamstrings can be considered as lying in a posterior compartment of the thigh. This compartment is limited anteriorly and laterally by . . .

A. A strong intermuscular septum, which extends from the linea aspera to the iliotibial tract, and separates the hamstring compartment from the vastus lateralis muscle. Medial to the linea aspera, the hamstring muscles lie on the posterior surface of the adductor magnus.

Q. The popliteal fossa is a rhomboid-shaped fossa posterior to the knee joint. Its superior boundaries are . . .

A. The semimembranosus muscle and the semitendinosus muscle, medially, and the biceps femoris muscle, laterally.

Q. Its inferior boundaries are . . .

A. The medial and lateral heads of the gastrocnemius muscle, on their respective sides.

Q. The floor (anterior wall) of the popliteal fossa is formed by . . .

A. The knee joint capsule, superiorly, and the popliteus muscle, covered by a thick layer of fascia, inferiorly.

Q. The action of the popliteus muscle, by its insertion into the lateral aspect of the lateral femoral condyle, is to . . .

A. Laterally rotate the femur on the tibia when the knee is extended. This slackens the ligaments and allows the knee to flex. Hence, the aphorisms "unlocking the knee joint" and "the popliteus muscle is the key that unlocks the knee joint."

Q. The nerve supply of the popliteus muscle is . . .

A. The tibial nerve. The nerve to the popliteus muscle runs across its posterior surface and then curves around its inferior border to enter its anterior surface.

Q. The popliteal artery enters the popliteal fossa through . . .

A. The adductor hiatus. As is to be expected, it travels in company with the popliteal vein.

Q. The relation of the popliteal artery to the popliteal vein as they enter the popliteal fossa is . . .

A. The artery is anteromedial to the vein. As they pass through the fossa, the artery gradually crosses back to the lateral side of the vein.

Q. As the tibial nerve descends through the popliteal fossa, it lies at first . . .

A. Superficial to the popliteal vessels. It then crosses them from the lateral to the medial side. Distally, at the lower border of the popliteus, where the popliteal artery divides into the anterior tibial and the posterior tibial arteries, the tibial nerve again crosses posteriorly to regain the lateral side of the posterior tibial artery and its venae comitantes.

Q. The tibial nerve leaves the popliteal fossa . . .

A. By passing deep to the uniting two heads of the gastrocnemius muscle. It then passes deep to the soleus muscle to continue down the leg deep to the deep transverse fascia of the leg, the transverse crural intermuscular septum.

Q. The popliteal artery has now given off the anterior tibial artery to become the posterior tibial artery, which leaves the popliteal fossa in company with, but deep to, . . .

A. The tibial nerve.

Q. The popliteal artery terminates at the lower border of . . .

A. The popliteus muscle.

Q. The popliteal artery terminates by dividing into . . .

A. The anterior and posterior tibial arteries.

Q. The anterior tibial artery enters the anterior compartment of the leg by passing . . .

A. Above the interosseous membrane to enter the anterior compartment of the leg. In the proximal third of the leg, the anterior tibial artery is joined by the deep fibular (deep peroneal) nerve.

Q. The deep fibular nerve enters the anterior compartment of the leg by passing through . . .

A. The anterior crural intermuscular septum.

Q. The branches of the popliteal artery in the popliteal fossa are . . .

A. The medial and lateral superior genicular arteries, the middle genicular artery, and the medial and lateral inferior genicular arteries. They constitute the anastomosis round the knee joint.

Q. In the popliteal fossa the common fibular (common peroneal) nerve follows . . .

A. The tendon of the biceps femoris muscle. It runs between it and the lateral head of the gastrocnemius muscle to reach the neck of the fibula, where it winds around the neck of the fibula to enter the lateral (peroneal) compartment of the leg.

Q. To enter the lateral compartment of the leg, the common fibular nerve passes through . . .

A. The posterior crural intermuscular septum.

Q. The muscle that is traversed by the common fibular nerve on entering the lateral compartment of the leg is . . .

A. The fibularis longus (peroneus longus) muscle.

Q. On the neck of the fibula, while in the substance of the fibularis longus (peroneus longus) muscle, the common fibular (common peroneal) nerve divides into its two terminal branches. They are . . .

A. The superficial fibular (superficial peroneal) nerve and the deep fibular (deep peroneal) nerve.

TRANSVERSE SECTIONS OF THE LEG

Q. In Figure 7-11, identify A.

A. The subcutaneous medial surface of the tibia. Its superficial position makes it vulnerable to direct trauma.

Q. In Figure 7-11, identify B.

A. The deep transverse intermuscular septum. It encloses the upper part of the tibialis posterior muscle in a separate deep compartment.

Q. In Figure 7-11, identify C.

A. The deep transverse fascia of the leg. It separates the soleus and the gastrocnemius muscles from the deeper muscle group. In some terminologies, the deep transverse intermuscular septum is not named. The deep transverse fascia of the leg can then alternatively be called the transverse crural intermuscular septum.

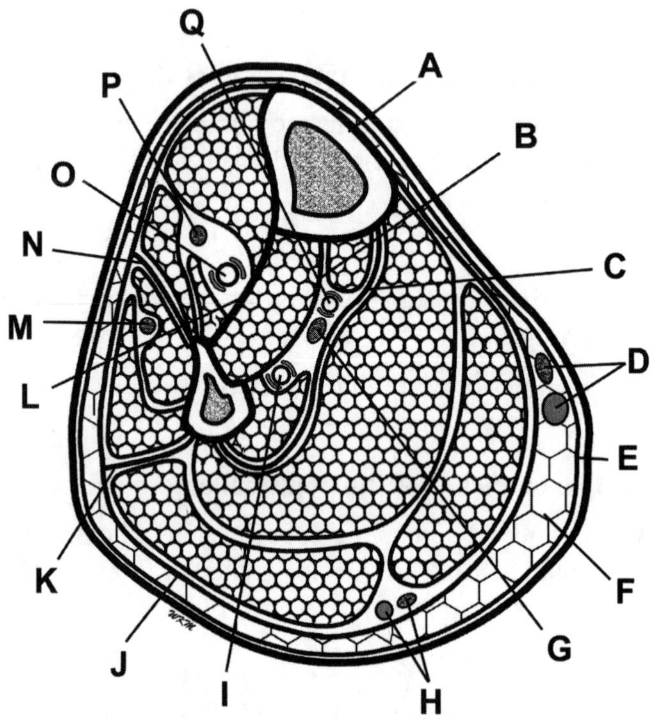

Figure 7-11 The Transverse Section of the Leg at Midcalf: Fascia, Vessels, and Nerves

Q. In Figure 7-11, identify D.

A. The saphenous nerve. It is a cutaneous branch of the femoral nerve to the medial side of the leg and foot. It is closely accompanied by the great, long, saphenous vein. The nerve is at risk during vein-stripping operations for varicose veins, and it also may be involved in the inflammation that accompanies thrombophlebitis of the vein.

Q. In Figure 7-11, identify E.

A. The thick superficial fascia. Its thickness makes percutaneous phlebotomy difficult in the leg. A cut-down procedure often is necessary.

Q. In Figure 7-11, identify F.

A. Subcutaneous fat. It is relatively thin in the leg.

Q. In Figure 7-11, identify G.

A. The tibial nerve. It supplies the deep muscles of the back of the leg and all of the muscles on the plantar aspect of the foot.

Q. In Figure 7-11, identify H.

A. The sural nerve and the small saphenous vein. They are closely associated. They both supply the lateral side of the leg and foot. The nerve often is in danger during vein-stripping and is often affected in the inflammation accompanying thrombophlebitis of the vein.

Q. In Figure 7-11, identify I.

A. The fibular (peroneal) vessels.

Q. In Figure 7-11, identify J.

A. The investing layer of deep fascia, the fascia cruris. Its strength and unyieldingness is one of the major causes of "compartment syndrome," pressure-induced ischemic muscle damage.

Q. In Figure 7-11, identify K.

A. The posterior crural intermuscular septum. The lateral compartment of the leg, which contains the fibular (peroneal) muscles and the superficial fibular (peroneal) nerve, lies between the anterior and posterior crural intermuscular septa.

Q. In Figure 7-11, identify L.

A. The interosseous membrane. It separates the anterior and posterior compartments of the leg.

Q. In Figure 7-11, identify M.

A. The superficial fibular (peroneal) nerve. It supplies the fibularis (peroneus) longus muscle and the fibularis (peroneus) brevis muscle before terminating by supplying cutaneous branches to the dorsum of the foot.

Q. In Figure 7-11, identify N.

A. The anterior crural intermuscular septum.

Q. In Figure 7-11, identify O.

A. The anterior tibial vessels.

Q. In Figure 7-11, identify P.

A. The deep fibular (peroneal) nerve. It supplies all of the muscles in the anterior compartment of the leg, the short muscles of the toes, and the skin between the big and the second toe.

Q. In Figure 7-11, identify Q.

A. The posterior tibial vessels.

Q. In Figure 7-12, identify A.

A. The extensor digitorum longus muscle. It is supplied by the deep fibular (peroneal) nerve, as are all of the muscles in the anterior compartment,.

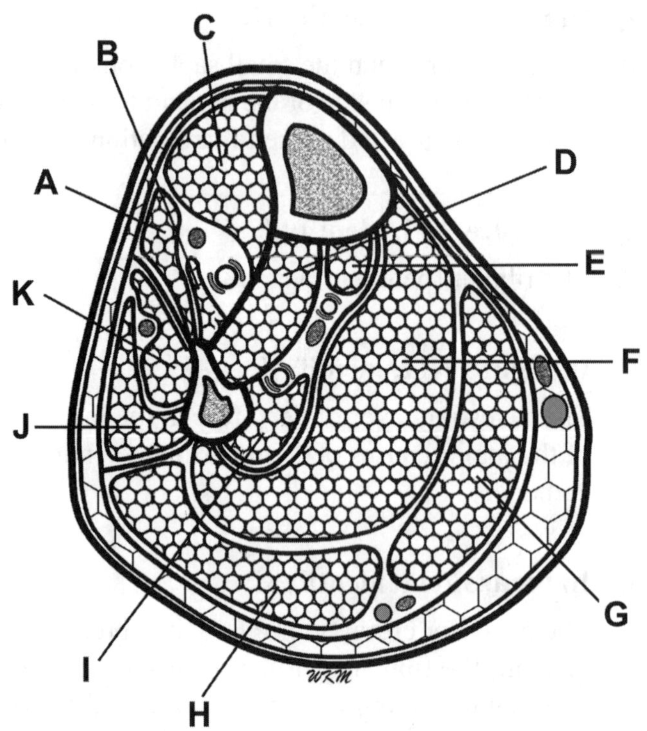

Figure 7-12 Transverse Section of the Leg at Midcalf: Muscles

Q. In Figure 7-12, identify B.

A. The extensor hallucis longus muscle. It arises from the middle two quarters of the anterior surface of the shaft of the fibula and from the interosseous membrane.

Q. In Figure 7-12, identify C.

A. The tibialis anterior muscle. It is the strongest of the muscles in the anterior compartment and is the main extensor (dorsiflexor) of the foot.

Q. In Figure 7-12, identify D.

A. The tibialis posterior. It is the largest of the three deep muscles of the leg that occupy the deep posterior compartment. It is a powerful inverter of the foot.

Q. In Figure 7-12, identify E.

A. The flexor digitorum longus muscle. In the sole of the foot, its tendon will cross, superficially, the tendon of the flexor hallucis longus muscle to reach the lateral four toes.

Q. In Figure 7-12, identify F.

A. The powerful soleus muscle. It is joined by the two heads of the gastrocnemius muscle to form the tendocalcaneus.

Q. In Figure 7-12, identify G.

A. The medial head of the gastrocnemius muscle.

Q. In Figure 7-12, identify H.

A. The lateral head of the gastrocnemius muscle. The gastrocnemius and soleus muscles, together with the much smaller, atavistic, plantaris muscle (not shown in this diagram), form the prominent calf of the leg. They occupy the superficial posterior compartment of the leg. This compartment is the least likely to suffer from compartment syndrome, because the investing layer of fascia is thinner posteriorly.

Q. In Figure 7-12, identify I.

A. The flexor hallucis longus muscle. Its tendon is the most lateral of the structures that cross the posterior surface of the medial malleolus.

Q. In Figure 7-12, identify J.

A. The fibularis (peroneus) longus muscle. Its tendon will cross the sole of the foot, deeply, to be inserted into the lateral side of the base of the first metatarsal bone and the medial cuneiform bone.

Q. In Figure 7-12, identify K.

A. The fibularis (peroneus) brevis muscle. It is anterior to the fibularis (peroneus) longus muscle, with which it shares a groove on the posterior surface of the lateral malleolus. It is inserted into a tubercle on the base of the 5th metatarsal bone. These two muscles lie in the lateral compartment of the leg.

THE LEG

Q. The four distinct compartments that can be identified in the leg are . . .

A. The anterior compartment, the lateral compartment, the deep compartment, and the superficial posterior compartment.

Q. The anatomical factor that renders a muscular compartment liable to "acute compartment syndrome"—muscular swelling with vascular compromise after excessive exercise or trauma—is . . .

A. The thickness and strength of the deep fascia, the fascia cruris. It cannot stretch to allow for swelling of the contents of the compartments that it encloses.

Q. The compartment that is most likely to be the subject of acute compartment syndrome is . . .

A. The anterior compartment.

Q. The walls of the anterior compartment of the leg are . . .

A. The fascia cruris, anteriorly; the tibia, medially; the anterior intermuscular septum, laterally; and the interosseous membrane and the fibula, posteriorly.

Q. The lateral compartment of the leg lies between . . .

A. The anterior and posterior intermuscular septa.

Q. The muscles in the lateral compartment of the leg are . . .

A. The fibularis (peroneus) longus muscle and the fibularis (peroneus) brevis muscle.

Q. The compartment that is the least likely to be affected by acute compartment syndrome is . . .

A. The posterior superficial compartment.

Q. The muscles in the anterior (extensor) compartment of the leg, from the medial to the lateral side, are . . .

A. The tibialis anterior muscle, the extensor hallucis longus muscle, and the extensor digitorum longus muscle. The fibularis (peroneus) tertius muscle is inferior to, and is really a part of, the extensor digitorum longus muscle.

Q. The muscle of the anterior compartment that arises from the tibia is . . .

A. The tibialis anterior muscle. The extensor digitorum muscle does gain a small attachment to the lateral side of the medial tibial condyle. However, its main origin is from the fibula.

Q. The tibialis anterior muscle is inserted into . . .

A. The medial side of the medial cuneiform bone and the base of the first metatarsal bone.

Q. The muscles of the anterior compartment that gain attachment to the interosseous membrane are . . .

A. The extensor hallucis longus muscle, the tibialis anterior muscle, and the extensor digitorum longus muscle. They all gain some attachment to the anterior surface of the interosseous membrane.

Q. The fibularis (peroneus) tertius muscle is inserted into . . .

A. The shaft of the 5th metatarsal bone. It assists the fibularis (peroneus) longus and the fibularis (peroneus) brevis muscles in everting the foot.

Q. All of the muscles of the anterior compartment are supplied by . . .

A. The deep fibular (deep peroneal) nerve, L4, L5.

Q. The action of the muscles of the anterior compartment is to . . .

A. Assist in extending (dorsiflexing) the ankle. The extensor hallucis longus muscle and the extensor digitorum longus muscle also extend the toes.

Q. The muscle that is most likely to be spared in a patient with a low meningomyelocele is . . .

A. The tibialis anterior muscle. Such patients, therefore, do not suffer from foot drop.

Q. The deep fibular (peroneal) nerve reaches the anterior compartment by . . .

A. Winding around the neck of the fibula.

Q. The fibular (peroneal) nerve is particularly susceptible to injury as it winds around the neck of the fibula. The most disabling consequence is . . .

A. Foot drop.

Q. The blood supply of the muscles of the anterior compartment is from . . .

A. The anterior tibial artery.

Q. The anterior tibial artery enters the anterior compartment of the leg from its origin from the popliteal artery in the posterior compartment of the leg by . . .

A. Passing above the interosseous membrane.

Q. The anterior tibial artery leaves the anterior compartment of the leg by passing deep to both . . .

A. The superior extensor retinaculum and the inferior extensor retinaculum medial to the deep fibular (deep peroneal) nerve. It remains in the interval between the extensor hallucis longus muscle and the tibialis anterior muscle.

Q. The anterior tibial artery terminates . . .

A. As it emerges from deep to the inferior extensor retinaculum. It is then renamed the dorsalis pedis artery. The dorsalis pedis artery immediately crosses deep to the extensor hallucis longus muscle to lie between it and the extensor digitorum longus muscle. It is commonly palpated at this point to determine the efficiency of the peripheral circulation in the leg and foot.

Q. The dorsalis pedis artery terminates by passing inferiorly between . . .

A. The two heads of the first dorsal interosseous muscle. It reaches the sole of the foot and completes the plantar arterial arch.

Q. The branches of the dorsal pedis artery are . . .

A. The medial and lateral tarsal arteries; the arcuate artery, its largest branch; and the 1st dorsal metatarsal artery, its terminal branch.

Q. The arcuate artery runs laterally across the foot. Its branches are . . .

A. The 2nd, 3rd, and 4th dorsal metacarpal arteries. They run to the clefts between the toes and then divide into dorsal digital branches to supply the dorsal surfaces of the toes.

Q. The deep fibular (peroneal) nerve enters the foot lateral to the dorsalis pedis artery. It then divides into medial and lateral branches. The lateral branch of the deep fibular (peroneal) nerve supplies . . .

A. The extensor digitorum brevis muscle.

Q. The medial branch of the deep fibular (peroneal) nerve supplies . . .

A. The adjacent sides of the first and second toes.

Q. The only muscle on the dorsum of the foot is the extensor digitorum brevis muscle. Its first tendon serves the big toe and is sometimes called the extensor hallucis brevis muscle. The extensor digitorum brevis muscle arises from . . .

A. The anterior part of the superior surface of the calcaneus. It assists in extension of the toes.

Q. The muscles that occupy the posterior deep compartment of the leg are . . .

A. The flexor digitorum longus muscle, the tibialis posterior muscle, and the flexor hallucis longus muscle, in order from the lateral to the medial side.

Q. The muscle in the deep posterior compartment of the leg that arises from the tibia, the fibula, and the interosseous membrane is . . .

A. The tibialis posterior muscle.

Q. The muscle in the deep posterior compartment that arises only from the tibia is . . .

A. The flexor digitorum longus muscle.

Q. The nerve supply of the muscles in the deep posterior compartment of the leg is . . .

A. The tibial nerve.

Q. The blood supply of the muscles in the deep posterior compartment of the leg comes from . . .

A. The posterior tibial artery. By its large fibular (peroneal) branch, it supplies the flexor hallucis longus muscle and the lateral part of the tibialis posterior muscle.

Q. The structures in the deep posterior compartment of the leg reach the foot by passing posterior to . . .

A. The medial malleolus of the tibia, deep to the flexor retinaculum.

Q. As the structures in the posterior compartment run across the posterior surface of the medial malleolus, deep to the flexor retinaculum, they are arranged in sequence from the medial to the lateral side as follows . . .

A. The tibialis posterior muscle; the flexor digitorum longus muscle; the posterior tibial artery with its venae comitantes; and finally, the flexor hallucis longus muscle. Note that the flexor digitorum longus muscle crosses the tibialis posterior muscle superficially and that the tibial nerve is now again on the lateral side of the artery.

Q. The tibialis posterior muscle is inserted into . . .

A. The tubercle of the navicular bone, with an extension to the medial cuneiform bone. To reach its insertion, the tendon crosses the plantar calcaneonavicular ligament, the "spring" ligament, inferiorly. Note that both the tibialis anterior muscle and the tibialis posterior muscle gain some attachment to the medial side of the medial cuneiform bone.

Q. The action of the tibialis posterior muscle is to . . .

A. Invert the foot. In fact, it is the major inverter of the foot. In practice, this ensures that the lateral side of the foot takes a major share of the body weight.

Q. The muscles occupying the superficial posterior compartment are . . .

A. The combining heads of the gastrocnemius muscle and the soleus muscle. The old name for the combined muscle was the triceps surae muscle. The small plantaris muscle, closely associated with the lateral head of the gastrocnemius muscle, is often absent.

Q. The origin of the gastrocnemius muscle is by medial and lateral heads from . . .

A. The posterior surface of the appropriate femoral condyles.

Q. The soleus muscle arises from . . .

A. The soleal line on the tibia and the superior one quarter of the posterior surface of the fibula.

Q. The soleus muscle and the combined heads of the gastrocnemius muscle form the very strong tendocalcaneus, which is inserted into . . .

A. The posterior surface of the calcaneus.

Q. The nerve supply of these three muscle bellies, the triceps surae muscle, is from . . .

A. The tibial nerve.

Q. The action of the triceps surae is to . . .

A. Powerfully flex the ankle. They are used in standing, walking, running, and jumping. Tears, usually only partial, of the tendocalcaneus itself are relatively common due to the combined strength of the three muscle bellies. Natural healing of even partial tears of this tendon is slow, due to the lack of a good blood supply. Complete tears require surgical intervention.

Q. The muscles that occupy the lateral compartment of the leg are . . .

A. The fibularis (peroneus) longus muscle and the fibularis (peroneus) brevis muscle.

Q. The origin of both the fibularis (peroneus) longus muscle and the fibularis (peroneus) brevis muscle is . . .

A. The lateral surface of the fibula. The fibularis longus muscle originates from the upper two-thirds of the fibula; the fibularis brevis muscle originates from the lower two-thirds of the fibula.

Q. The nerve supply of the fibularis (peroneus) longus and fibularis (peroneus) brevis muscles is from . . .

A. The superficial fibular (peroneal) nerve.

Q. The blood supply of the fibularis (peroneus) longus and fibularis (peroneus) brevis muscles is from . . .

A. The fibular (peroneal) branch of the posterior tibial artery.

Q. These two fibularis (peroneus) muscles reach the foot by passing posterior to . . .

A. The lateral malleolus, deep to the superior fibular (peroneal) retinaculum. Then they pass through individual osseoaponeurotic canals, deep to the inferior fibular (peroneal) retinaculum.

Q. The fibularis (peroneus) longus muscle lies posterior to the fibularis (peroneus) brevis muscle. Reaching the lateral side of the cuboid bone, it turns medially to run across the sole of the foot in a groove on the inferior surface of . . .

A. The cuboid bone.

Q. The groove in the cuboid bone for the tendon of the fibularis (peroneus) longus muscle is converted into an osseoaponeurotic tunnel by . . .

A. The long plantar ligament.

Q. The fibularis longus muscle is inserted into . . .

A. The lateral side of the medial cuneiform bone and the base of the 1st metatarsal bone.

Q. The fibularis brevis muscle is inserted into . . .

A. The styloid process, a subcutaneous tubercle, on the base of the 5th metatarsal bone. This tubercle forms a prominent landmark on the lateral border of the foot, where it can be readily palpated. Continuous pressure on this bony prominence from poorly fitting shoes or a tight bandage or cast can be very painful.

Q. The fibularis (peroneus) longus muscle and the fibularis (peroneus) brevis muscle act together as . . .

A. Everters of the foot. Therefore, they help to keep the foot plantigrade. Acting from their attachments to the foot, they help to provide balance when the body is in the standing position.

THE VEINS OF THE LOWER EXTREMITY

Q. The lower extremity has three sets of veins, all with valves. These sets of veins are . . .

A. The superficial, the great and small (long and short) saphenous veins; the deep veins, which accompany the arteries; and a set of perforating veins, which connect the superficial veins to the deep veins in the leg.

Q. Normally, valves in the perforating veins allow blood to flow only from . . .

A. The superficial veins to the deep veins.

Q. Many of the deep veins are venae comitantes. The change from venae comitantes to a single vein for each artery occurs . . .

A. At the level of the knee joint.

Q. The veins with the most valves are . . .

A. The deep veins of the leg.

Q. In Figure 7-13, identify A.

A. The margin of the saphenous opening. This opening in the deep fascia is closed by the thin cribriform fascia. It is traversed by the great saphenous vein and its proximal tributaries.

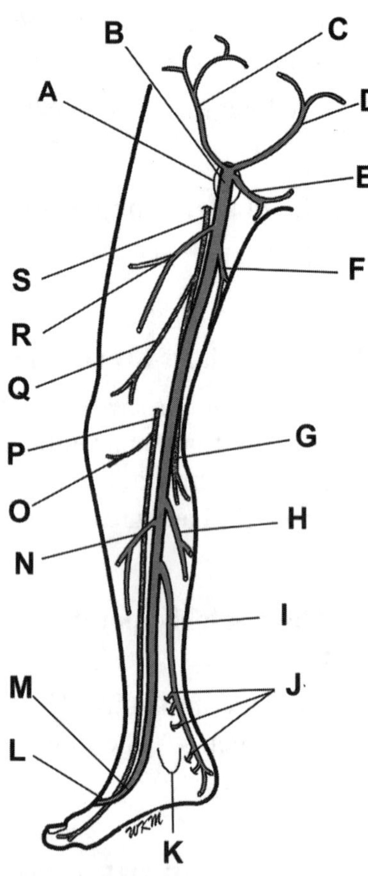

Figure 7-13 The Great Saphenous Vein and Its Accompanying Nerves

Q. In Figure 7-13, identify B.

A. The great saphenous vein. It passes through the saphenous opening to enter the femoral vein. Its entrance into the femoral vein is guarded by a valve. Varicosity of the proximal segment of the great saphenous vein may be misdiagnosed as a femoral hernia.

Q. In Figure 7-13, identify C.

A. The superficial circumflex iliac vein. Its course parallels the inguinal ligament.

Q. In Figure 7-13, identify D.

A. The superficial epigastric vein.

Q. In Figure 7-13, identify E.

A. The superficial external pudendal vein. Note that all three of these superficial veins—the superficial circumflex iliac vein, the superficial epigastric vein, and the superficial external pudendal vein—open into the great saphenous vein. They may provide unwanted collateral circulation if the great saphenous vein is ligated too low during an operation for varicose veins.

Q. In Figure 7-13, identify F.

A. The posteromedial vein of the thigh, the accessory saphenous vein.

Q. In Figure 7-13, identify G.

A. The posterior branch of the medial femoral cutaneous nerve. Note its proximity to the great saphenous vein.

Q. In Figure 7-13, identify H.

A. The posterior crural branch of the great saphenous vein.

Q. In Figure 7-13, identify I.

A. The malleolar vein. It is connected to the deep veins by numerous perforating veins.

Q. In Figure 7-13, identify J.

A. The perforating veins. Valves in these veins permit flow of blood only from the superficial to the deep veins. Failure of these valves is the cause of varicose ulceration of the skin.

Q. In Figure 7-13, identify K.

A. The medial malleolus.

Q. In Figure 7-13, identify L.

A. The dorsal venous arch. It connects the commencement of the small, short, and the great, long, saphenous systems.

Q. In Figure 7-13, identify M.

A. The medial marginal vein of the foot. It is the commencement of the great saphenous vein.

Q. In Figure 7-13, identify N.

A. The anterior crural tributary to the great saphenous vein.

Q. In Figure 7-13, identify O.

A. The infrapatellar branch of the saphenous nerve.

Q. In Figure 7-13, identify P.

A. The saphenous nerve as it pierces the deep fascia to become superficial. Note its subsequent contiguity with the great saphenous vein. Thrombophlebitis of the vein often involves the saphenous nerve, causing referred pain along the medial margin of the foot.

Q. In Figure 7-13, identify Q.

A. The suprapatellar branch of the medial femoral cutaneous nerve.

Q. In Figure 7-13, identify R.

A. The anterior femoral vein.

Q. In Figure 7-13, identify S.

A. The medial femoral cutaneous nerve.

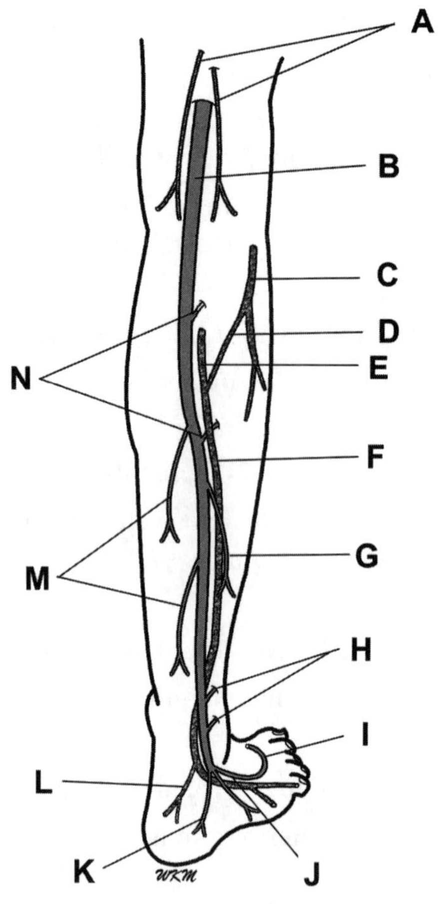

Figure 7-14 The Small Saphenous Vein and Its Accompanying Nerves

Q. In Figure 7-14, identify A.

A. The terminal branches of the posterior femoral cutaneous nerve. Note their close proximity to the small saphenous vein.

Q. In Figure 7-14, identify B.

A. The short saphenous vein. It pierces the deep fascia to terminate in the popliteal vein 2 inches above the knee joint.

Q. In Figure 7-14, identify C.

A. The lateral sural cutaneous nerve. It is a branch of the common fibular nerve.

Q. In Figure 7-14, identify D.

A. The sural communicating nerve. It is a branch of the lateral sural nerve.

Q. In Figure 7-14, identify E.

A. The medial sural cutaneous nerve. It is a branch of the tibial nerve.

Q. In Figure 7-14, identify F.

A. The sural nerve. It is formed by the union of the medial sural nerve and the sural communicating nerve.

Q. In Figure 7-14, identify G.

A. A lateral crural tributary of the small saphenous vein.

Q. In Figure 7-14, identify H.

A. Malleolar perforating branches of the small saphenous vein.

Q. In Figure 7-14, identify I.

A. The dorsal venous arch. It connects the origins of the lateral and medial marginal veins.

Q. The lateral marginal vein continues as . . .

A. The small saphenous vein.

Q. The medial marginal vein continues as . . .

A. The great saphenous vein.

Q. In Figure 7-14, identify J.

A. The lateral marginal vein.

Q. In Figure 7-14, identify K.

A. A calcaneal tributary to the small saphenous vein.

Q. In Figure 7-14, identify L.

A. The calcaneal branch of the sural nerve.

Q. In Figure 7-14, identify M.

A. Posterior crural tributaries of the small saphenous vein.

Q. In Figure 7-14, identify N.

A. Crural perforating branches of the small saphenous vein.

Q. Varicose ulcers are more common on the medial side of the ankle than on the lateral side because . . .

A. The venous pressure at the ankle is higher in the great saphenous vein, particularly in the presence of varicosities, which are much more common in the great saphenous system.

Q. When standing at ease, the venous pressure in the dorsal venous arch is approximately . . .

A. 100 mm of mercury.

Q. The pressure in the dorsal venous arch rapidly falls on activity due to the action of the so-called . . .

A. Muscle pump. Contraction of the muscles in the tightly enclosed fascial compartments of the leg compresses the deep veins and, when the deep valves are competent, drives the blood upward toward the heart.

THE DORSUM OF THE FOOT

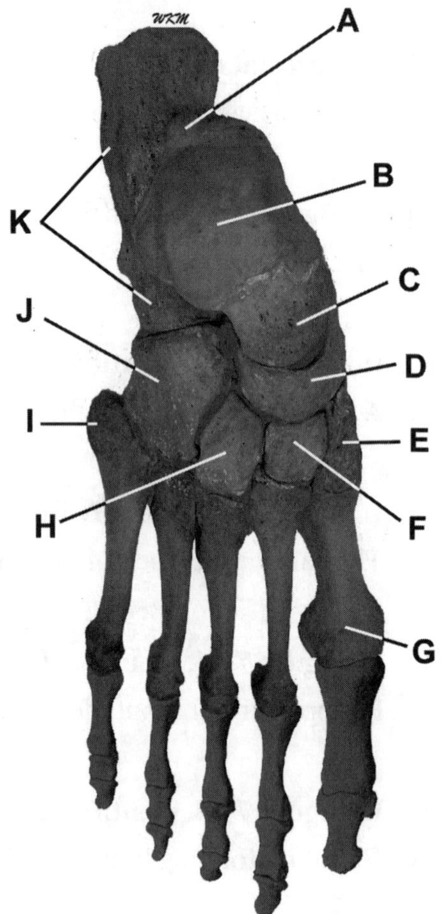

Figure 7-15 The Dorsum of the Foot: Bones

Q. In Figure 7-15, identify A.

A. The posterior tubercle of the talus.

Q. In Figure 7-15, identify B.

A. The trochlear surface of the talus.

Q. In Figure 7-15, identify C.

A. The head of the talus.

Q. In Figure 7-15, identify D.

A. The navicular bone.

Q. In Figure 7-15, identify E.

A. The medial cuneiform bone.

Q. In Figure 7-15, identify F.

A. The intermediate cuneiform bone.

Q. In Figure 7-15, identify G.

A. The head of the 1st metatarsal bone.

Q. In Figure 7-15, identify H.

A. The lateral cuneiform bone.

Q. In Figure 7-15, identify I.

A. The tuberosity, the styloid process, on the base of the 5th metatarsal bone. The fibularis brevis is inserted into it.

Q. In Figure 7-15, identify J.

A. The cuboid bone.

Q. In Figure 7-15, identify K.

A. The calcaneus.

Q. In Figure 7-16, identify A and B.

A. The superior band and the inferior band of the inferior extensor retinaculum, respectively.

Q. In Figure 7-16, identify C.

A. The tendon of the tibialis anterior muscle.

Q. In Figure 7-16, identify D.

A. The tendon of the extensor hallucis longus muscle. It crosses the dorsalis pedis artery superficially.

Q. In Figure 7-16, identify E.

A. The dorsalis pedis artery. After giving off its arcuate branch, it passes between the two heads of the first dorsal interosseous muscle to complete the plantar arterial arch.

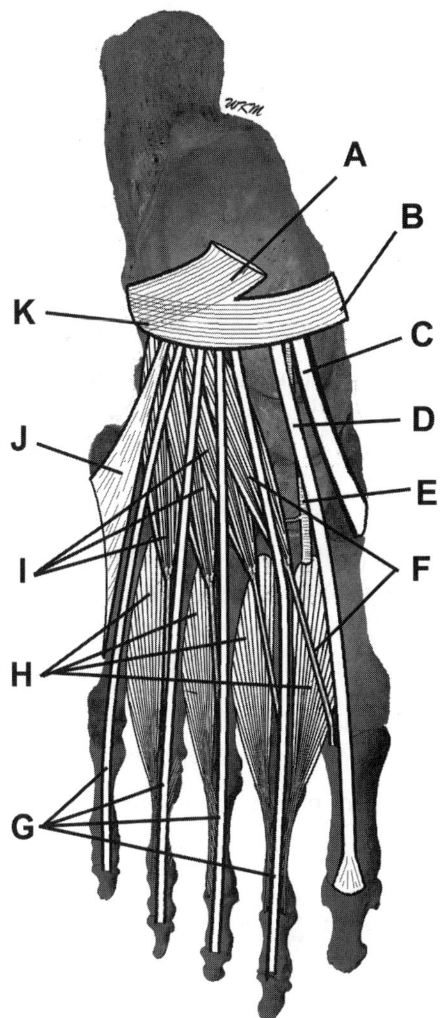

Figure 7-16 The Dorsum of the Foot: Muscles and Tendons

Q. In Figure 7-16, identify F.

A. The extensor hallucis brevis muscle.

Q. In Figure 7-16, identify G.

A. The tendons of the extensor digitorum longus muscle.

Q. In Figure 7-16, identify H.

A. The dorsal interosseous muscles.

Q. In Figure 7-16, identify I.

A. The belly of the extensor digitorum muscle.

Q. In Figure 7-16, identify J.

A. The insertion of the fibularis tertius muscle.

Q. In Figure 7-16, identify K.

A. The stem of the inferior extensor retinaculum. It forms a loop around the tendons of the fibularis tertius muscle and the four tendons of the extensor digitorum longus muscle before it divides into superior and inferior bands.

THE SOLE OF THE FOOT

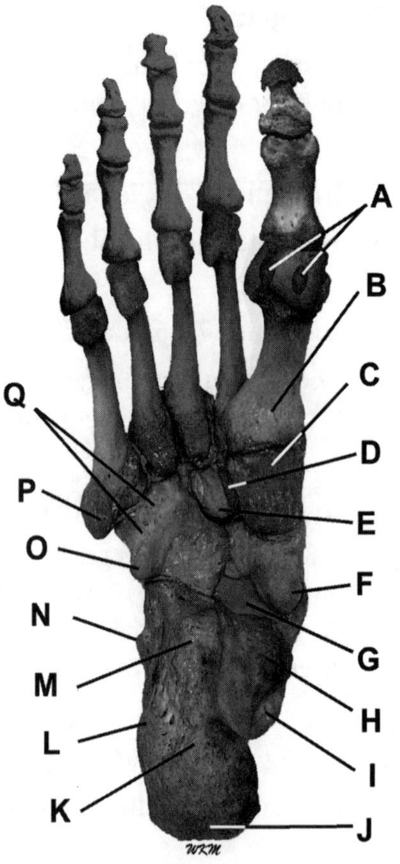

Q. In Figure 7-17, identify A.

A. The sesamoid bones in the tendons of the flexor hallucis brevis muscle.

Q. In Figure 7-17, identify B.

A. The stout base of the 1st metatarsal bone. It provides insertions for the tibialis anterior muscle and for the fibularis longus muscle.

Q. In Figure 7-17, identify C.

A. The medial cuneiform bone. In addition to the tibialis posterior muscle, proximally, it provides attachment for the tibialis anterior muscle on its medial aspect, distally, and for the fibularis longus muscle, laterally.

Q. In Figure 7-17, identify D.

A. The intermediate cuneiform bone. It is seen more easily on the dorsum of the foot.

Figure 7-17 The Plantar Surface of the Foot: Bones

Q. In Figure 7-17, identify E.

A. The lateral cuneiform bone. Together with the majority of the surrounding bones, it provides an additional insertion for the tibialis posterior muscle.

Q. In Figure 7-17, identify F.

A. The tubercle of the navicular bone. Together with the medial cuneiform bone, it provides the major insertion for the tibialis posterior muscle.

Q. In Figure 7-17, identify G.

A. The head of the talus bone. It articulates with the sustentaculum tali of the calcaneus, with the plantar calcaneonavicular (spring) ligament, and with the navicular bone.

Q. In Figure 7-17, identify H.

A. The sustentaculum tali. It is grooved inferiorly by the tendon of flexor hallucis longus muscle. The plantar calcaneonavicular (spring) ligament is attached to its anterior surface.

Q. In Figure 7-17, identify I.

A. The body of the talus. It articulates inferiorly with the calcaneus and superiorly with the tibia.

Q. In Figure 7-17, identify J.

A. The calcaneal tuberosity. It provides attachment to the tendo calcaneus.

Q. In Figure 7-17, identify K.

A. The medial process of the calcaneal tuberosity. Superficially, it provides attachment for the plantar aponeurosis. The abductor hallucis brevis muscle and the flexor digitorum brevis muscle arise from it, deep to the plantar aponeurosis.

Q. In Figure 7-17, identify L.

A. The lateral process of the calcaneal tuberosity. It gives origin to the abductor digiti minimi muscle.

Q. In Figure 7-17, identify M.

A. The tubercle of the calcaneus. It marks the distal end of the attachment of the long plantar ligament to the inferior surface of the calcaneus. Distally, the tubercle gives attachment to the short plantar (plantar calcaneocuboid) ligament.

Q. In Figure 7-17, identify N.

A. The fibular (peroneal) trochlea. It separates the tendons of the fibularis brevis muscle, which grooves the calcaneus above it, and the fibularis longus muscle, which grooves the lateral side of the calcaneus inferior to it. Both pass beneath the inferior fibular retinaculum.

Q. In Figure 7-17, identify O.

A. The lateral end of the ridge of the cuboid bone. It gives attachment to the deeper fibers of the long plantar ligament. The superficial fibers of the ligament continue to the bases of the 2nd, 3rd, and 4th metatarsal bones. Proximal to the ridge, the roughened inferior surface of the cuboid bone gives attachment to the short plantar ligament.

Q. In Figure 7-17, identify P.

A. The tubercle, the styloid process, on the base of the 5th metatarsal bone. It provides insertion for the tendon of the fibularis brevis muscle.

Q. In Figure 7-17, identify Q.

A. The groove on the cuboid bone for the tendon of the fibularis longus muscle.

Q. The sole of the foot is described as having four layers of intrinsic muscles. The deepest layer consists of . . .

A. The four dorsal interossei muscles and the three plantar interossei muscles.

Q. The action of the dorsal interossei muscles is to . . .

A. Abduct the digits, as in the hand. However, when considering abduction and adduction of the toes, the 2nd toe is considered to be the midline of the foot.

Q. The 2nd toe, therefore, has . . .

A. Two dorsal interossei muscles, one on each side. It can only be abducted from the anatomical position. The 3rd and 4th toes have one each, situated on their lateral sides.

Q. In Figure 7-18, identify A.

A. The 1st and 2nd dorsal interosseous muscles.

Q. The plantar interosseous muscles, unlike the dorsal interosseous muscles, each arise from only one metatarsal bone. Their action is to . . .

A. Adduct the toes. The 3rd, 4th, and 5th toes each have a plantar interosseous muscle.

Q. In Figure 7-18, identify B.

A. The three plantar interosseous muscles.

Q. All of the interossei are inserted into . . .

A. The dorsal expansions of the extensor digitorum tendons.

Q. In Figure 7-18, identify C.

A. The tendon of the fibularis longus muscle. It lies in a fibroaponeurotic canal in a groove on the inferior surface of the cuboid bone.

Q. In Figure 7-18, identify D.

A. The insertion of the fibularis brevis.

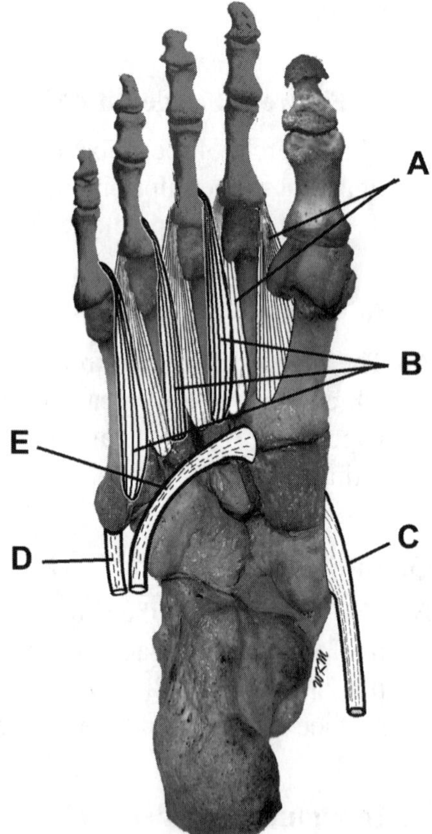

Figure 7-18 The Plantar Surface of the Foot: The Fourth Layer of Muscles

Q. The three muscles that constitute the third layer of the muscles of the foot are . . .

A. The flexor hallucis brevis muscle, the adductor hallucis muscle, and the flexor digiti minimi brevis muscle.

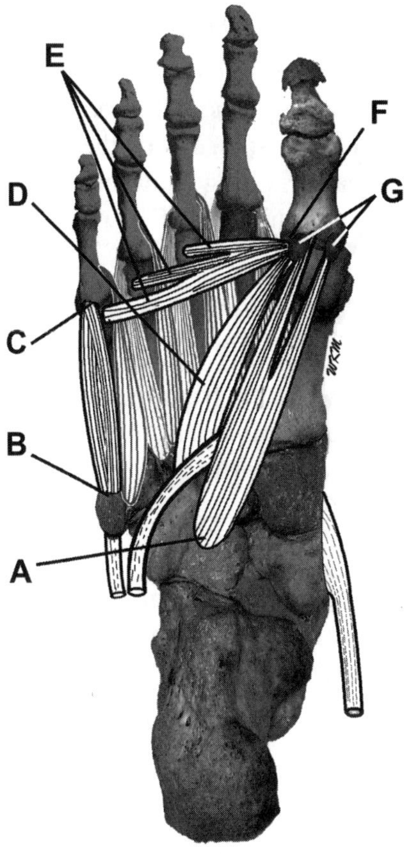

Figure 7-19 The Plantar Surface of the Foot: The Third Layer of Muscles

Q. In Figure 7-19, the proximal attachment of the flexor hallucis brevis muscle, A, is to . . .

A. The plantar surface of the cuboid bone.

Q. In Figure 7-19, the origin of the flexor digiti minimi brevis muscle, B, is from . . .

A. The base of the 5th metatarsal bone.

Q. In Figure 7-19, the insertion of the flexor digiti minimi muscle, C, is into . . .

A. The lateral side of the base of the proximal phalanx of the little toe. It is inserted with the tendon of the abductor digiti minimi muscle.

Q. In Figure 7-19, the proximal attachment of the oblique head of the adductor hallucis muscle, D, is . . .

A. The bases of the 2nd, 3rd, and 4th metatarsal bones and the sheath of the fibularis longusmuscle.

Q. In Figure 7-19, the transverse head of the adductor hallucis muscle, E, arises from . . .

A. The plantar metatarsophalangeal ligaments of the 3rd, 4th, and 5th metatarsal bones.

Q. In Figure 7-19, the distal attachment of the adductor hallucis muscle, F, is . . .

A. The lateral sesamoid bone of the hallux, and hence to the lateral side of the proximal phalanx of the big toe.

Q. In Figure 7-19, distally, the flexor hallucis brevis muscle divides to form two tendons, each of which contains a sesamoid bone, G. Each tendon inserts into . . .

A. Its own side of the base of the proximal phalanx of the great toe.

Q. The function of sesamoid bones is . . .

A. Not known for certain. They may have different functions in different places. These functions may include changing the line of pull of a tendon, reducing friction, and modifying or preventing pressure on vessels or muscles.

Q. The intrinsic muscles of the foot that constitute the second layer of muscles are . . .

A. The lumbrical muscles and the quadratus plantae muscle (the flexor digitorum accessorius muscle). The latter can be considered as part of the flexor digitorum longus muscle, which was "displaced" by the calcaneus from the leg to the foot. The long tendons of the flexor hallucis longus muscle and of the flexor digitorum longus muscle also can be considered to be in this layer. They are not, however, intrinsic muscle of the foot.

Q. The proximal attachments of the flexor digitorum accessorius muscle (the quadratus plantae muscle) are by . . .

A. Two heads from the inferior surface of the calcaneus, one from each side of the long plantar ligament. It is, of course, attached distally to the tendon of the flexor digitorum longus muscle. Its action is to correct the line of pull of the tendons of the flexor digitorum muscle.

Q. The lumbrical muscles arise, as do those in the hand, from the tendons of the long flexor muscles. They are inserted into . . .

A. The dorsal digital expansion of the lateral four toes.

Q. In Figure 7-20, identify A.

A. The first lumbrical muscle. Note that it is the only lumbrical muscle to arise from only one tendon of the flexor digitorum longus and that it is the only lumbrical muscle supplied by the medial plantar nerve.

Q. In Figure 7-20, identify B.

A. The 2nd, 3rd, and 4th lumbrical muscles.

Q. In Figure 7-20, identify C.

A. The tendon of the extensor digitorum longus muscle.

Q. In Figure 7-20, identify D.

A. The quadratus plantae muscle.

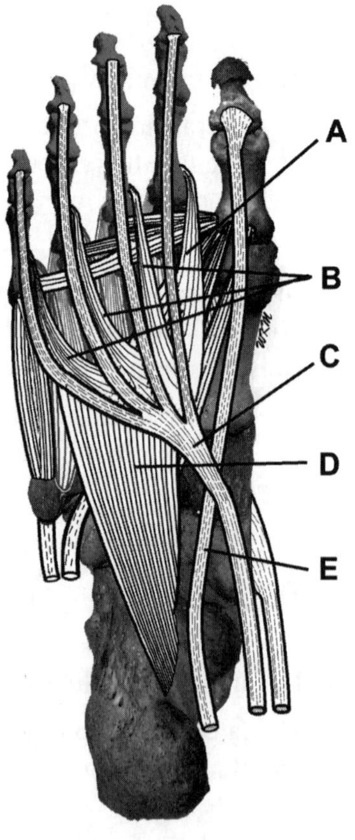

Figure 7-20 The Plantar Surface of the Foot: The Second Layer of Muscles

Q. In Figure 7-20, identify E.

A. The tendon of the flexor hallucis longus muscle. The posterior tibial vessels and the tibial nerve enter the foot in the interval between the tendon of the flexor hallucis longus muscle and the tendon of the flexor digitorum longus muscle.

Q. The muscles of the first, the most superficial, layer of the muscles of the foot are . . .

A. The abductor hallucis muscle, the flexor digitorum brevis muscle, and the abductor digiti minimi muscle.

Q. The proximal attachments of the abductor hallucis muscle are to . . .

A. The surface of the flexor retinaculum and the medial process of the calcaneal tuberosity. Distally, it is attached to the medial side of the proximal phalanx of the great toe.

Q. In Figure 7-21, identify A.

A. The abductor hallucis muscle.

Q. The proximal attachment of the flexor digitorum brevis muscle is to . . .

A. The medial process of the calcaneal tuberosity. Distally, like the flexor digitorum superficialis muscle in the hand, its tendons split to allow perforation by the tendons of the flexor digitorum longus muscle. They are attached to the sides of the middle phalanges of the toes.

Q. In Figure 7-21, identify B.

A. The belly and the four tendons of the flexor digitorum brevis muscle.

Q. The proximal attachment of the abductor digiti minimi muscle is to . . .

A. The lateral process of the calcaneal tuberosity.

Q. In Figure 7-21, identify C.

A. The abductor digiti minimi muscle.

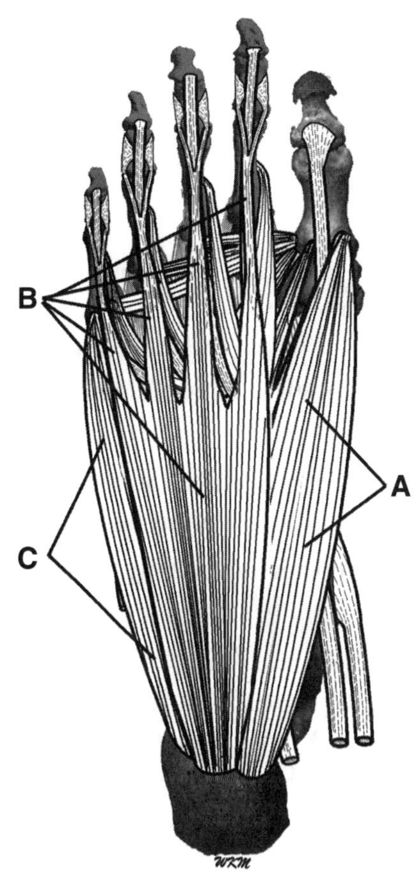

Figure 7-21 The Plantar Surface of the Foot: The First Layer of Muscles

Q. The abductor digiti minimi muscle is inserted distally to . . .

A. The lateral side of the base of the proximal phalanx of the little toe.

Q. The deep fascia superficial to the flexor digitorum brevis muscle is much thickened and firmly adherent to the skin. It is . . .

A. The plantar aponeurosis.

Q. The proximal attachment of the plantar aponeurosis is to . . .

A. The medial process of the calcaneal tuberosity.

Q. Distally, the plantar aponeurosis divides into five thick bands, one for each toe. Each of these bands . . .

A. Gives off two septa that pass upward, one on each side of the corresponding flexor tendon, to fuse with the deep transverse metatarsal ligaments.

Q. The medial and lateral parts of the plantar fascia that cover the two abductor muscles are much thinner, except over . . .

A. The proximal part of the abductor digiti minimi muscle, where it again becomes aponeurotic.

Q. The attachments of the aponeurotic part of the thickened, proximal, lateral plantar fascia are to . . .

A. The lateral process of the calcaneal tuberosity, proximally, and the tubercle on the base of the 5th metatarsal bone base, distally.

Q. The subcutaneous superficial plantar fascia attaches the skin firmly to the underlying plantar aponeurosis. Strong connective tissue binds them both to the . . .

A. Superficial first layer of muscles.

Q. The fourth layer of muscles, the interossei, lie between the metatarsal bones. The muscles of the third layer—the flexor hallucis brevis muscle, the adductor hallucis brevis muscle, and the flexor digiti minimi brevis muscle—are applied closely to the metatarsal bones. Therefore, the vessels and nerves must travel on both surfaces of . . .

A. The second layer of muscles.

Q. The tibial nerve enters the sole of the foot by passing deep to the flexor retinaculum, where it divides into . . .

A. The medial and lateral plantar nerves.

Q. The medial plantar nerve, lying lateral to the medial plantar artery, runs forward, deep to . . .

A. The abductor hallucis muscle.

Q. The medial plantar nerve becomes superficial between the abductor hallucis muscle and . . .

A. The flexor digitorum brevis muscle, at the medial edge of the plantar aponeurosis.

Q. The final terminal branches of the medial plantar nerves are . . .

A. The proper digital branches to the medial three and a half toes.

Q. The muscles supplied by the medial plantar nerve are . . .

A. The abductor hallucis muscle, the flexor hallucis brevis muscle, the flexor digitorum brevis muscle, and the first lumbrical muscle.

Q. The nerve that supplies the remaining 14 muscles of the foot is . . .

A. The lateral plantar nerve.

Q. The lateral plantar nerve arises, together with the medial plantar nerve, from the tibial nerve, deep to the flexor retinaculum. They both pass deep to the abductor hallucis muscle. The lateral plantar nerve then continues across the sole of the foot between . . .

A. The flexor digitorum brevis muscle and the quadratus plantae muscle (the flexor digitorum accessorius muscle).

Q. The relationship of the lateral plantar artery to the lateral plantar nerve is that . . .

A. The lateral plantar artery lies lateral to the lateral plantar nerve.

Q. The lateral plantar nerve divides into its superficial and deep branches at the lateral border of . . .

A. The flexor digitorum brevis muscle.

Q. The superficial branch of the lateral plantar nerve becomes superficial at . . .

A. The lateral border of the plantar aponeurosis, between the flexor digitorum brevis muscle and the abductor digiti minimi muscle.

Q. The final terminal branches of the superficial branch of the lateral plantar nerve are . . .

A. Three proper digital branches to the sides of the lateral one and a half toes.

Q. The deep branch of the lateral plantar nerve accompanies . . .

A. The lateral plantar artery passing medially between the second and third layers of muscles. It terminates by supplying the adductor hallucis muscle. It branches to the 2nd and the 3rd lumbrical muscles, passing deep to the transverse head of the adductor hallucis muscle before looping around it to reach these two lumbrical muscles.

Q. The lateral plantar artery passes through the interval between the bases of the 1st and 2nd metatarsal bones to anastomose with . . .

A. The terminal branch of the dorsalis pedis artery.

Q. The lateral plantar artery, as it crosses the foot medially at the level of the bases of the metatarsal bones, forms . . .

A. The plantar arch. It is completed by the dorsalis pedis artery. Note that there is only one plantar arch in the foot. In the hand, there are two palmar arches: the superficial and the deep palmar arches.

Q. The artery in the hand that is homologous with the dorsalis pedis artery is . . .

A. The radial artery.

Q. The arterial arch in the hand that is homologous with the plantar arch is . . .

A. The deep palmar arch.

Q. The nerve in the hand that is homologous with the lateral plantar nerve is . . .

A. The ulnar nerve.

Q. The nerve in the hand that is homologous with the medial plantar nerve is . . .

A. The median nerve.

THE HIP JOINT

Q. The hip joint is classified as . . .

A. A triaxial, diarthrodial synovial joint. It is between the round head of the femur and the deep acetabular fossa of the innominate bone, the hip bone.

Q. Movements that take place at the hip joint are . . .

A. Flexion, extension, abduction, adduction, and rotation.

Q. The major factor in maintaining the stability of the hip joint is . . .

A. The acetabular fossa and its labrum. It almost completely encloses the head of the femur.

Q. The already deep acetabular fossa is increased in depth by . . .

A. The acetabular labrum, a triangular fibrocartilaginous labrum around the acetabular rim.

Q. The perimeter of the acetabular fossa is incomplete. There is a wide acetabular notch that lies . . .

A. Inferiorly, above the obturator membrane.

Q. The acetabular labrum is carried across the acetabular notch by . . .

A. The transverse acetabular ligament.

Q. The acetabular fossa is not completely lined by cartilage. The cartilage is . . .

A. Horseshoe shaped, with a central deficiency continuous with the acetabular notch.

Q. The acetabular cartilage is thickest . . .

A. Superiorly. This is the area that is normally under pressure during standing and walking.

Q. The femoral head also is not completely covered by cartilage. It has a deficiency . . .

A. In its center, the fovea capitis femoris. The ligamentum teres femoris is attached to it.

Q. The function of the ligamentum teres femoris, the round ligament of the head of the femur, during intrauterine life and early childhood is to . . .

A. Carry a small but important artery, a branch of the obturator artery, to supply blood to the proximal side of the growth plate of the head of the femur. In adult life, the growth plate is no longer present, and therefore this artery has disappeared. Fractures of the neck of the femur in the adult are therefore slow to unite, because the only blood supply to the femoral head is along the neck of the femur. The vessels travel in bands of fibrous tissue, the retinacula. This supply is disrupted by a fracture.

Q. The capsular ligament is thick anteriorly but thinner posteroinferiorly. It is lined by synovial membrane. It is attached to the innominate bone, the os coxa, by . . .

A. The acetabular labrum and the adjacent bone of the acetabular margin.

Q. The capsular ligament is attached distally to . . .

A. The intertrochanteric line of the femur, anteriorly, and to the neck of the femur, posteriorly.

Q. The three ligaments that strengthen the capsule are . . .

A. The iliofemoral ligament, the pubofemoral ligament, and the ischiofemoral ligament. All are triangular. Of the three, only the iliofemoral ligament has its base on the femur and its apex attached to the hipbone.

Q. In Figure 7-22, identify A.

A. The anterior superior iliac spine.

Q. In Figure 7-22, identify B.

A. The anterior inferior iliac spine. Both the iliofemoral ligament and the straight head of the rectus femoris are attached to it.

Q. In Figure 7-22, identify C.

A. The lateral band of the iliofemoral ligament.

Q. In Figure 7-22, identify D.

A. The greater trochanter of the femur.

Q. In Figure 7-22, identify E.

A. The intertrochanteric line on the femur.

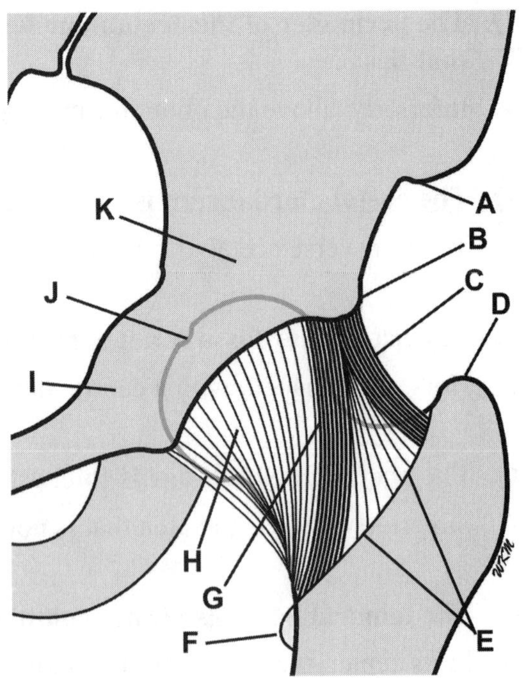

Figure 7-22 The Hip Joint: Anterior Ligaments

Q. In Figure 7-22, identify F.

A. The lesser trochanter of the femur.

Q. In Figure 7-22, identify G.

A. The medial band of the iliofemoral ligament.

Q. In Figure 7-22, identify H.

A. The pubofemoral ligament. It is also a triangular ligament, but its base is at the acetabular rim. Its apex is at the lesser trochanter. Its major attachments, superiorly, are to the pubic part of the acetabular rim. It is the thinnest of the three major ligaments of the hip joint.

Q. In Figure 7-22, identify I.

A. The pubic contribution to the acetabulum.

Q. In Figure 7-22, identify J.

A. The fovea capitis femoris. It marks the attachment of the ligament of the head of the femur.

Q. In Figure 7-22, identify K.

A. The iliac contribution to the acetabulum.

Q. In Figure 7-23, identify A.

A. The ischial tuberosity.

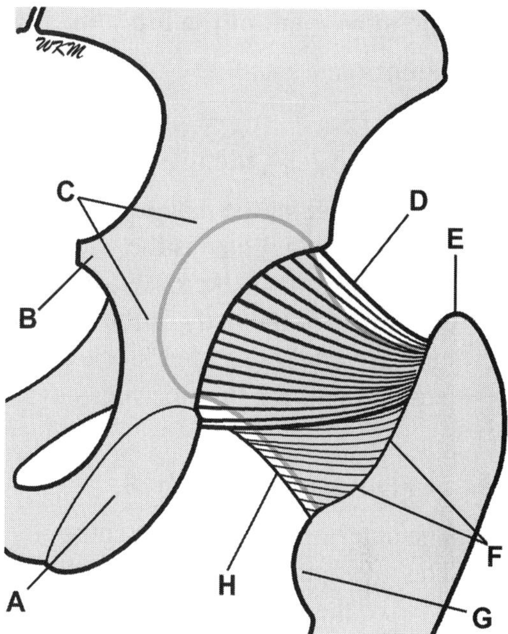

Figure 7-23 The Hip Joint: Posterior Ligaments

Q. In Figure 7-23, identify B.

A. The ischial spine.

Q. In Figure 7-23, identify C.

A. The ischial contribution to the acetabulum.

Q. In Figure 7-23, identify D.

A. The thick ischiofemoral ligament. Its fibers spiral upward and laterally from their broad attachment to the acetabular labrum, across the back of the femoral neck, to the base of the greater trochanter of the femur. It limits extension of the joint.

Q. In Figure 7-23, identify E.

A. The greater trochanter.

Q. In Figure 7-23, identify F.

A. The intertrochanteric crest.

Q. In Figure 7-23, identify G.

A. The lesser trochanter.

Q. In Figure 7-23, identify H.

A. The thin, inferior pubofemoral ligament.

Q. The attachments of the pubofemoral ligament are . . .

A. Proximally, to the iliopubic eminence and the acetabular extremity of the superior ramus of the pubis. Distally, it fuses with the medial band of the iliofemoral ligament.

Q. The strongest of the ligaments of the hip joint is . . .

A. The iliofemoral ligament, the Y-shaped ligament of Bigelow. Superiorly, it is attached to the anterior inferior iliac spine. Inferiorly, it has two immensely strong bands that diverge. They are attached to either end of the intertrochanteric line of the femur. The central part of the ligament is relatively thin.

Q. The movement of the hip joint that is limited by the iliofemoral ligament is . . .

A. Extension.

Q. In Figure 7-24, identify A.

A. The tubercle of the iliac crest. The intertubercular plane is the widest part of the pelvis. It crosses the upper part of the body of the 5th lumbar vertebra and marks the beginning of the inferior vena cava.

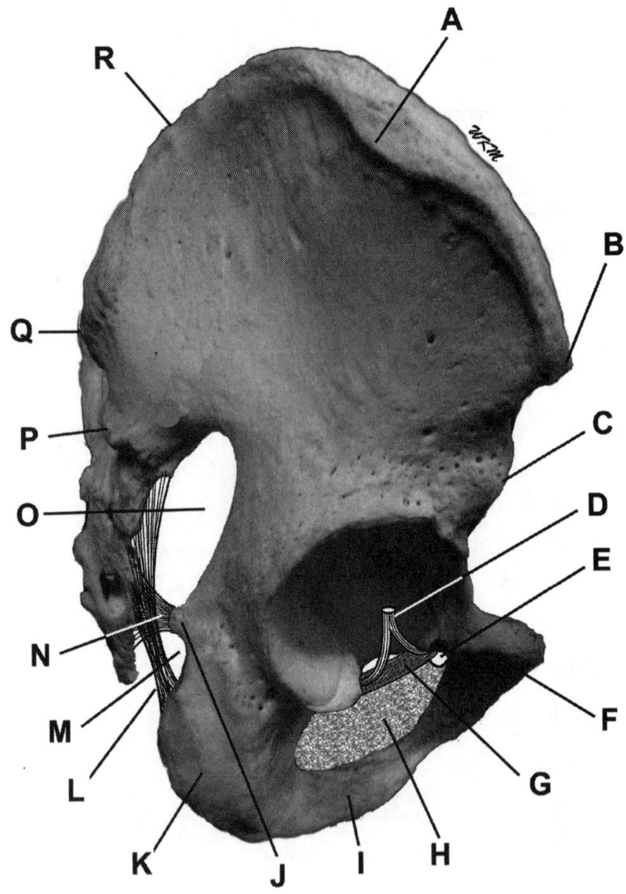

Figure 7-24 The Hip Joint, Lateral Aspect: Bones and Ligaments

Q. In Figure 7-24, identify B.

A. The anterior superior iliac spine. The interspinous plane marks the level of the sacral promontory.

Q. In Figure 7-24, identify C.

A. The anterior inferior iliac spine. It cannot be palpated.

Q. In Figure 7-24, identify D.

A. The ligament of the head of the femur. It carries a small artery to the head of the femur from either a branch of the medial circumflex femoral artery, a branch of the obturator artery, or of their anastomosis. These arteries reach the ligament by traversing the space between the transverse acetabular ligament and the acetabular notch.

Q. In Figure 7-24, identify E.

A. The obturator canal. The obturator nerve and the obturator vessels enter the thigh through the obturator canal.

Q. In Figure 7-24, identify F.

A. The body of the pubis.

Q. In Figure 7-24, identify G.

A. The transverse acetabular ligament. The glenoidal labrum is completed along its margin.

Q. In Figure 7-24, identify H.

A. The obturator membrane.

Q. In Figure 7-24, identify I.

A. The ramus of the ischium.

Q. In Figure 7-24, identify J.

A. The spine of the ischium.

Q. In Figure 7-24, identify K.

A. The ischial tuberosity.

Q. In Figure 7-24, identify L.

A. The sacrotuberous ligament.

Q. In Figure 7-24, identify M.

A. The lesser sciatic foramen.

Q. In Figure 7-24, identify N.

A. The sacrospinous ligament.

Q. In Figure 7-24, identify O.

A. The greater sciatic foramen.

Q. In Figure 7-24, identify P.

A. The posterior inferior iliac spine.

Q. In Figure 7-24, identify Q.

A. The posterior superior iliac spine.

Q. In Figure 7-24, identify R.

A. The iliac crest.

Q. In Figure 7-25, identify A.

A. The gluteus minimus muscle.

Q. In Figure 7-25, identify B.

A. The reflected head of the rectus femoris muscle.

Q. In Figure 7-25, identify C.

A. The straight head of the rectus femoris muscle.

Q. In Figure 7-25, identify D.

A. The iliopsoas muscle. It is inserted into the lesser trochanter of the femur.

Q. In Figure 7-25, identify E.

A. The pectineus muscle.

Q. In Figure 7-25, identify F.

A. The obturator externus muscle. It is inserted into the greater trochanter of the femur.

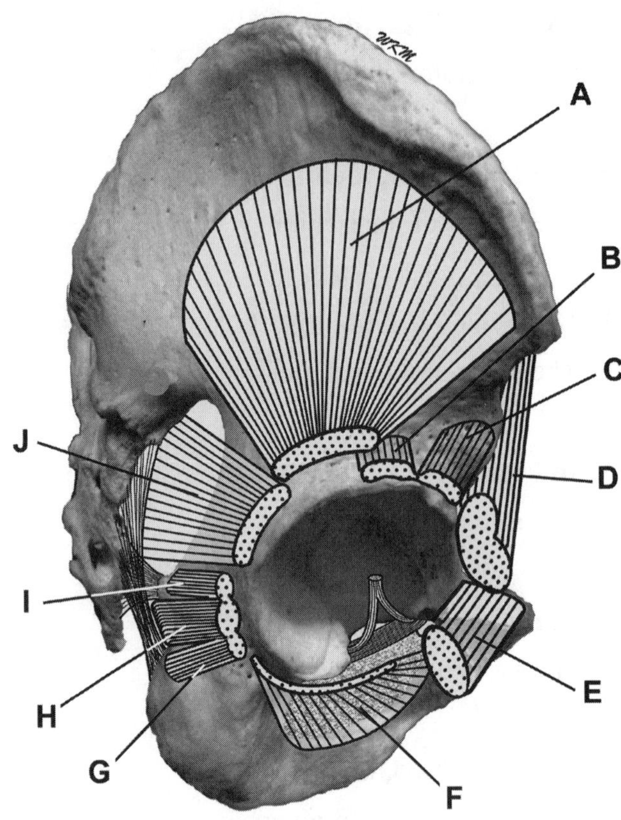

Figure 7-25 The Hip Joint, Lateral Aspect: The Inner Ring of Muscles

Q. In Figure 7-25, identify G.

A. The inferior gemellus muscle.

Q. In Figure 7-25, identify H.

A. The obturator internus muscle. It arises from the medial surface of the obturator membrane and the surrounding bone and is inserted into the greater trochanter of the femur.

Q. In Figure 7-25, identify I.

A. The superior gemellus muscle.

Q. In Figure 7-25, identify J.

A. The piriformis muscle. It arises from the anterior surface of the sacrum between the sacral foramina. It is inserted into the tip of the greater trochanter of the femur.

Q. In Figure 7-26, identify A.

A. The quadratus femoris muscle.

Q. In Figure 7-26, identify B.

A. The gluteus maximus muscle.

Q. In Figure 7-26, identify C.

A. The gluteus medius muscle.

Q. In Figure 7-26, identify D.

A. The tensor fasciae latae muscle.

Q. In Figure 7-26, identify E.

A. The sartorius muscle.

Q. In Figure 7-26, identify F.

A. The adductor longus muscle.

Q. In Figure 7-26, identify G.

A. The adductor brevis muscle.

Q. In Figure 7-26, identify H.

A. The gracilis muscle.

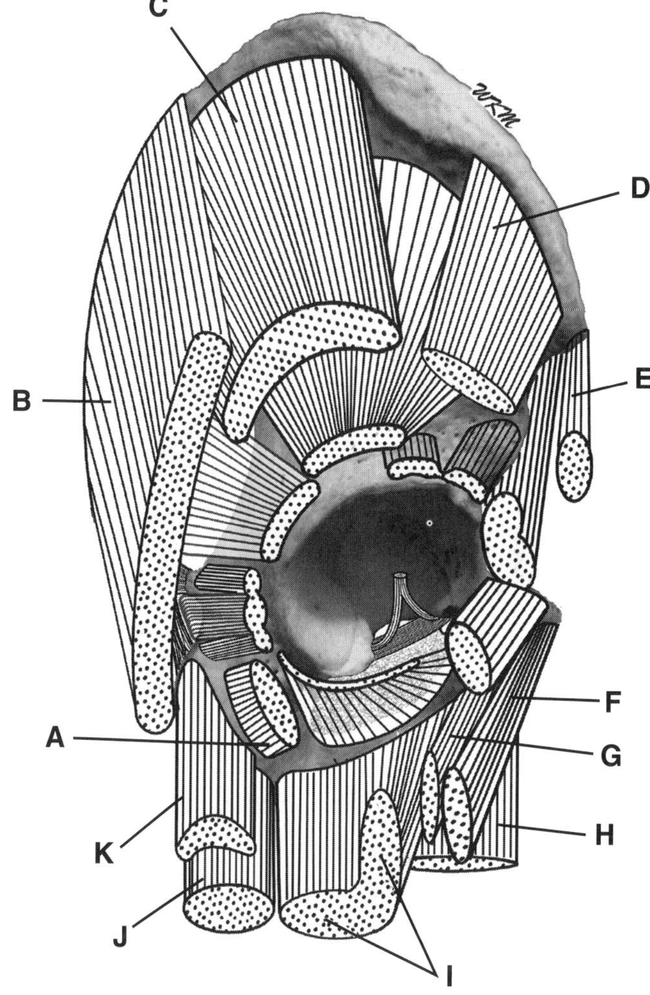

Figure 7-26 The Hip Joint, Lateral Aspect: The Outer Ring of Muscles

Q. In Figure 7-26, identify I.

A. The adductor and the hamstring parts of the adductor magnus muscle.

Q. In Figure 7-26, identify J.

A. The common tendinous origin of the long head of the biceps femoris muscle and the semitendinosus muscle.

Q. In Figure 7-26, identify K.

A. The semimembranosus muscle.

Q. The actions of the muscles that move the hip joint, as in all joints, are determined by their attachments. The action of the medial group of muscles (e.g., the adductor longus muscle, the adductor brevis muscle and the adductor magnus muscle) is . . .

A. Adduction of the hip.

Q. The action of the lateral group of muscles (e.g., the gluteus medius muscle and the gluteus minimus muscle) is . . .

A. Abduction of the hip.

Q. The anterior muscles are flexors of the hip. They are . . .

A. The iliopsoas muscle, the rectus femoris muscle, and the sartorius muscle.

Q. The posterior muscles are extensors of the hip. They are . . .

A. The gluteus maximus muscle and the hamstring muscles: the semitendinosus muscle, the semimembranosus muscle, and the biceps femoris muscle.

Q. Medial rotation of the hip is relatively weak. The muscles involved are . . .

A. The anterior fibers of the gluteus minimus muscle, the anterior fibers of the gluteus medius muscles, and, in some positions of the joint, the iliopsoas muscle.

Q. Lateral rotation of the hip involves a number of muscles. They include . . .

A. The piriformis muscle, the obturator internus muscle, and the quadratus femoris muscle. The adductor muscles are both adductors and lateral rotators.

Q. The major factor in maintaining the stability of the hip joint is . . .

A. The shape of the bone ends.

Q. The most important ligament in stabilizing the hip joint is . . .

A. The iliofemoral ligament. In contrast to the rotator cuff muscles in the shoulder, the muscles surrounding the hip play an insignificant role in preventing dislocation of the hip joint.

Q. In congenital dysplasia (dislocation) of the hip, the acetabulum is shallow and the ligaments are softened by the placental passage of . . .

A. The maternal hormone relaxin to the fetus. Maternal production of relaxin occurs in late pregnancy to "soften" the maternal pelvic ligaments.

Q. In congenital dysplasia of the hip, the head of the femur is displaced . . .

A. Upward due to muscle overaction. Maintenance of 90° of abduction of the hip from birth continued for the early months of extrauterine life allows the ligaments to recover and the acetabulum to form properly. Improper treatment or absence of treatment allows the resulting deformity to become extreme. If treatment is delayed until after the child starts to walk, major surgery is required for a good result.

Q. Congenital dislocation of the hip is much more common in . . .

A. Females, American Indians, and the Mediterranean races.

THE KNEE JOINT

Q. In Figure 7-27, identify A.

A. The shaft of the femur. Note that its long axis is deviated laterally from the vertical line of the tibia.

Q. In Figure 7-27, identify B.

A. The adductor tubercle. It is the attachment of the hamstring portion of the adductor magnus muscle.

Q. In Figure 7-27, identify C.

A. The medial epicondyle of the femur.

Q. In Figure 7-27, identify D.

A. The rounded medial condyle of the femur.

Q. In Figure 27, identify E.

A. The flattened medial condyle of the tibia.

Q. In Figure 7-27, identify F.

A. The medial intercondylar tubercle.

Q. In Figure 7-27, identify G.

A. The apex of the patella.

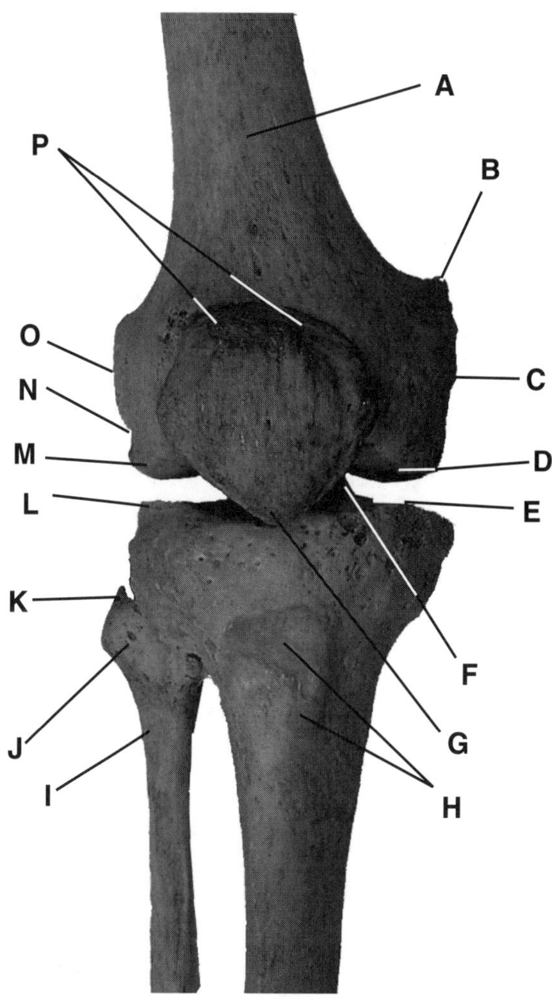

Figure 7-27 The Right Knee Joint, Anterior Aspect: Bones

Q. In Figure 7-27, identify H.

A. The tibial tuberosity. The superior smooth area of the tuberosity is for the attachment of the ligamentum patellae. The roughened lower part of the tibial tuberosity is separated from the skin by the subcutaneous infrapatellar bursa.

Q. In Figure 7-27, identify I.

A. The neck of the fibula.

Q. The nerve that winds around the neck of the fibula is . . .

A. The common fibular (peroneal) nerve. It is vulnerable to direct trauma at this point.

Q. In Figure 7-27, identify J.

A. The head of the fibula.

Q. The joint between the head of the fibula and the lateral condyle of the tibia, the superior tibiofibular joint, is a . . .

A. Diarthrodial synovial joint.

Q. The inferior tibiofibular joint is a . . .

A. Syndesmosis. It is a fibrous joint that lacks a synovial cavity.

Q. In Figure 7-27, identify K.

A. The apex, styloid process, of the fibula. The fibular collateral ligament of the knee joint is attached to the head of the fibula immediately anterior to the apex of the bone.

Q. In Figure 7-27, identify L.

A. The flattened lateral tibial condyle.

Q. In Figure 7-27, identify M.

A. The curved lateral femoral condyle.

Q. In Figure 7-27, identify N.

A. The groove for the tendon of the popliteus muscle. The tendon separates the fibular collateral ligament from the lateral meniscus.

Q. In Figure 7-27, identify O.

A. The lateral epicondyle of the femur.

Q. In Figure 7-27, identify P.

A. The upper border of the patella.

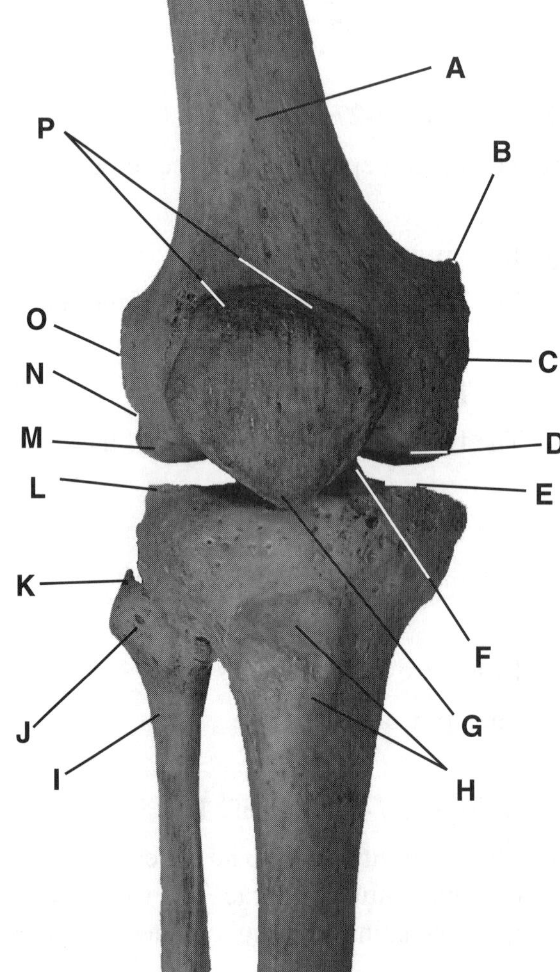

Figure 7-27 The Right Knee Joint, Anterior Aspect: Bones

Q. The muscles inserted into the upper border of the patella are . . .

A. The deeper vastus intermedius muscle and the more superficial rectus femoris muscle.

Q. In Figure 7-28, identify A.

A. The medial collateral ligament of the knee joint. Note its attachment to the periphery of the medial meniscus.

Q. In Figure 7-28, identify B.

A. The medial meniscus. It is much thicker at its peripheral margin.

Q. In Figure 7-28, identify C.

A. The central part of the ligamentum patellae.

Q. In Figure 7-28, identify D.

A. The interosseous membrane.

Q. In Figure 7-28, identify E.

A. Opening for the anterior tibial vessels. The nerve to the muscles in the anterior compartment of the leg is the deep branch of the common fibular nerve.

Q. In Figure 7-28, identify F.

A. The thickened anterior part of the capsule of the superior tibiofibular joint.

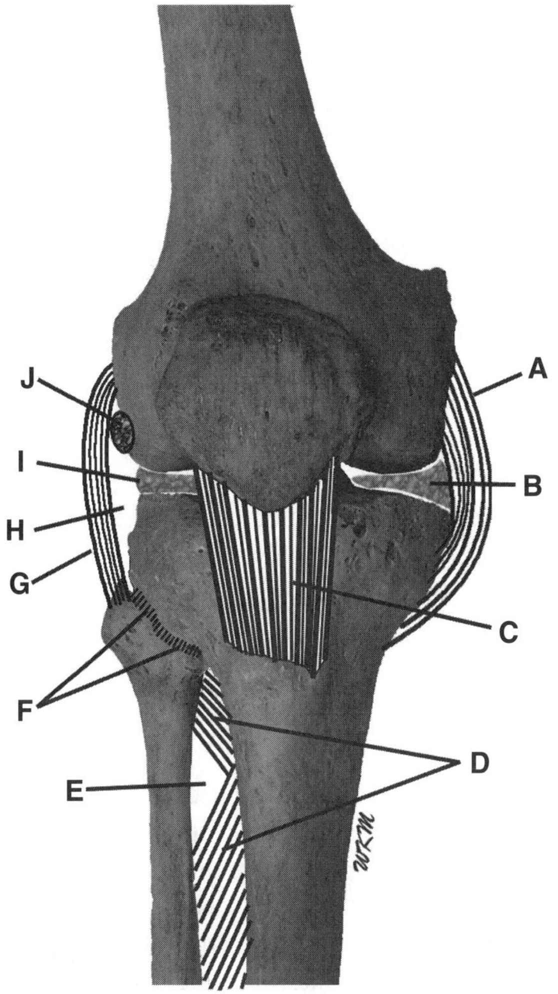

Figure 7-28 The Right Knee Joint, Anterior Aspect: Ligaments and Cartilages

Q. In Figure 7-28, identify G.

A. The lateral (fibular) collateral ligament of the knee joint. Note that it is *not* attached to the lateral meniscus.

Q. In Figure 7-28, identify H.

A. The interval through which the lateral inferior genicular vessels pass.

Q. In Figure 7-28, identify I.

A. The lateral meniscus. It is not attached to the fibular collateral ligament.

Q. In Figure 7-28, identify J.

A. The tendon of the popliteus muscle.

Q. In Figure 7-29, identify A.

A. The tendon of the biceps femoris muscle.

Q. In Figure 7-29, identify B.

A. The iliotibial tract.

Q. In Figure 7-29, identify C.

A. The vastus lateralis muscle.

Q. In Figure 7-29, identify D.

A. The vastus intermedius muscle.

Q. In Figure 7-29, identify E.

A. The rectus femoris muscle.

Q. In Figure 7-29, identify F.

A. The vastus medialis muscle. Note the oblique direction of its lower fibers. This part of the muscle is sometimes called the vastus obliquus medialis. It serves to reduce the possibility of lateral dislocation of the patella.

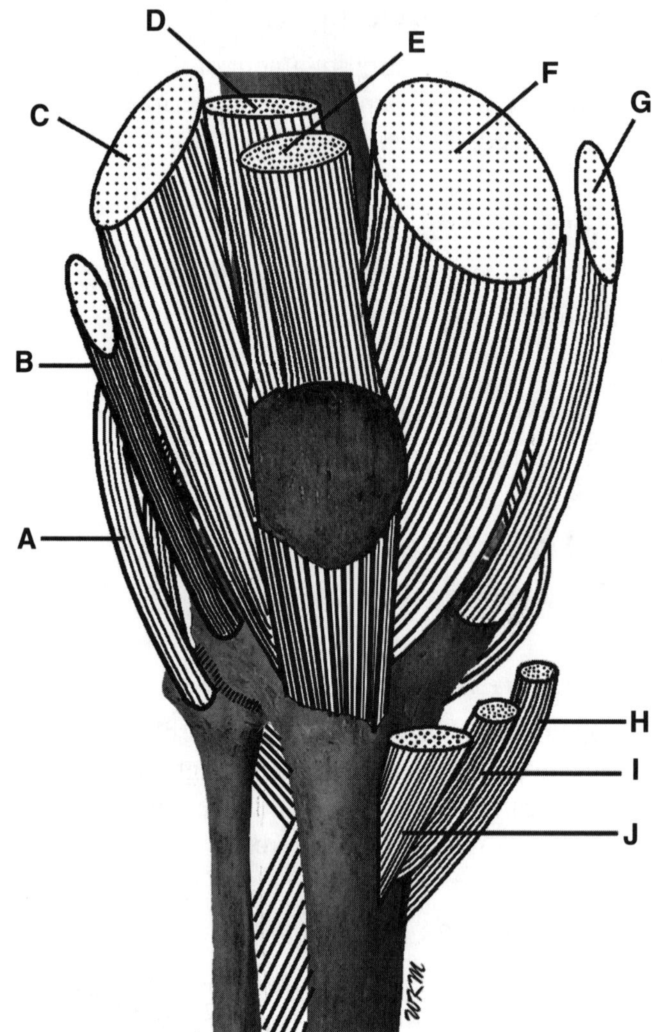

Figure 7-29 The Right Knee Joint, Anterior Aspect: Muscles and Tendons

Q. In Figure 7-29, identify G.

A. The semimembranosus muscle.

Q. In Figure 7-29, identify H.

A. The semitendinosus muscle.

Q. In Figure 7-29, identify I.

A. The gracilis muscle.

Q. In Figure 7-29, identify J.

A. The sartorius muscle. The insertions of the sartorius muscle, the gracilis muscle, and the semitendinosus muscle are collectively called the *pes anserinus*, "the foot of the duck."

Q. In Figure 7-30, identify A.

A. The soleal line. The popliteus muscle arises from the tibia from an area above and medial to this ridge. The ridge gives attachment to the tibial origin of the soleus muscle.

Q. In Figure 7-30, identify B.

A. The groove on the medial condyle of the tibia. It separates the attachment of the tibial collateral ligament, superiorly, from the attachment of the semimembranosus muscle, inferiorly.

Q. In Figure 7-30, identify C.

A. The medial intercondylar tubercle.

Q. In Figure 7-30, identify D.

A. The medial epicondyle. The tibial (medial) collateral ligament gains attachment to it.

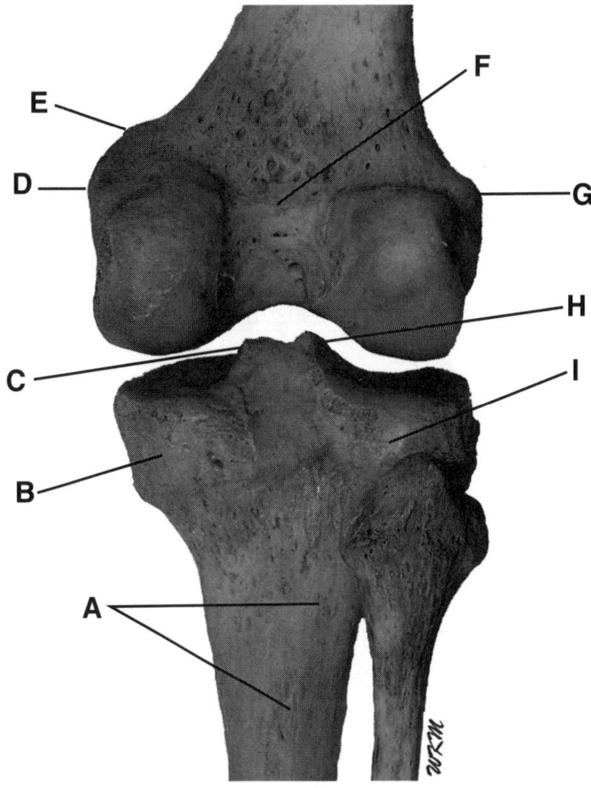

Figure 7-30 The Right Knee Joint, Posterior Aspect: Bones

Q. In Figure 7-30, identify E.

A. The adductor tubercle.

Q. In Figure 7-30, identify F.

A. The intercondylar line. It separates the intercondylar area from the posterior surface of the femur.

Q. In Figure 7-30, identify G.

A. The lateral epicondyle. The interepicondylar distance is the greatest width of the bone.

Q. In Figure 7-30, identify H.

A. The lateral intercondylar tubercle. The anterior and posterior attachments of the lateral meniscus are immediately anterior and posterior to the lateral intercondylar tubercle, respectively.

Q. In Figure 7-30, identify I.

A. The groove for the tendon of the popliteus muscle.

Q. In Figure 7-31, identify A.

A. The tendon of the semimembranosus muscle.

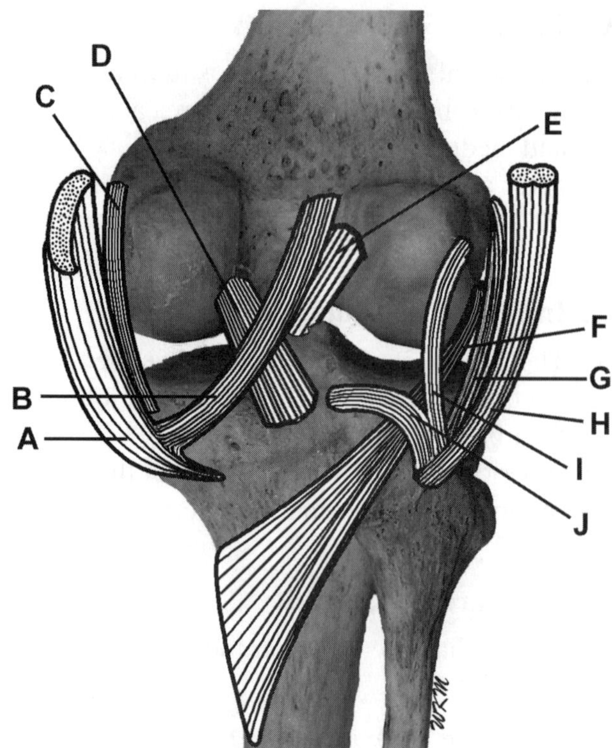

Figure 7-31 The Right Knee Joint, Posterior Aspect: Ligaments and Tendons
Note: The menisci and the capsule have been omitted for the sake of clarity.

Q. In Figure 7-31, identify B.

A. The oblique popliteal ligament. It is an expansion of the tendon of insertion of the semimembranosus muscle.

Q. In Figure 7-31, identify C.

A. The tibial collateral ligament.

Q. In Figure 7-31, identify D.

A. The posterior cruciate ligament. It prevents posterior displacement of the tibia on the femur.

Q. In Figure 7-31, identify E.

A. The anterior cruciate ligament. It prevents anterior displacement of the tibia on the femur.

Q. In Figure 7-31, identify F.

A. The tendon of the popliteus muscle.

Q. In Figure 7-31, identify G.

A. The fibular collateral ligament.

Q. In Figure 7-31, identify H.

A. The tendon of the biceps femoris muscle.

Q. In Figure 7-31, identify I.

A. The anterior limb of the arcuate popliteal ligament. It is sometimes called the short lateral genual ligament.

Q. In Figure 7-31, identify J.

A. The posterior limb of the arcuate popliteal ligament.

Q. In Figure 7-32, identify A.

A. The adductor hiatus.

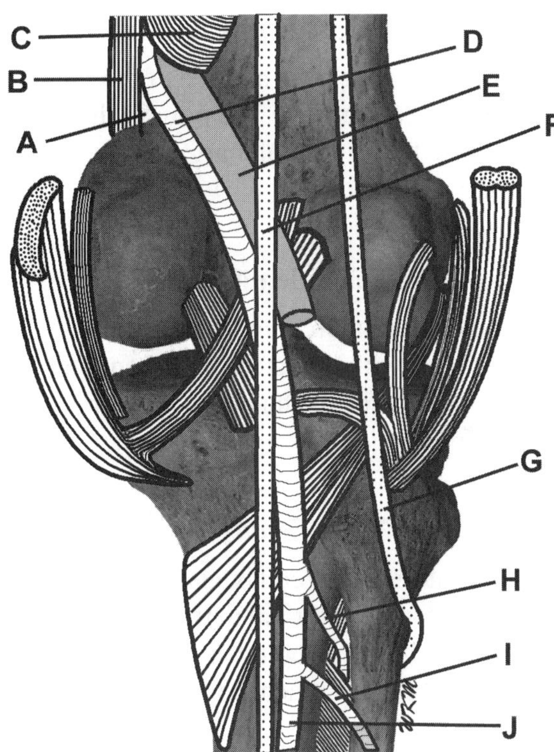

Figure 7-32 The Right Knee Joint, Posterior Aspect: Vessels and Nerves
Note: The menisci and the capsule have been omitted for the sake of clarity.

Q. In Figure 7-32, identify B.

A. The hamstring part of the adductor magnus muscle. It is supplied by a branch of the tibial nerve.

Q. In Figure 7-32, identify C.

A. The adductor part of the adductor magnus muscle. It is supplied by the posterior division of the obturator nerve.

Q. In Figure 7-32, identify D.

A. The popliteal artery. It is the continuation of the femoral artery.

Q. In Figure 7-32, identify E.

A. The popliteal vein.

Q. In Figure 7-32, identify F.

A. The tibial nerve.

Q. In Figure 7-32, identify G.

A. The common fibular (common peroneal) nerve.

Q. In Figure 7-32, identify H.

A. The anterior tibial artery. The tibial artery supplies the muscle in the anterior compartment of the leg. It reaches the anterior compartment by passing above the main part of the interosseous membrane. In the anterior compartment, it is accompanied by the deep fibular nerve, a branch of the common fibular nerve.

Q. In Figure 7-32, identify I.

A. The fibular (peroneal) artery. It supplies the muscles in the lateral compartment of the leg. The corresponding nerve is the superficial fibular branch of the common fibular nerve.

Q. In Figure 7-32, identify J.

A. The posterior tibial artery.

Q. In Figure 7-33, identify A.

A. The weight-bearing surface of the medial condyle of the tibia. The point indicated is close to the medial margin of the medial meniscus.

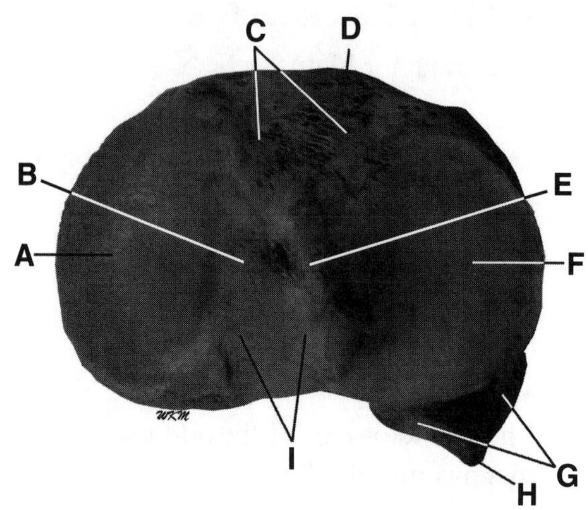

Figure 7-33 The Proximal Surface of the Right Tibia and Fibula: Bone Markings

Q. In Figure 7-33, identify B.

A. The medial intercondylar tubercle. Together with the lateral intercondylar tubercle, it forms the intercondylar eminence.

Q. In Figure 7-33, identify C.

A. The anterior intercondylar area. The inferior end of the anterior cruciate ligament and the anterior horns of both the medial and lateral menisci are all attached to this area.

Q. In Figure 7-33, identify D.

A. The tuberosity of the tibia.

Q. In Figure 7-33, identify E.

A. The lateral intercondylar tubercle. The anterior and posterior horns of the lateral lemniscus are attached to the small depressions on its anterior and posterior slopes.

Q. In Figure 7-33, identify F.

A. The weight-bearing surface of the lateral condyle of the tibia. The point indicated is close to the thin medial margin of the lateral meniscus.

Q. In Figure 7-33, identify G.

A. The head of the fibula.

Q. In Figure 7-33, identify H.

A. The apex, the styloid process, of the fibula.

Q. In Figure 7-33, identify I.

A. The posterior intercondylar area of the tibia. The inferior end of the posterior cruciate ligament, the posterior horn of the medial meniscus, and the posterior horn of the lateral meniscus are all attached to this area.

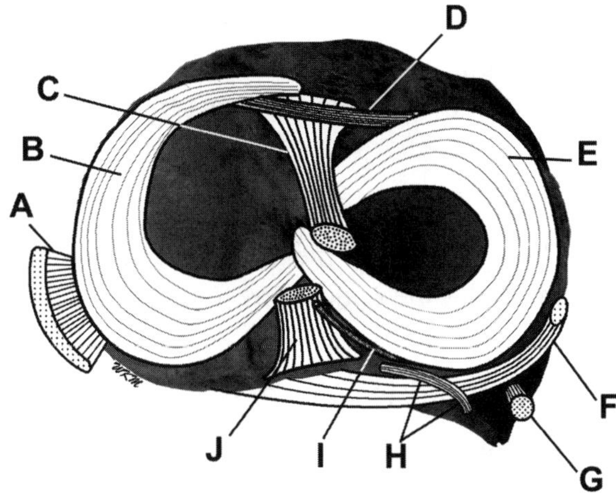

Figure 7-34 The Proximal Surface of the Right Tibia and Fibula: Menisci and Ligaments

Q. In Figure 7-34, identify A.

A. The tibial collateral ligament.

Q. In Figure 7-34, identify B.

A. The medial meniscus. Note that it fuses with the tibial collateral ligament.

Q. In Figure 7-34, identify C.

A. The anterior cruciate ligament. It is attached superiorly to the posterior part of the medial surface of the lateral condyle of the femur. When the knee is weight-bearing, the medial meniscus is trapped between the tibia and the femur. Force applied to the lateral side of the knee will tighten the tibial collateral ligament. When the force is excessive and the knee is weight-bearing, the medial meniscus often is torn.

Q. In Figure 7-34, identify D.

A. The transverse, the meniscomeniscal, ligament.

Q. In Figure 7-34, identify E.

A. The lateral meniscus. Note that it is *not* fused with the fibular collateral ligament. It is only rarely torn.

Q. In Figure 7-34, identify G.

A. The fibular collateral ligament. It is separated from the lateral meniscus by the tendon of the popliteus.

Q. In Figure 7-34, identify H.

A. The posterior limb of the arcuate popliteal ligament.

Q. In Figure 7-34, identify I.

A. The posterior meniscofemoral ligament.

Q. In Figure 7-34, identify J.

A. The posterior cruciate ligament. It is attached superiorly to the anterior part of the lateral surface of the medial condyle of the femur. It prevents posterior dislocation of the tibia on the femur.

Q. The stability of any joint depends on three factors. They are . . .

A. The configuration of the bone ends, the strength of the ligaments, and the strength and condition of the muscles that move the joint.

Q. The stability of the knee joint depends on . . .

A. The ligaments of the joints and the strength and condition of the muscles of the joint, in particular the quadriceps femoris muscle.

Q. Anterior dislocation of the knee results in tearing of . . .

A. The anterior cruciate ligament.

Q. Posterior dislocation of the knee results in tearing of . . .

A. The posterior cruciate ligament.

Q. A tear of the tibial collateral ligament is usually caused by . . .

A. A blow on the lateral side of the knee joint when the foot is planted.

Q. It is often accompanied by a tear of . . .

A. The medial meniscus. The medial meniscus is attached to the tibial collateral ligament.

Q. The lateral meniscus is much less frequently torn because . . .

A. It is separated from the fibular collateral ligament by the tendon of the popliteus muscle.

THE ANKLE JOINT AND THE TARSAL JOINTS

Q. The ankle joint is the joint between . . .

A. The tibia, the fibula, and the talus.

Q. The movements that occur at the ankle joint are . . .

A. Flexion and extension. A small amount of rotation is possible when the joint is in extreme plantar flexion. This is one of the reasons that very high-heeled shoes allow increased inversion and eversion, resulting in an unstable and characteristic gait.

Q. The stability of the ankle joint depends on . . .

A. The configuration of the bones and the strength of the ligaments of the joint.

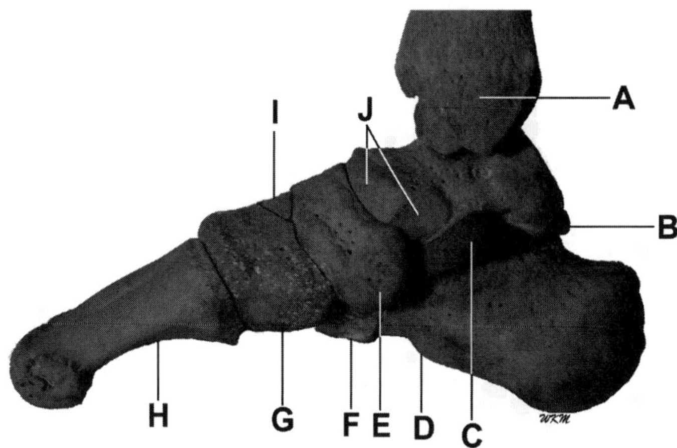

Figure 7-35 The Ankle and the Tarsal Joints, Medial Aspect: Bones

Q. In Figure 7-35, identify A.

A. The medial malleolus of the tibia.

Q. In Figure 7-35, identify B.

A. The medial tubercle of the talus.

Q. In Figure 7-35, identify C.

A. The sustentaculum tali of the calcaneus.

Q. In Figure 7-35, identify D.

A. The tubercle of the calcaneus.

Q. In Figure 7-35, identify E.

A. The tuberosity of the navicular bone. It is readily palpable on the medial border of the foot.

Q. In Figure 7-35, identify F.

A. The crest of the cuboid bone.

Q. In Figure 7-35, identify G.

A. The medial cuneiform bone.

Q. In Figure 7-35, identify H.

A. The 1st metatarsal bone.

Q. In Figure 7-35, identify I.

A. The intermediate cuneiform bone.

Q. In Figure 7-35, identify J.

A. The head of the talus bone. It is separated from the body of the talus, which articulates with the tibia and fibula, by a slightly constricted region, the neck.

Q. In Figure 7-36, identify A.

A. The anterior tibiotalar ligament.

Q. In Figure 7-36, identify B.

A. The tibionavicular ligament. It fuses with the medial margin of the plantar calcaneonavicular (spring) ligament.

Q. In Figure 7-36, identify C.

A. The tibiocalcaneal ligament. It is attached to the sustentaculum tali.

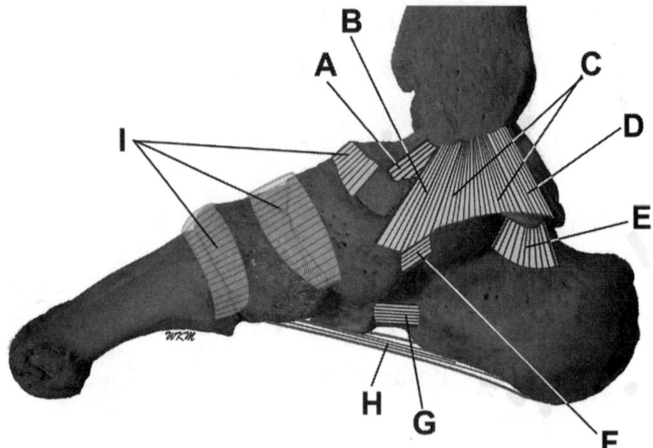

Figure 7-36 The Ankle and the Tarsal Joints, Medial Aspect: Ligaments

Q. In Figure 7-36, identify D.

A. The posterior tibiotalar ligament. It is attached to the medial tubercle of the talus. **A**, **B**, **C**, and **D** constitute the deltoid ligament.

Q. In Figure 7-36, identify E.

A. The medial talocalcaneal ligament.

Q. In Figure 7-36, identify F.

A. The plantar calcaneonavicular (spring) ligament. It articulates with and supports the head of the talus.

Q. In Figure 7-36, identify G.

A. The short plantar ligament.

Q. In Figure 7-36, identify H.

A. The long plantar ligament. It is attached, anteriorly, to the bases of the 2nd, 3rd, and 4th metatarsal bones.

Q. In Figure 7-36, identify I.

A. The thin dorsal intertarsal ligaments and the first dorsal tarsometatarsal ligament.

Q. In Figure 7-37, identify A.

A. The lateral malleolus of the fibula.

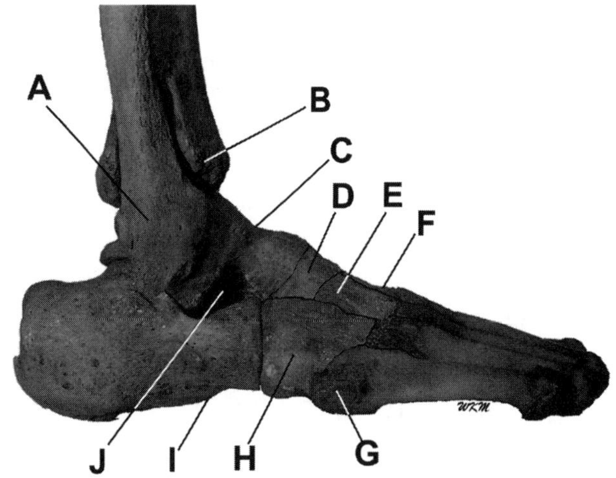

Figure 7-37 The Ankle and Tarsal Joints, Lateral Aspect: Bones

Q. In Figure 7-37, identify B.

A. The distal end of the tibia.

Q. In Figure 7-37, identify C.

A. The neck of the talus bone.

Q. In Figure 7-37, identify D.

A. The navicular bone.

Q. In Figure 7-37, identify E.

A. The lateral cuneiform bone. Note that it articulates mainly with the 3rd metatarsal bone, although it does have a small facet for the 4th metatarsal bone.

Q. In Figure 7-37, identify F.

A. The intermediate cuneiform bone. It articulates with the 2nd metatarsal bone.

Q. In Figure 7-37, identify G.

A. The tuberosity, the styloid process, of the base of the 5th metatarsal bone. It forms a prominent landmark on the lateral margin of the foot, and it is the bone of the foot most likely to be fractured by indirect violence.

Q. In Figure 7-37, identify H.

A. The cuboid bone. It articulates distally with the 4th and 5th metatarsal bones.

Q. In Figure 7-37, identify I.

A. The tubercle of the calcaneus.

Q. In Figure 7-37, identify J.

A. The sinus tarsi. It is formed by the sulcus tarsi, superiorly, and the sulcus calcanei, inferiorly. It separates the anterior and posterior talocalcaneal joints. Movement of the subtalar joints is necessary for inversion and eversion of the foot.

Q. In Figure 7-38, identify A.

A. The anterior talofibular ligament.

Q. In Figure 7-38, identify B.

A. The lateral calcaneofibular ligament.

Q. In Figure 7-38, identify C.

A. The posterior talofibular ligament. Compare **A**, **B**, and **C**, with the similar components of the deltoid ligament on the medial side of the ankle. They are frequently torn in inversion injuries.

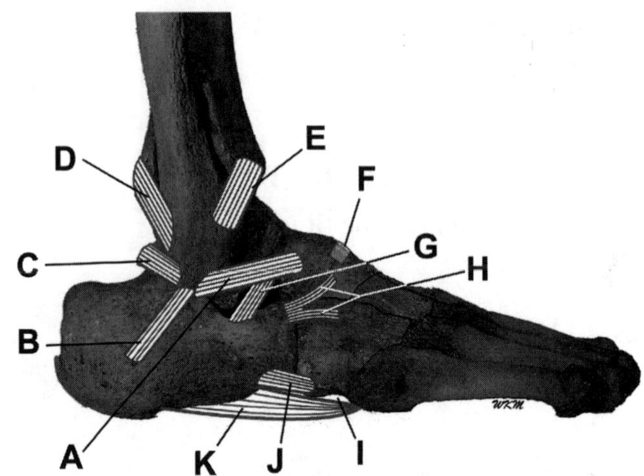

Figure 7-38 The Ankle and the Tarsal Joints, Lateral Aspect: Ligaments

Q. In Figure 7-38, identify D and E.

A. The posterior and the anterior tibiofibular ligaments.

Q. In Figure 7-38, identify F.

A. The thin dorsal talonavicular ligament.

Q. In Figure 7-38, identify G.

A. The interosseous talocalcaneal ligament. It occupies the sinus tarsi between the talocalcaneal joint and the calcaneotalonavicular joints.

Q. In Figure 7-38, identify H.

A. The calcaneonavicular and the calcaneocuboid bands of the bifurcate ligament.

Q. In Figure 7-38, identify I.

A. The aperture for the tendon of the fibularis longus (peroneus longus) muscle.

Q. In Figure 7-38, identify J.

A. The short plantar ligament.

Q. In Figure 7-38, identify K.

A. The long plantar ligament. It attaches distally to the bases of the 2nd, 3rd, and 4th metatarsal bones. Its attachment is here hidden by the base of the 5th metatarsal bone.

RADIOLOGY OF THE LOWER LIMB

Q. In Figure 7-39, identify A.

A. The sacral promontory.

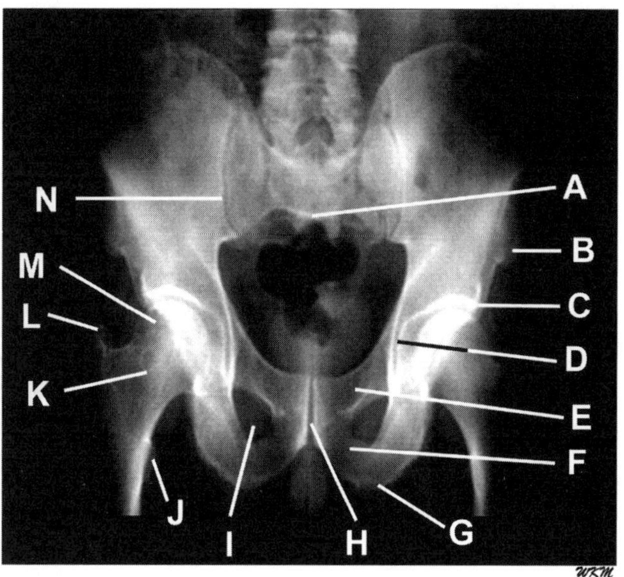

Figure 7-39 PA X-ray of the Male Pelvis

Q. In Figure 7-39, identify B.

A. The anterior superior iliac spine. It gives origin to the sartorius muscle.

Q. In Figure 7-39, identify C.

A. The anterior inferior iliac spine. It gives origin to the straight head of the rectus femoris muscle.

Q. In Figure 7-39, identify D.

A. The thin acetabular floor.

Q. In Figure 7-39, identify E.

A. The superior ramus of the pubis.

Q. In Figure 7-39, identify F.

A. The ischiopubic ramus.

Q. In Figure 7-39, identify G.

A. The ischial tuberosity.

Q. In Figure 7-39, identify H.

A. The pubic symphysis. Note the soft-tissue shadow of the penis in the background.

Q. In Figure 7-39, identify I.

A. The obturator foramen.

Q. In Figure 7-39, identify J.

A. The lesser trochanter of the femur.

Q. In Figure 7-39, identify K.

A. The neck of the femur.

Q. In Figure 7-39, identify L.

A. The greater trochanter.

Q. In Figure 7-39, identify M.

A. The head of the femur.

Q. In Figure 7-39, identify N.

A. The sacroiliac joint.

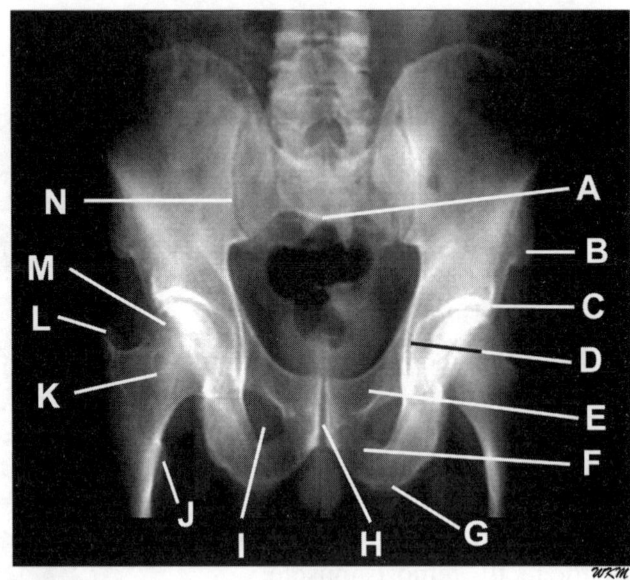

Figure 7-39 PA X-ray of the Male Pelvis

Q. In Figure 7-40, identify A.

A. The ischiopubic ramus.

Q. In Figure 7-40, identify B.

A. The obturator foramen.

Q. In Figure 7-40, identify C.

A. The superior ramus of the pubis.

Q. In Figure 7-40, identify D.

A. The bony floor of the acetabulum. Note the thinness of the bone.

Q. In Figure 7-40, identify E.

A. The head of the femur.

Q. In Figure 7-40, identify F.

A. The neck of the femur.

Q. In Figure 7-40, identify G.

A. The greater trochanter of the femur.

Q. In Figure 7-40, identify H.

A. The lesser trochanter of the femur.

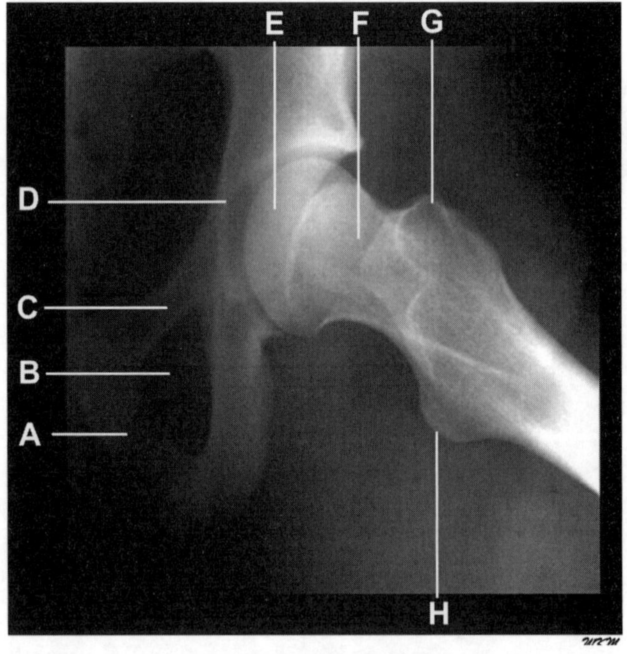

Figure 7-40 AP X-ray of Flexed, Abducted Hip Joint

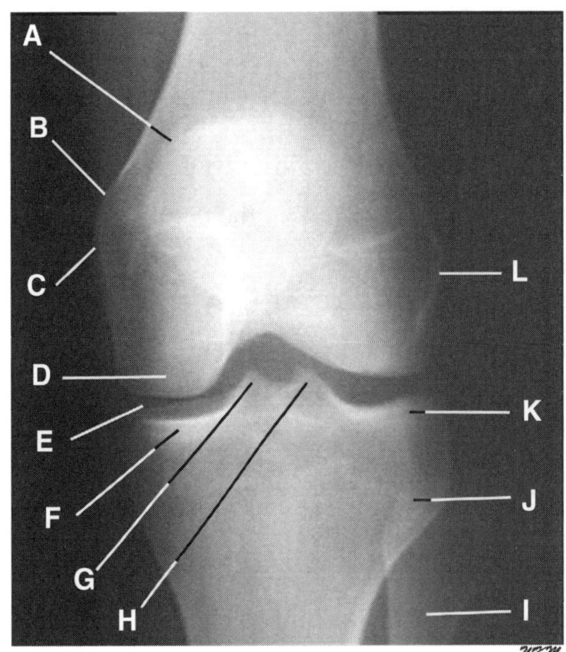

Figure 7-41 AP X-ray of the Knee Joint

Q. In Figure 7-41, identify A.
A. The edge of the patella.

Q. In Figure 7-41, identify B.
A. The adductor tubercle.

Q. In Figure 7-41, identify C.
A. The medial epicondyle.

Q. In Figure 7-41, identify D.
A. The medial femoral condyle.

Q. In Figure 7-41, identify E.
A. The space occupied by the medial meniscus.

Q. In Figure 7-41, identify F.
A. The medial condyle of the tibia.

Q. In Figure 7-41, identify G.
A. The medial intercondylar tubercle. It is part of the intercondylar eminence.

Q. In Figure 7-41, identify H.
A. The lateral intercondylar tubercle. It is part of the intercondylar eminence.

Q. In Figure 7-41, identify I.
A. The neck of the fibula. The common fibular nerve winds around it at this point.

Q. In Figure 7-41, identify J.
A. The apex of the fibular head. It is the inferior attachment of the fibular collateral ligament.

Q. In Figure 7-41, identify K.
A. The lateral condyle of the tibia.

Q. In Figure 7-41, identify L.
A. The lateral epicondyle of the femur.

Q. In Figure 7-42, identify A.

A. The lateral femoral condyle.

Q. In Figure 7-42, identify B.

A. An oblique view of the patella.

Q. In Figure 7-42, identify C.

A. The adductor tubercle on the superior aspect of the medial femoral condyle.

Q. In Figure 7-42, identify D.

A. The medial condyle of the femur.

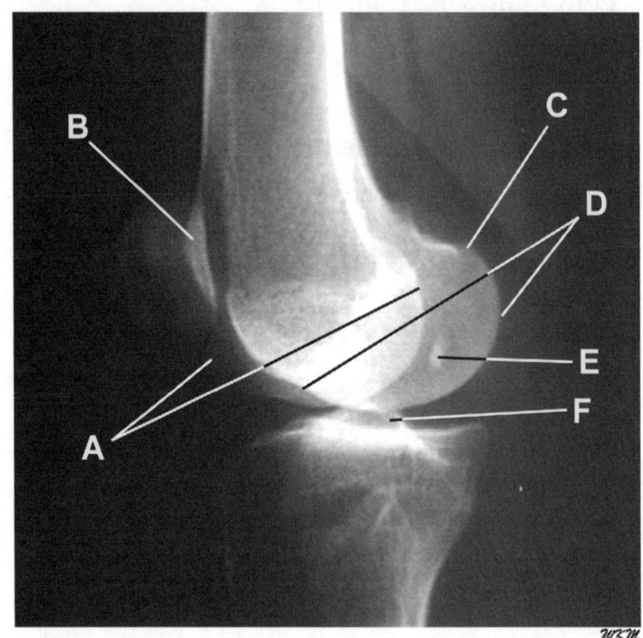

Figure 7-42 Lateral X-ray of the Knee Joint

Q. In Figure 7-42, identify E.

A. The fabella. This is a sesamoid bone in the tendon of the lateral head of the gastrocnemius muscle at the point where it crosses the posterior surface of the lateral femoral condyle.

Q. In Figure 7-42, identify F.

A. The intercondylar eminence of the tibia.

Q. In Figure 7-43, identify A.

A. The articular surface of the lateral femoral condyle.

Q. In Figure 7-43, identify B.

A. The lateral articular facet on the patella. It is slightly larger than the medial facet.

Q. In Figure 7-43, identify C.

A. The medial articular facet on the patella.

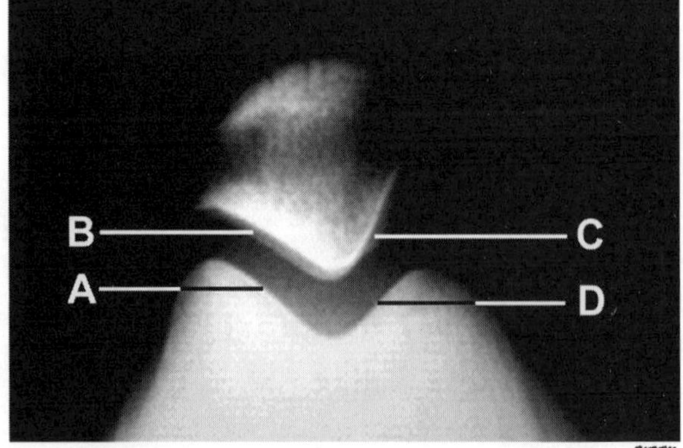

Figure 7-43 Vertical View of the Patella with the Knee Flexed

Q. In Figure 7-43, identify D.

A. The articular facet on the medial femoral condyle. The angle between the two condyles is more acute than would be expected, due to the degree of flexion of the knee and the angle from which the X-ray was taken.

Q. The ankle joint, the talocrural joint, depends for its stability on . . .

A. The mortise configuration of the bone ends and the strength of the medial and lateral collateral ligaments.

Q. The only significant movement that can take place at the talocrural joint is . . .

A. Flexion and extension. A small amount of rotation can occur when the ankle is plantar flexed. Plantar flexion is the most usual term for this movement, which is anatomically named flexion.

Q. In Figure 7-44, identify A.

A. The shaft of the fibula.

Q. In Figure 7-44, identify B.

A. The shaft of the tibia.

Q. In Figure 7-44, identify C.

A. The medial malleolus.

Q. The major ligament attached to the medial malleolus is . . .

A. The deltoid ligament.

Q. In Figure 7-44, identify D.

A. The talus bone.

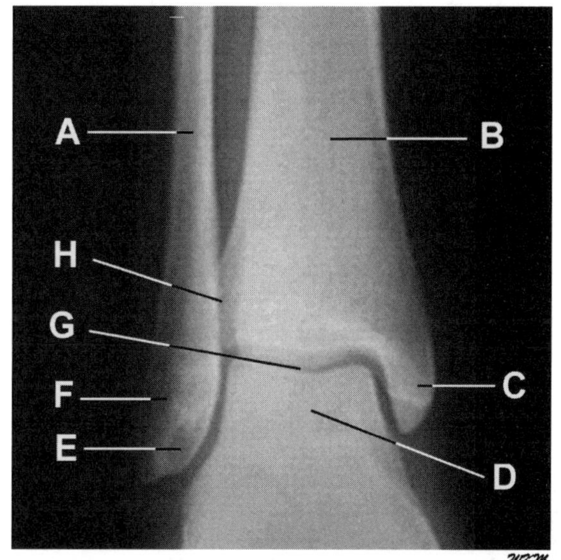

Figure 7-44 AP X-ray of the Talocrural Joint

Q. In Figure 7-44, identify E.

A. The malleolar fossa on the fibula. The posterior tibiofibular ligament is attached to it.

Q. In Figure 7-44, identify F.

A. The lateral malleolus.

Q. In Figure 7-44, identify G.

A. The trochlear surface of the talus bone.

Q. In Figure 7-44, identify H.

A. The inferior tibiofibular joint. It is a syndesmosis, fibrous, joint. The superior tibiofibular joint is a diarthrodial, synovial joint.

Q. In Figure 7-45, identify A.

A. The lower end of the shaft of the tibia. The medial malleolus cannot be seen in this view.

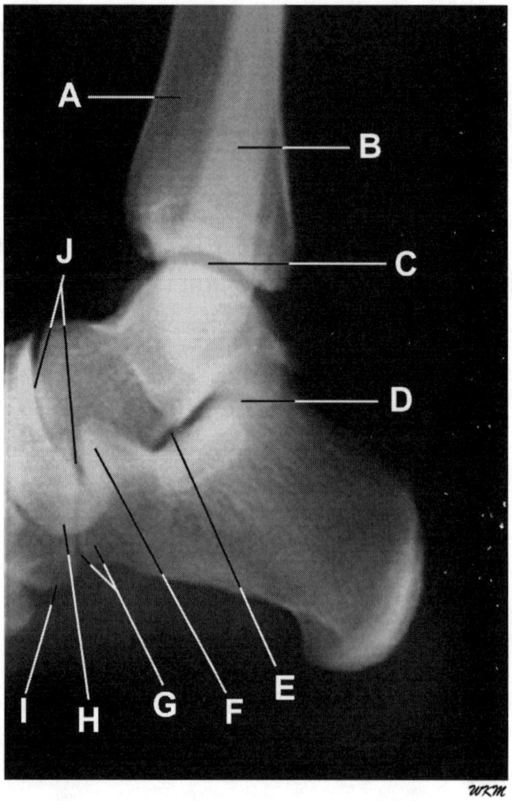

Q. In Figure 7-45, identify B.

A. The lower end of the shaft of the fibula. It can be seen continuing inferiorly into the lateral malleolus.

Q. In Figure 7-45, identify C.

A. The talocrural joint.

Q. In Figure 7-45, identify D.

A. The talocalcaneal, posterior subtalar, joint.

Q. In Figure 7-45, identify E.

A. The sinus tarsi.

Q. In Figure 7-45, identify F.

A. The sustentaculum tali.

Figure 7-45 Lateral X-ray of the Talocrural and Subtalar Joints

Q. In Figure 7-45, identify G.

A. The calcaneocuboid joint and the anterior end of the calcaneus.

Q. In Figure 7-45, identify H.

A. The tuberosity of the navicular bone.

Q. In Figure 7-45, identify I.

A. The ridge on the cuboid bone.

Q. In Figure 7-45, identify J.

A. The talocalcaneonavicular, the anterior subtalar, joint.

Q. Inversion and eversion of the foot take place mainly at two joints. They are . . .

A. The talocalcaneal joint and the talocaneonavicular joint. The twisting movement of the calcaneus on the talus is essential for inversion and eversion of the foot.

Q. In Figure 7-46, identify A.

A. The tip of the lateral malleolus.

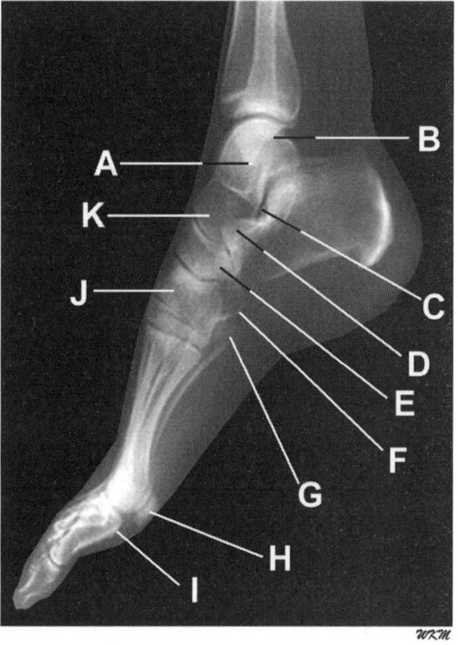

Figure 7-46 Lateral X-ray of the Foot

Q. In Figure 7-46, identify B.

A. The tip of the medial malleolus. It is difficult to see. Notice that it is about 1 cm higher than the tip of the lateral malleolus.

Q. In Figure 7-46, identify C.

A. The sinus tarsi. It lies between the anterior subtalar (talocalcaneonavicular) joint and the posterior subtalar (talocalcaneal) joint.

Q. In Figure 7-46, identify D.

A. The sustentaculum tali of the calcaneus bone.

Q. In Figure 7-46, identify E.

A. The tuberosity of the navicular bone.

Q. In Figure 7-46, identify F.

A. The ridge on the cuboid bone.

Q. In Figure 7-46, identify G.

A. The tuberosity of the base of the 5th metatarsal bone.

Q. In Figure 7-46, identify H.

A. Sesamoid bones. They are in the medial and lateral insertions of the flexor hallucis brevis muscle.

Q. In Figure 7-46, identify I.

A. The bases of the proximal phalanges.

Q. In Figure 7-46, identify J.

A. The medial cuneiform bone. Its shadow is superimposed on the shadows of the intermediate cuneiform bone, the lateral cuneiform bones, and the cuboid bones.

Q. In Figure 7-46, identify K.

A. The head of the talus bone.

Q. In Figure 7-47, identify A.

A. The tuberosity of the calcaneus bone.

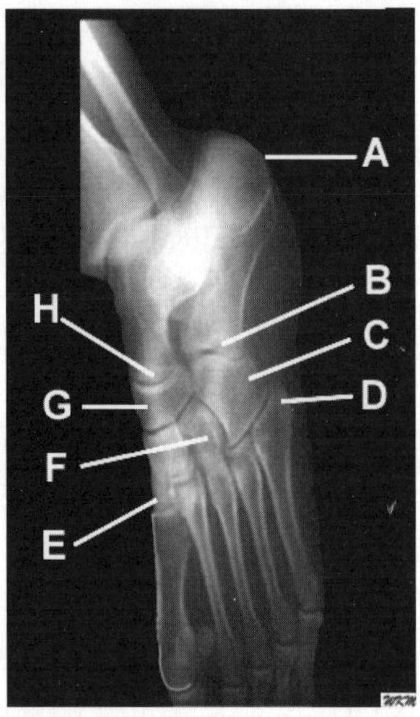

Figure 7-47 Oblique X-ray of the Foot

Q. In Figure 7-47, identify B.

A. The anterior end of the calcaneus bone. It articulates with the cuboid bone, forming the calcaneocuboid joint.

Q. In Figure 7-47, identify C.

A. The cuboid bone.

Q. In Figure 7-47, identify D.

A. The tuberosity on the base of the 5th metatarsal bone. It is the attachment of the fibularis brevis muscle.

Q. In Figure 7-47, identify E.

A. The medial cuneiform bone.

Q. In Figure 7-47, identify F.

A. The lateral cuneiform bone.

Q. In Figure 7-47, identify G.

A. The navicular bone.

Q. In Figure 7-47, identify H.

A. The head of the talus bone. It articulates with the navicular bone to form the talonavicular joint. The talonavicular joint is only one part of the talocalcaneonavicular joint.

Q. The two joints that comprise the midtarsal (transverse tarsal) joint are . . .

A. The calcaneocuboid and the talonavicular joints.